Clinical
Procedures
in Veterinary
Nursing

For Elsevier:

Commissioning Editor: Rita Demetriou-Swanwick
Development Editor: Louisa Welch
Project Manager: Frances Affleck
Designer: Charles Gray
Illustration Manager: Merlyn Harvey
Illustrator: Samantha Elmhurst

Clinical Procedures in Veterinary Nursing

SECOND EDITION

Edited by

Victoria Aspinall
BVSc, MRCVS

Director, Abbeydale Vetlink Veterinary Training Ltd, Gloucester, UK

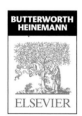

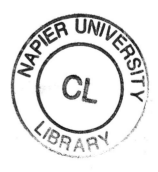

EDINBURGH   LONDON   NEW   YORK   OXFORD   PHILADELPHIA   ST LOUIS
SYDNEY   TORONTO   2008

BUTTERWORTH
HEINEMANN
ELSEVIER

ELSEVIER BUTTERWORTH-HEINEMANN

First published 2008

ISBN 978-0-08-045266-1

British Library Cataloguing in Publication Data
A catalogue record for this book is available from the British Library

Library of Congress Cataloging in Publication Data
A catalog record for this book is available from the Library of Congress

Printed in China

Contents

Contributors vii
Foreword ix
Preface xi
Acknowledgements xii

1. Handling and restraint   1

Victoria Aspinall

2. Measuring clinical parameters   25

Richard Aspinall

3. Medical nursing procedures   41

Jo Masters

4. Administration of fluid therapy   67

Carole Martin

5. Provision of nutritional support   87

Carole Martin

6. Anaesthetic procedures   105

Pip Millard

7. Theatre practice   135

Pip Millard

8. Surgical nursing procedures   163

Trish Scorer

9. First aid procedures   187

Trish Scorer

10. Diagnostic imaging   213

Suzanne Easton

11. Diagnostic laboratory techniques   243

Jennifer Davis

12. Treatment of exotic species   277

Rachel Mowbray

13. Preparing for the veterinary nursing exams   323

Justine Dunstone and Sarah Cottingham

Index   337

Contributors

Victoria Aspinall BVSc MRCVS
Director of Abbeydale Vetlink Veterinary Training
Ltd, Gloucester UK. Course Leader for Veterinary
Nursing, Filton College, Bristol, UK

Richard Aspinall BVSc MRCVS
Partner in Aspinall, Auld and Stevenson, The
Animal Hospital, 20 Glevum Way, Abbeydale,
Gloucester, UK

Sarah Cottingham BSc (Hons) PG Dip CABC PGCEVN
Programme Leader for Veterinary Nursing,
Plumpton College, Ditchling Road, Plumpton,
nr Lewes, Sussex, UK

Jennifer Davis MRIPH
Laboratory Manager, Wood Veterinary Group,
Bristol Road, Quedgeley, Gloucester, UK

Justine Dunstone Cert Ed VN
Lecturer in Veterinary Nursing, Plumpton College,
Ditchling Road, Plumpton, nr Lewes, Sussex, UK.
RCVS VN Examiner

Suzanne Easton MSc BSc (Hons) PGCE
Senior Lecturer in Diagnostic Imaging, Faculty of
Health and Social Care, University of the West of
England, Bristol, UK

Carole Martin Dip AVN (Surgical) VN
Head Veterinary Nurse and Practice Supervisor,
Clifton Villa Veterinary Services Ltd, Truro,
Cornwall, UK. RCVS VN Examiner

Jo Masters Cert Ed VN
Practice Supervisor, Langport Veterinary Centre,
Langport, Somerset, UK. RCVS VN Examiner

Pip Millard, VN
Lecturer in Veterinary Nursing, Practice Manager,
Woodlands Veterinary Clinic, Cheltenham,
Glocestershire, UK

Rachel Mowbray BVSc MRCVS
Veterinary Surgeon, Vale Vets, The Animal
Hospital, Stinchcombe, Dursley, Glocestershire, UK

Trish Scorer VN
Internal Verifier, Abbeydale Vetlink Veterinary
Training Ltd, Gloucester, UK. RCVS VN examiner

Foreword

Veterinary nursing has undergone much change over the last few years, including changes in Syllabus, Occupational Standards, practical examinations and a greater emphasis on a competence based approach. The second edition of Clinical Procedures in Veterinary Nursing goes a huge way to capture the procedures that are carried out in veterinary practice. This publication is intended for those working in veterinary practice, preparing for examinations and those teaching in colleges or universities. Effectively it is written for anyone who wants to know how to carry out a particular clinical procedure.

Whilst the basic elements of veterinary nursing education remain the same, changes in public expectations and technology, and the recent introduction of professional regulation, mean that the book could not have been published at a more relevant time, this book will act as a resource for those who have to teach and assess veterinary nurses.

Clinical Procedures in Veterinary Nursing will assist students in the development of their skills and will be useful later as a quick reference guide for up to date information on clinical procedures. The book will also be an invaluable aid for those returning to veterinary practice after a career break.

This book is based on the Veterinary Nursing Curriculum, however the content and presentation are intended to have a practical application for all those involved. Furthermore, the authors have presented topics in a way that will guide the student veterinary nurse, providing them with a rationale for each action taken.

Students preparing for their examinations will find Chapter 13 particularly useful. The authors have clearly identified the clinical procedures which are of fundamental importance in the preparation and continuing education of veterinary nurses.

Barbara Cooper Hon Assoc RCVS Cert Ed Lic IPD DTM VN

The College of Animal Welfare

Preface

Over the past few years the first edition of *Clinical Procedures in Veterinary Nursing* has become a 'standard' textbook and may be found on the shelves of hundreds of veterinary practices. Research shows that it is used by a wide range of people from students and qualified veterinary nurses, degree nurses, students of animal care and even by some veterinary surgeons!

However veterinary science is not a static discipline and techniques have changed or been replaced making it important to update the text. Many of the procedures have been rewritten and new ones have been added. In addition, we have added new diagrams and increased the number of photographs, many of which are used to expand and explain the information in the diagrams.

The practical exams which form part of the professional qualification in veterinary nursing have for a long time been a cause of great anxiety to the candidates and *Clinical Procedures* has been used to help with revision. In this edition, a new chapter has been added to assist student veterinary nurses with their exam preparation. It has been written by two people who have wide experience in the subject and have written extensively on learning theory and revision techniques. It is my great hope that all students using this book will pass their exams first time but above all that it helps to reduce that incapacitating panic!

Victoria Aspinall
2008

Acknowledgements

As with the previous edition, this book would not have been possible without the support of my long-suffering husband and family and the team at Elsevier, particularly Rita Demetriou-Swanwick and Louisa Welch who are always there when I need them. I would also like to thank all my students who give me inspiration and act as a testing ground for new ideas even though they may not realise what is happening!

Chapter 1

Handling and restraint

Victoria Aspinall

CHAPTER CONTENTS

Introduction 2

Dogs 2
Tying a tape muzzle 2
Lifting dogs up to 15 kg bodyweight 3
Lifting dogs over 20 kg bodyweight 4
Lifting small dogs with spinal damage 4
Lifting large dogs with spinal damage 5

Restraint for general examination 6
To examine the cranial end of the body 6
To examine the caudal end of the body or take
    the rectal temperature 6
To examine the dog on its side or to provide
    stronger control 6
To examine or restrain the dog on its back 7

Restraint for the administration of drugs 8
Administering a tablet 8
Administering a liquid feed or medication 8
Applying ear medication 9
Applying eye medication 9
Restraint for a subcutaneous injection 10
Restraint for an intramuscular injection 10
Restraint for an intravenous injection using the
    cephalic vein 11
Restraint for an intravenous injection using the
    lateral saphenous vein 12
Restraint for an intravenous injection using the
    jugular vein 13

Cats 14
Lifting a friendly cat used to being handled –
    method 1 14
Lifting a friendly cat used to being handled –
    method 2 15
Lifting a frightened or aggressive cat 15
Carrying a cat 15

Restraint for general examination 16
To examine a friendly cat 16
To examine a fractious cat 16

Restraint for the administration of drugs 17
Administering a tablet 17
Administering a liquid feed or medication 18
Applying ear medication 18
Applying eye medication 19
Restraint for a subcutaneous injection 19
Restraint for an intramuscular injection 20
Restraint for an intravenous injection using the
    cephalic vein 21
Restraint for an intravenous injection using the
    lateral saphenous vein 22
Restraint for an intravenous injection using the
    jugular vein – method 1 22
Restraint for an intravenous injection using the
    jugular vein – method 2 23

INTRODUCTION

No matter which procedure is to be performed, correct restraint of the patient is essential for the safety and welfare of both the animal and the handler. An animal that is securely and comfortably restrained will suffer less stress and will be less inclined to struggle and escape.

Most animals brought into a veterinary practice are used to being handled, but you may encounter stray dogs and feral cats which are wary of human contact. Their reaction to restraint may be unpredictable and even dangerous and you must protect your own safety.

It is important when handling any species of animal that you approach quietly and confidently and perform the technique correctly at the first attempt not at the third or fourth attempt – nothing upsets an animal more than clumsy inept handling. You must know how to carry out the procedure, have all the equipment ready to hand and organise assistance if you think you are going to need it. It is also important to feel confidence in yourself. Animals are very sensitive to your mood and may detect your fear and bite you.

(For the purposes of description, the veterinary nurse restrains the patient, while the veterinary surgeon performs the task. In many cases two nurses or a nurse and the animal's owner can perform the task.)

DOGS

Procedure: Tying a tape muzzle (Fig. 1.1)

This prevents the dog from biting the handler and diverts its attention away from the procedure being carried out.

1. **Action:** Place the dog in a sitting position on the floor.

   Rationale: In this position the dog is less likely to wriggle or bite. If the dog is small, it may be easier to place it on a table – avoid being bitten while you lift it onto the table.

2. **Action:** Ask an assistant to stand astride the dog and grasp the scruff on either side of the head just behind the ears.

   Rationale: If the dog moves its head around, the muzzle cannot be tied quickly. Be careful when scruffing a brachycephalic breed as there is a risk of prolapsing the eyes.

3. **Action:** Using a length of cotton tape or bandage, tie a loop in it.

   Rationale: Any long strip of material can be used, e.g. a tie or even a stocking, but it must be strong enough to hold the jaws together.

4. **Action:** Approach the dog slowly and deliberately, crouching down to its level.

   Rationale: Crouching low helps to prevent fear aggression; standing over the dog may provoke it to jump up and bite.

5. **Action:** Place the looped tape over the nose and tighten quickly and firmly with the knot over the nose.

   Rationale: Any delay in tightening the loop may allow the dog to shake its head free.

6. **Action:** Bring the long ends of the tape down and cross over under the chin.

   Rationale: Further throws around the nose before finally crossing over will strengthen the muzzle.

7. **Action:** Take the two ends of the tape backwards and tie them in a bow behind the ears.

   Rationale: A bow allows a quick release if the dog becomes distressed.

8. **Action:** Ask the assistant holding the dog to keep the head pressed downwards.

   Rationale: This position prevents the dog from lifting its forefeet to pull off the muzzle.

9. **Action:** If the dog is a brachycephalic or short-nosed breed, insert another piece of tape under the loop over the nose and under the piece at the back of the head.

   Rationale: This prevents the muzzle from slipping off over the short nose.

10. **Action:** Bring the two ends of this piece together and tie into a bow on the bridge of the nose.

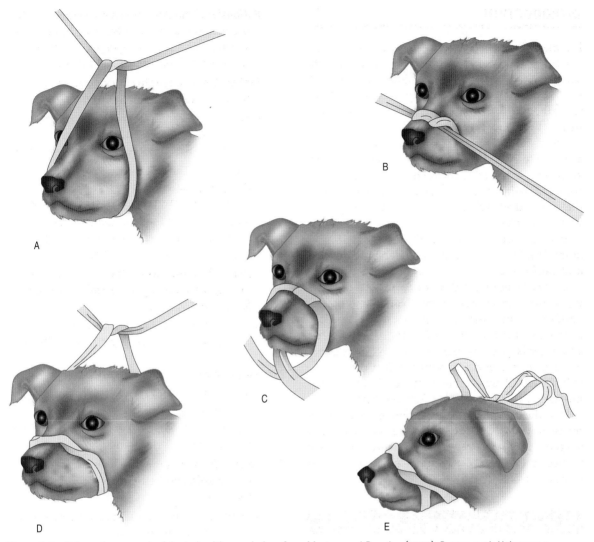

Figure 1.1 Tying a tape muzzle. Adapted, with permission, from Masters and Bowden (2001), Butterworth Heinemann.

Rationale: The dog must be carefully observed as pressure over the nose may lead to respiratory distress.

11. **Action:** Never leave a muzzled animal unattended.

   Rationale: There is a risk of asphyxiation by vomit or saliva.

Procedure: Lifting dogs up to 15 kg bodyweight

(For example, cocker spaniels, beagles, etc.)

1. **Action:** Keep your back straight and with your legs slightly apart, bend your knees.

   Rationale: This ensures that the weight of the dog is borne by your spine and your pelvic girdle.

2. **Action:** Place one arm around the front of the dog's chest and the other around its back end, over the tail.

3. **Action:** Hold the dog close to your chest.

   Rationale: This will prevent the dog from struggling as it is lifted.

4. **Action:** Straighten your legs, so raising the dog off the ground.

5. **Action:** Place it firmly on the table.

6. **Action:** Do not leave the animal unattended while it is on the table.

    Rationale: The dog may attempt to jump off the table, injuring itself, and it may then escape.

Procedure: Lifting dogs over 20 kg bodyweight (Fig. 1.2)

(For example, labradors, springer spaniels, etc.)

1. **Action:** Arrange for another person to assist you.

    Rationale: Never attempt to lift a heavy dog by yourself. You may do permanent damage to your back!

2. **Action:** Both people stand on the same side of the dog.

3. **Action:** Keep your back straight and with your legs slightly apart, bend your knees.

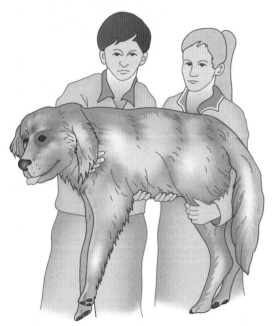

Figure 1.2 Lifting a large dog. Redrawn from Lane and Cooper (1994), Butterworth-Heinemann.

Rationale: This ensures that the weight of the dog is borne by your spine and your pelvic girdle.

4. **Action:** You take the head end by placing one hand under the chest and the other under the neck.

    Rationale: If possible, the person lifting the head should be familiar to the dog, e.g. the owner. This reduces the risk of anyone being bitten.

5. **Action:** Hold the head close to your chest.

    Rationale: If the head is held close to you the dog cannot turn its head round to bite.

6. **Action:** Instruct your assistant to adopt the safe lifting position.

7. **Action:** Instruct your assistant to place one hand under the abdomen and the other around the back end over the tail.

8. **Action:** At the same time both people straighten their legs and lift the dog onto the table.

Procedure: Lifting small dogs with spinal damage (Fig. 1.3)

(This can also be used for cats.)

1. **Action:** Approach the animal quietly and with care.

    Rationale: It may be frightened and in extreme pain, leading to unpredictable behaviour.

2. **Action:** If appropriate, apply a tape muzzle.

    Rationale: This will prevent the dog biting you as you lift it.

3. **Action:** With a straight back and bent knees, place your arms around the chest.

4. **Action:** Straighten your knees and lift the animal, allowing the legs to hang downwards.

    Rationale: This position prevents compression of the spine, which would cause acute pain and further damage.

5. **Action:** Gently place the animal on its side on a suitable non-slip surface ready for examination.

    Rationale: Care must be taken to avoid causing further pain.

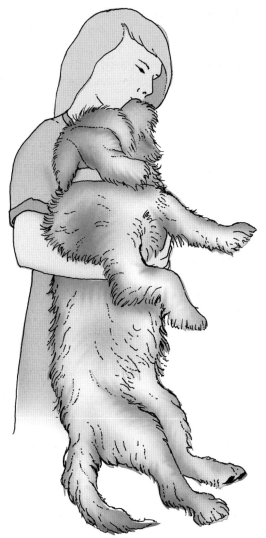

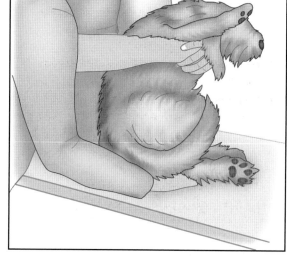

Figure 1.3   Lifting a small dog with spinal damage.

Procedure: Lifting large dogs with spinal damage (Fig. 1.4)

1. **Action:** Arrange for another person to assist you.

   Rationale: Do not attempt to lift a large injured dog by yourself. You may damage your back, get bitten or may cause the condition of the patient to deteriorate.

2. **Action:** Find something that can be used as a 'stretcher' such as a blanket or sheet, an ironing board or a solid plank of wood.

   Rationale: The dog must be supported on something that prevents compression of the spine. This would cause acute pain and further damage.

3. **Action:** Approach the animal quietly and with care.

   Rationale: It may be frightened and in extreme pain, leading to unpredictable behaviour.

4. **Action:** If appropriate, apply a tape muzzle.

   Rationale: This will prevent the dog biting you as you lift it.

5. **Action:** With the help of your assistant and adopting the correct lifting position, lift the dog onto the blanket or plank.

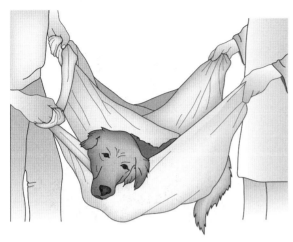

Figure 1.4   Lifting a large dog with spinal damage.

6.   **Action:** If using a plank, tie the dog onto it using tapes or bandages.

    Rationale: This will prevent the dog from falling or jumping off the 'stretcher' as you lift it, with the risk of further injury.

7.   **Action:** Gently carry the dog to the table and place it on the table, still on the blanket or plank.

    Rationale: The 'stretcher' can be removed from under the dog later on.

RESTRAINT FOR GENERAL EXAMINATION

Procedure: To examine the cranial end of the body

1.   **Action:** Using the correct procedure, lift the dog onto a stable examination table covered in a non-slip mat.

    Rationale: If the table does not shake and the dog's paws do not slip, the dog will feel secure and be less inclined to try and jump off the table.

2.   **Action:** Stand to one side of the dog.

3.   **Action:** Place one arm under the dog's neck and pull the head close to your chest with your hand.

    Rationale: If the head is held firmly against your chest , the dog cannot move to bite you.

4.   **Action:** Place the other arm over the dog's back with your elbow pointing towards the far side.

5.   **Action:** Apply pressure with your elbow and forearm along the spine, making the dog sit down.

    Rationale: In a sitting position the dog will feel secure.

Procedure: To examine the caudal end of the body or take the rectal temperature

(Continuing from the previous procedure.)

1.   **Action:** Keep one arm under the neck pulling the head close to your chest.

    Rationale: If the head is held firmly against your chest, the dog cannot move to bite you.

2.   **Action:** Move the other arm and place it under the abdomen, gently lifting the dog into a standing position.

3.   **Action:** Pull the body close to your chest by bringing your forearm up under the abdomen.

    Rationale: This position holds the dog securely against you, reducing the risk of your being bitten and preventing it from moving during the examination.

4.   **Action:** If you are required to restrain the dog for a long period of time, move your hand to lie over the spine, but be careful that the dog does not sit down again.

    Rationale: This position may be more comfy for you, while still maintaining control over the dog.

5.   **Action:** If the dog starts to move or object to the examination, quickly return to the previous position.

    Rationale: You must be aware of the dog's 'mood' and respond quickly to prevent anyone being bitten.

Procedure: To examine the dog on its side or to provide stronger control (Fig. 1.5)

1.   **Action:** Apply a tape muzzle if appropriate.

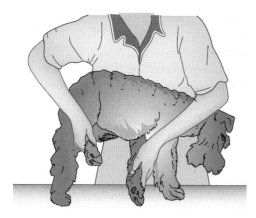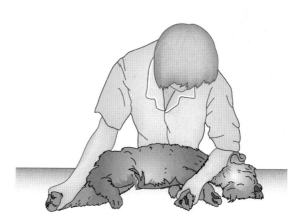

Figure 1.5 Restraining a dog on its side.

Rationale: This method is used to restrain more difficult dogs and you should be prepared for an aggressive response.

2. Action: Using the correct lifting procedure, lift the dog and place it on a stable table covered in a non-slip mat.

   Rationale: If the table does not shake and the dog's paws do not slip, the dog will feel secure and be less inclined to struggle and escape.

3. Action: With the dog in a standing position, stand to one side of the dog.

4. Action: Reach over the dog and grasp the foreleg and hind leg furthest away from you at the level of the radius and tibia.

   Rationale: It may be difficult to reach over the back of larger dogs, especially if you are short or the table is high.

5. Action: As quickly and as firmly as possible, pull the legs away from you, supporting the dog's spine against your chest.

   Rationale: This move must be done quickly before the dog begins to struggle and change position.

6. Action: Gently lower the body down to the table.

   Rationale: Avoid letting the body drop to the table as it may injure or frighten the animal.

7. Action: Place your arm across the chest and neck and apply firm pressure to keep the dog's head on the table.

   Rationale: Most dogs will become submissive in this position, but some will try to stand up again and you must be prepared. With large dogs, you may have to lean quite heavily but you must always observe the condition of the animal.

Procedure: To examine or restrain the dog on its back

1. Action: Place the dog on its side as previously described.

2. Action: Ask an assistant to hold both the back legs and you hold both the forelegs.

   Rationale: If the dog is small, this may be performed by one person.

3. Action: Roll the dog over until it is lying on its back.

4. Action: Extend the forelegs and hind legs presenting the ventral abdomen for examination.

5. Action: The sides of the neck can be grasped between the forelegs to give greater restraint if necessary.

   Rationale: Most dogs will feel quite comfortable in this position and will only struggle if they feel insecure or are in pain.

RESTRAINT FOR THE ADMINISTRATION OF DRUGS

Procedure: Administering a tablet (Fig. 1.6)

1. **Action:** Place the dog in a sitting position or in sternal recumbency on a suitable non-slip surface.

   Rationale: If the dog feels secure it will be less inclined to attempt to escape. Select a surface of a suitable height for you. Bending over for long periods may injure your back – place small dogs on a table, but larger dogs can be dosed on the floor.

2. **Action:** If necessary ask an assistant to hold the tail end of the dog.

   Rationale: This will prevent the dog from standing up or moving backwards.

3. **Action:** Place one hand over the top of the muzzle and, using your fingers and thumb, gently raise the head and open the mouth.

   Rationale: Raising the head makes the lower jaw relax, making it easier to open.

4. **Action:** Hold the tablet in the fingers of your other hand and with your forefinger pull down the lower jaw.

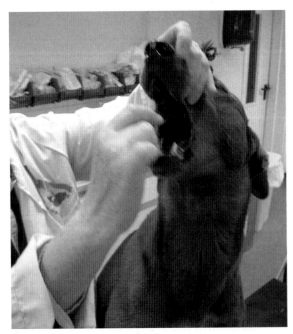

Figure 1.6 Administering a tablet to a dog.

5. **Action:** Place the tablet on the back of the tongue.

   Rationale: If the tablet is placed as far back on the tongue as possible, the swallowing reflex is initiated and the dog cannot spit it out.

6. **Action:** Close the mouth and hold it closed with one hand.

   Rationale: This also prevents the dog from spitting the tablet out.

7. **Action:** Stroke the neck until you feel the dog swallow the tablet.

   Rationale: The dog may hold the tablet in the side of its mouth and spit it out as soon as you relax your grip. If swallowing has occurred, the tablet should be passing down the oesophagus!

Procedure: Administering a liquid feed or medication

1. **Action:** Place the dog in a sitting position or in sternal recumbency on a suitable non-slip surface.

   Rationale: If the dog feels secure it will be less inclined to attempt to escape. Select a surface of a suitable height for you. Bending over for long periods may injure your back – place small dogs on a table, but larger dogs can be dosed on the floor.

2. **Action:** If necessary ask an assistant to hold the tail end of the dog.

   Rationale: This will prevent the dog from standing up or moving backwards.

3. **Action:** Place one hand over the top of the muzzle and, using your fingers and thumb, gently tilt the head upwards and to one side.

   Rationale: This position restrains the head while encouraging the jaw to relax and open.

4. **Action:** Open the mouth slightly, creating a pocket at the angle of the jaw.

   Rationale: The pocket holds the liquid as it runs into the main part of the oral cavity.

5. **Action:** Using a syringe filled with the liquid, insert it into the side of the mouth.

Rationale: Try to avoid scraping the syringe over the gums as you may damage the mucous membranes.

6. **Action:** Slowly depress the plunger so that the liquid trickles into the back of the mouth.

   Rationale: If you depress the plunger too quickly the liquid will squirt out over you and the dog.

7. **Action:** Continue until the syringe is empty and repeat as necessary.

8. **Action:** When the procedure is complete, wipe the mouth clean and wipe up any spillage on the dog's coat.

   Rationale: Never leave the dog covered in liquid as it will become wet and cold and in summer dried food may attract flies.

Procedure: Applying ear medication

1. **Action:** Place the dog in a sitting position or in sternal recumbency on a suitable non-slip surface.

   Rationale: If the dog feels secure it will be less inclined to attempt to escape. Select a surface of a suitable height for you. Bending over for long periods may injure your back – place small dogs on a table, but larger dogs can be dosed on the floor.

2. **Action:** If necessary apply a tape muzzle.

   Rationale: Some dogs may object to the application of ear medication.

3. **Action:** Stand to one side of the dog.

4. **Action:** Place one arm under the dog's neck and over the muzzle. Pull the head towards your chest.

   Rationale: This prevents the head from moving suddenly when the medication is applied. Avoid holding the head in the area of the ear as this will interfere with the treatment.

5. **Action:** Place the other arm over the dog's back with your elbow pointing towards the far side.

   Rationale: If the dog starts to struggle you can apply extra pressure by pressing your elbow closer to your side.

6. **Action:** The veterinary surgeon will stand on the other side of the dog and apply the medication to the nearest ear.

   Rationale: The applicator is introduced down the vertical part of the ear canal and squeezed.

7. **Action:** The ear is gently massaged to disperse the drops or ointment.

8. **Action:** To treat the other ear exchange places.

NB. Many dogs do not object to the application of ear medication and can be treated single-handedly.

Procedure: Applying eye medication

1. **Action:** Place the dog in a sitting position or in sternal recumbency on a suitable non-slip surface.

   Rationale: If the dog feels secure it will be less inclined to attempt to escape. Select a surface of a suitable height for you. Bending over for long periods may injure your back – place small dogs on a table, but larger dogs can be dosed on the floor.

2. **Action:** If necessary apply a tape muzzle.

   Rationale: Some dogs may object to the application of eye medication.

3. **Action:** Stand to one side of the dog.

4. **Action:** Place one arm under the dog's neck and over the muzzle. Pull the head towards your chest.

   Rationale: This prevents the head from moving suddenly when the medication is applied. Avoid holding the head in the area of the eye as this will interfere with the treatment.

5. **Action:** Place the other arm over the dog's spine with your elbow pointing towards the far side.

   Rationale: If the dog starts to struggle you can apply extra pressure by pressing your elbow closer to your side.

6. **Action:** The veterinary surgeon should stand in front of the dog and cup the head in both hands. Using the thumb of one hand the lower eyelid can be pulled down and the medication can be applied around the edge of the conjunctiva.

Rationale: You must ensure that the head is held firmly as sudden movement may result in damage to the eye.

7. **Action:** Release the tension on the eyelid and close the eyelids over the medication.

   Rationale: This allows the medication to spread over the tissues of the eye and eyelid.

8. **Action:** As you relax your hold on the dog, make sure that it does not rub at its eye with its paws or rub its head on the ground.

   Rationale: After about a minute most medication will have dispersed and will no longer cause any discomfort.

NB. Eye medication may be applied single-handedly, but if the dog moves suddenly, there is a risk of damaging the eye.

Procedure: Restraint for a subcutaneous injection

1. **Action:** Place the dog in a sitting position or in sternal recumbency on an examination table with a non-slip surface.

   Rationale: If the dog feels secure and comfortable it will be less inclined to move or try to escape.

2. **Action:** Apply a tape muzzle if necessary.

   Rationale: This is usually a quick and painless procedure, but some dogs may object and should be muzzled to prevent you being bitten.

3. **Action:** Grasp the scruff firmly with one hand.

   Rationale: This restrains the head and tents the skin ready for injection.

4. **Action:** Using the other hand insert the point of the needle with the bevel uppermost into the raised skin of the scruff.

   Rationale: Be careful to avoid pushing the point of the needle through the skin on the opposite side of the raised scruff.

5. **Action:** Inject the contents of the syringe into the subcuticular space and withdraw the needle.

   Rationale: If you wish, you may draw back on the syringe, before injecting, to check that you have not penetrated a small blood

capillary, but the blood supply to this area is relatively poor and the risk is low.

6. **Action:** Gently massage the site of injection to disperse the drug.

   Rationale: Absorption from this site takes about 30–45 minutes.

NB. If the dog is likely to object to this procedure, it may be safer to arrange for an assistant to restrain the dog.

Procedure: Restraint for an intramuscular injection

1. **Action:** The dog should be placed in a standing position on the floor or on a suitable table with a non-slip surface.

   Rationale: If the dog feels secure it will be less inclined to attempt to escape. Select a surface of a suitable height for you. Bending over for long periods may injure your back – place small dogs on a table, but larger dogs can be injected on the floor.

2. **Action:** Apply a tape muzzle if necessary.

   Rationale: This injection may be slightly painful and some dogs may object.

3. **Action:** Stand to one side of the dog.

4. **Action:** Place one arm under the neck and pull the head close to your chest.

   Rationale: If the head is firmly restrained, the dog cannot move suddenly or turn to bite.

5. **Action:** Place your other arm over the dog's chest.

   Rationale: Be prepared to restrain the dog firmly in this position as sudden movement may cause damage and pain at the site of injection.

6. **Action:** The veterinary surgeon will stand to one side of the dog and towards the hind end of the body.

7. **Action:** The quadriceps group of muscles lies on the cranial aspect of the femur and the veterinary surgeon will fix them between the fingers and thumb of the hand lying closest to the caudal end of the dog.

Rationale: The quadriceps group is the most common site for intramuscular injections but the lumbodorsal muscles and the triceps of the forelimb can also be used.

8. **Action:** Using the other hand, the needle should be introduced through the skin and the muscle mass in a direction running towards the femur and almost at right angles to the lateral aspect of the thigh.

    Rationale: At this angle the needle is unlikely to penetrate any major blood vessels or nerves.

9. **Action:** Draw back slightly on the plunger to ensure that a blood vessel has not been penetrated.

    Rationale: Muscle tissue has a good blood supply and there is a risk of vascular penetration.

10. **Action:** If there is no blood present in the needle, inject the contents slowly.

    Rationale: Muscle tissue is very dense and rapid injections of any volume of fluid may be very painful. Avoid giving any more than 2 ml at a time.

11. **Action:** Withdraw the needle and massage the site gently.

    Rationale: Gentle massage will help to disperse the drug into the bloodstream. The effect usually takes about 20–30 minutes.

Procedure: Restraint for an intravenous injection using the cephalic vein (Fig. 1.7)

(Assume that the skin has been clipped and sterilised ready for venepuncture.)

The cephalic vein runs over the dorsal aspect of the lower foreleg.

1. **Action:** Place the dog in sternal recumbency on a stable examination table with a non-slip surface.

    Rationale: If the dog feels secure it will be less inclined to attempt to escape. Select a surface of a suitable height for you – bending over for long periods may injure your back.

2. **Action:** Apply a tape muzzle if necessary.

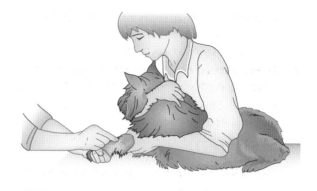

A

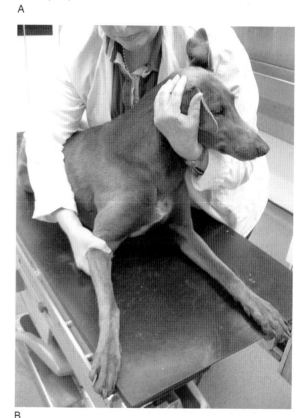

B

Figure 1.7 Holding a dog for intravenous injection using the cephalic vein.

   Rationale: Some dogs will object to this procedure and a tape muzzle will protect you and the veterinary surgeon from being bitten. It also diverts the dog's attention from the injection.

3. **Action:** Stand to one side of the dog.

4. **Action:** Place one arm under the dog's chin and around the head, holding the head close to your chest.

    Rationale: If the head is held firmly and as close to you as possible, the dog is less likely to be able to bite you or the veterinary surgeon.

5. **Action:** Using your other hand, extend the foreleg on the opposite side towards the veterinary surgeon.

    Rationale: Your hand can rest on the table, ensuring that the foreleg is supported and held firmly.

6. **Action:** Cup the elbow in the palm of your hand, bringing the thumb across the crook of the elbow.

7. **Action:** Apply gentle pressure with your thumb and rotate your hand slightly outwards.

    Rationale: This pressure acts as a tourniquet, trapping blood passing up the foreleg and resulting in dilation of the vein – referred to as 'raising the vein'.

8. **Action:** Maintain this pressure while the veterinary surgeon inserts the needle through the skin and into the underlying cephalic vein.

    Rationale: The cephalic vein should be clearly visible lying just under the skin.

9. **Action:** The veterinary surgeon should draw back on the syringe to check that the vein has been penetrated.

    Rationale: Perivascular injection may lead to tissue damage and a check must be made that the vein has been penetrated before attempting the injection.

10. **Action:** If blood appears at the hub of the needle, raise your thumb a little and the veterinary surgeon will slowly inject the contents of the syringe into the vein.

    Rationale: Releasing the pressure allows the drug to flow into the vein.

11. **Action:** When the procedure is complete, and the needle has been slowly withdrawn, you should apply gentle pressure to the injection site for about 30 seconds.

    Rationale: This prevents haemorrhage into the area around the vein.

NB. If a blood sample is to be collected, maintain pressure on the vein until enough blood is in the syringe.

Procedure: Restraint for an intravenous injection using the lateral saphenous vein (Fig. 1.8)

(Assume that the skin has been clipped and sterilised ready for venepuncture.)

The lateral saphenous vein runs over the lateral aspect of the hock.

1. **Action:** Apply a tape muzzle if necessary.

    Rationale: Some dogs may object to this procedure and should be muzzled. This must be done before putting the dog into lateral recumbency.

2. **Action:** Place the dog in lateral recumbency on a stable examination table with a non-slip surface.

    Rationale: If the dog feels secure and comfortable it will be less inclined to struggle and attempt to escape.

3. **Action:** Stand on the dorsal side of the dog, so that the legs are directed away from you.

4. **Action:** Using the arm closest to the head, place your forearm across the dog's neck and use this hand to hold both forepaws.

    Rationale: In this position you can use the weight of your body to hold the cranial end of the body onto the table.

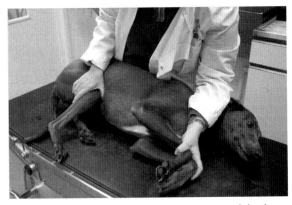

Figure 1.8   Restraining a dog for an intravenous injection using the saphenous vein.

5. **Action:** Place the other hand around the uppermost hind leg at the level of the mid-tibia/fibula.

    Rationale: The lateral saphenous vein collects blood from the hind paw and runs superficially on the caudal aspect of the hock and distal tibia. Pressure applied around the distal tibia acts as a tourniquet, trapping venous blood and causing the vein to dilate – known as 'raising the vein'.

6. **Action:** Stretch out the leg and apply gentle pressure.

7. **Action:** Maintain this pressure while the veterinary surgeon inserts the needle through the skin and into the underlying saphenous vein.

    Rationale: The saphenous vein should be clearly visible lying just under the skin.

8. **Action:** The veterinary surgeon should draw back on the syringe to check that the vein has been penetrated.

    Rationale: Perivascular injection may lead to tissue damage and a check must be made that the vein has been penetrated before attempting the injection.

9. **Action:** If blood appears at the hub of the needle, raise your thumb a little and the veterinary surgeon will slowly inject the contents of the syringe into the vein.

    Rationale: Releasing the pressure allows the drug to flow into the vein.

10. **Action:** When the procedure is complete, and the needle has been slowly withdrawn, you should apply gentle pressure to the injection site for about 30 seconds.

    Rationale: This prevents haemorrhage into the area around the vein.

NB. If a blood sample is to be collected, maintain pressure on the vein until enough blood is in the syringe.

Procedure: Restraint for an intravenous injection using the jugular vein (Fig. 1.9)

(Assume that the skin has been clipped and sterilised ready for venepuncture.)

The jugular veins run in the jugular furrow on either side of the trachea.

1. **Action:** Place the dog in a sitting position on a stable examination table with a non-slip surface.

    Rationale: If the dog feels secure and comfortable it will be less inclined to struggle and attempt to escape.

2. **Action:** Apply a tape muzzle if necessary.

    Rationale: Some dogs may object to this procedure.

3. **Action:** Stand to one side of the dog and place one hand under the dog's chin, raising the head and bringing it close to your chest.

    Rationale: Firm restraint is essential for this procedure to prevent the dog moving suddenly and causing injury to itself or to you.

4. **Action:** Place your other arm over the dog's back and round to the front of its chest, holding it close to your body.

5. **Action:** The veterinary surgeon will stand in front of the dog and apply pressure at the base of the jugular furrow with the fingers of one hand.

    Rationale: The jugular vein on each side of the trachea runs in a groove known as the jugular furrow. It collects venous blood from the head and carries it towards the heart. Pressure applied at the base of the vein will prevent the flow of blood towards the heart, causing the vein to dilate – known as 'raising the vein'.

6. **Action:** Using the other hand the veterinary surgeon should insert the needle through the skin into the underlying vein.

    Rationale: The jugular vein should be clearly visible lying just under the skin.

7. **Action:** The veterinary surgeon should draw back on the syringe to check that the vein has been penetrated.

    Rationale: Perivascular injection may lead to tissue damage and a check must be made that the vein has been penetrated before attempting the injection.

8. **Action:** If blood appears at the hub of the needle, raise your thumb a little and the

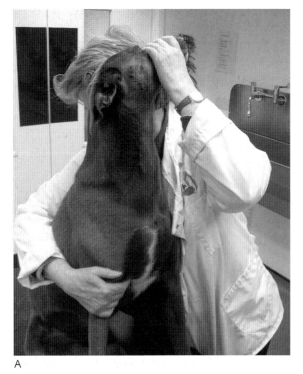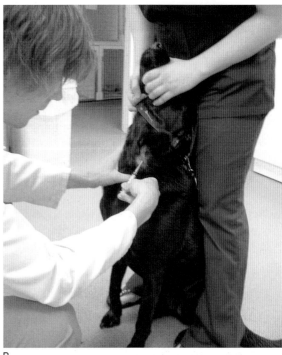

A   B

Figure 1.9   Restraining a dog for an intravenous injection using the jugular vein.

veterinary surgeon will slowly inject the contents of the syringe into the vein.

Rationale: Releasing the pressure allows the drug to flow into the vein.

9. **Action:** When the procedure is complete, and the needle has been slowly withdrawn, you should apply gentle pressure to the injection site for about 30 seconds.

    Rationale: This prevents haemorrhage into the area around the vein.

NB. If a blood sample is to be collected, maintain pressure on the vein until enough blood is in the syringe. This vein is rarely used in the dog as the other veins are more convenient and usually provide a sufficient volume of blood.

CATS

Most cats are used to being handled and will respond to being stroked and spoken to quietly. These cats do not pose much of a problem but some, particularly feral cats, can be extremely difficult to handle and you must be prepared to exercise varying degrees of restraint depending on the individual. It is important to remember that cats have five weapons of assault – four sets of claws and a set of sharp teeth!

Procedure: Lifting a friendly cat used to being handled – method 1

1. **Action:** Approach the cat calmly and confidently, talking to it quietly.

    Rationale: Most cats are used to human noise and will be reassured by a low quiet tone of voice.

2. **Action:** Assess whether the cat is safe to stroke.

    Rationale: A frightened or aggressive cat will warn you by hissing or growling as you approach, while a friendly cat may rub itself against your hand and even purr!

3. **Action:** If safe, gently stroke the top of the head and run your hand along its back.

    Rationale: This will reassure the cat, and may elicit a purr. If the cat hisses, use another method of lifting and restraint.

4. **Action:** Gently but firmly grasp the scruff of the neck with one hand and lift the cat.

   Rationale: Picking a cat up by the scruff mimics the way in which the queen carries her kittens. It initiates an innate relaxation response, which in the 'wild' would enable the queen to move the kittens safely from place to place without the risk of them struggling and escaping.

5. **Action:** Place the other hand under the sternum and support the cat.

   Rationale: Kittens and smaller cats may be lifted by the scruff, but heavier cats need added support.

6. **Action:** Place the cat on a stable non-slip surface.

   Rationale: If the cat feels insecure, it may try to scratch, bite or escape.

Procedure: Lifting a friendly cat used to being handled – method 2

1. **Action:** Approach the cat calmly and confidently, talking to it quietly.

   Rationale: Most cats are used to human noise and will be reassured by a low, quiet tone of voice.

2. **Action:** Assess whether the cat is safe to stroke.

   Rationale: A frightened or aggressive cat will warn you by hissing or growling as you approach.

3. **Action:** If safe, stroke the cat and gently run one hand over the chest and under the sternum.

4. **Action:** Place the other hand under the abdomen to support it from the other side.

   Rationale: In this position the cat feels supported and secure and is unlikely to struggle.

5. **Action:** Lift the cat onto a stable examination table with a non-slip surface.

Procedure: Lifting a frightened or aggressive cat (Fig. 1.10)

1. **Action:** Grasp the scruff of the cat quickly and firmly.

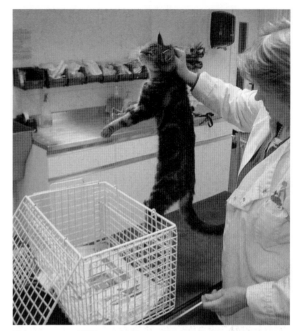

Figure 1.10   Lifting a frightened or aggressive cat.

   Rationale: If you do not take enough scruff or make any mistake in handling you are likely to get bitten or scratched.

2. **Action:** Lift the cat by the scruff letting the hind end of the body hang down.

   Rationale: Do not leave the cat 'hanging' for more than a few seconds as this is unpleasant for the cat, particularly if large.

3. **Action:** Place the cat on a table and restrain in an appropriate way.

   Rationale: Aggressive cats may have to be restrained using such equipment as a crusher cage or a restraining bag.

Procedure: Carrying a cat (Fig. 1.11)

1. **Action:** Place the body of the cat under one elbow and forearm, holding it close to your side. Let the hind legs gently dangle.

   Rationale: The body is supported by the angle of your arm, but the hind legs are unable to push the cat's body up in order to escape. Watch out for the hind legs getting caught in side pockets.

2. **Action:** Hold the forepaws together between the thumb and fingers of the hand on that side.

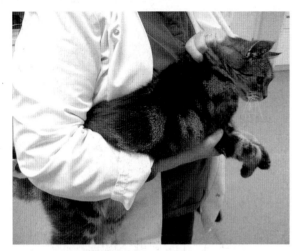

Figure 1.11   Carrying a cat.

Rationale: This prevents the forelegs from scratching you.

3. **Action:** Hold the scruff of the cat firmly with your free hand.

   Rationale: In this position, the cat feels secure and comfortable. If it tries to escape, you have control of the head via the scruff and you can apply stronger pressure to the body with your elbow.

NB. Avoid carrying aggressive or frightened cats around in your arms as their movements are often unpredictable. They should be carried in a wire cat basket which allows them to see out whilst providing you with clear visibility of their condition.

RESTRAINT FOR GENERAL EXAMINATION

Cats that are used to being handled respond to minimal restraint, but you should be prepared to use firmer methods on more difficult cats, particularly if you are single-handed.

Procedure: To examine a friendly cat

1. **Action:** Place the cat on a stable examination table in a sitting position.

   Rationale: The cat will feel secure and comfortable and will be less inclined to try and escape.

2. **Action:** Stand to one side of the cat.

3. **Action:** Run the hand closest to the cat over its back and under the cat's jaw, gently raising the head up a little.

   Rationale: If the cat is relaxed this hand can be placed on the chest, but you should be ready to move to restrain the head if necessary.

4. **Action:** Place the other hand over the forelegs.

   Rationale: This prevents the cat from raising its forepaws to scratch.

5. **Action:** If the cat begins to struggle or object to examination, move the hand from under the chin and grasp the scruff.

   Rationale: This controls the head, allowing examination of the body.

6. **Action:** Use the elbow on this side to press the cat's body firmly against your side.

   Rationale: In this position, the cat is unable to move or gain enough grip to make an escape. It may be more comfortable to lift the cat supporting it against your body rather than leaning over the examination table.

7. **Action:** Use the other hand to hold the forelegs firmly down on to the table.

   Rationale: This controls the forepaws and prevents scratching.

NB. This position uses minimal restraint, allowing examination of the whole body and enabling the rectal temperature to be taken safely.

Procedure: To examine a fractious cat

1. **Action:** Firmly grasp the scruff of the cat with one hand.

   Rationale: Some fractious cats seem to have the ability to 'use up' their scruffs by hunching their shoulders and letting their heads sink down, making the scruff very difficult to grasp. Adult toms also have thickened scruffs which are difficult to hold for any length of time.

2. **Action:** Pick up the cat and, with the other hand, grasp its hind legs.

3. **Action:** Place the cat on the table in lateral recumbency, extending its head and hind legs.

   Rationale: The cat is unable to move against the strength of the handler's arms, but a really angry cat will continue to attempt to escape and a great deal of growling and miaowing will be heard!

4. **Action:** As the cat struggles, make sure that you keep your arms wide apart to maintain the position.

    Rationale: As the forelegs are not restrained you must be careful to avoid being scratched.

This position allows examination of most of the body, but it is inadvisable to use it to take the rectal temperature, as the cat may struggle and damage itself. For the welfare of the cat, another method of restraint should be adopted as soon as possible.

Restraint equipment available for use with more aggressive cats includes crusher cages, cat grabbers and cat bags out of which the head or legs can be extended while the rest of the body is retained inside. Wrapping an aggressive cat in a towel and extending the head or a leg is also a useful means of restraint. Chemical restraint is widely used, but some form of contact with the cat will still be necessary to administer the drug.

RESTRAINT FOR THE ADMINISTRATION OF DRUGS

Procedure: Administering a tablet (Fig. 1.12)

1. **Action:** Place the cat in a sitting position on a suitable non-slip surface.

    Rationale: The cat will feel secure and less inclined to escape.

2. **Action:** Grasp the cat's head by placing one hand over the head and your thumb and forefinger at the angle of the jaw.

    Rationale: Be aware that the cat may raise its forepaws at this point.

3. **Action:** Apply gentle pressure at the angle of the jaw.

4. **Action:** Gently but firmly, tilt the head backwards.

    Rationale: As the head is tilted the jaw will naturally relax and the mouth should be easier to open.

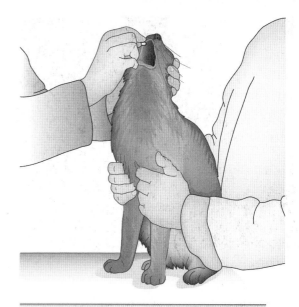

Figure 1.12   Administering a tablet.

5. **Action:** Hold the tablet between the thumb and forefinger of your other hand.

6. **Action:** Use your second and third fingers to apply gentle downward pressure to the cat's lower jaw.

    Rationale: At the first attempt the jaws should open easily. At later attempts, the cat may clench its jaws tightly closed, making the procedure more difficult – an experience often reported by owners!

7. **Action:** As the jaw opens, place or drop the tablet onto the back of the tongue.

    Rationale: If the tablet is placed as far back as possible on the tongue, the swallowing reflex will be induced.

8. **Action:** Keeping the head tilted vertically, close the mouth and hold it closed with your hand.

    Rationale: It is important to hold the mouth closed as this prevents the cat from spitting the tablet out.

9. **Action:** Gently stroke the throat until the cat is seen to swallow.

    Rationale: Some cats may learn to hold the tablet in the side of their cheeks until the head is released, when they then spit the tablet out!

NB. If you have an assistant, the cat can be further restrained by holding the forelegs while you administer the tablet as described (Fig. 1.12).

Procedure: Administering a liquid feed or medication (Fig. 1.13)

1. **Action:** Sit on a chair with a towel or other absorbent material covering your knees.

    Rationale: This procedure can be messy and the towel will absorb any spilt liquids.

2. **Action:** Take the cat onto your knee with its head pointing away from you.

    Rationale: In this position, the cat will be comfortable and easy to restrain.

3. **Action:** Grasp the cat's head with one hand, with your thumb and forefinger at the angle of the jaw, and slightly tilt the head to one side.

    Rationale: If the cat raises its forepaws, ask an assistant to hold them down or wrap them in the towel.

4. **Action:** Open the mouth slightly, creating a pocket at the angle of the jaw.

    Rationale: This pocket holds the liquid as it runs into the main part of the oral cavity.

5. **Action:** Using a small syringe filled with the liquid, gently insert the end of the barrel into the mouth at the angle of the jaw.

    Rationale: Be as gentle as possible – rough handling can easily damage the mouth.

6. **Action:** Slowly depress the plunger so that the liquid trickles into the mouth.

    Rationale: If you depress the plunger too quickly, the liquid may squirt out over you and the cat.

7. **Action:** Continue until the syringe is empty and repeat as necessary.

8. **Action:** When the procedure is complete, clean the cat's mouth, paws and any other parts which are wet or covered in liquid.

    Rationale: Never leave the cat covered in liquid as it will become wet and cold. Drying food may attract flies.

Procedure: Applying ear medication (Fig. 1.14)

1. **Action**: Place the cat in a sitting position on a stable examination table with a non-slip surface.

    Rationale: The cat will feel secure and less inclined to escape.

2. **Action:** Standing to one side, place your hands on either side of the cat bringing them forward to restrain the forelegs on the table.

    Rationale: Cats used to being handled prefer minimal restraint. This procedure does not usually cause too much discomfort and the cat is unlikely to struggle. However, if struggling does occur, be prepared to hold

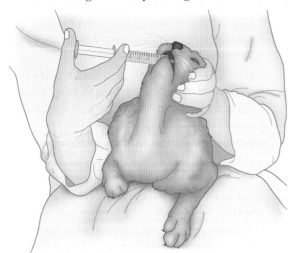

Figure 1.13   Administering a liquid feed or medication.

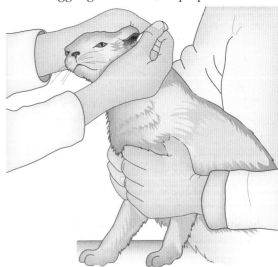

Figure 1.14   Applying ear medication. Redrawn from Lane and Cooper (1994), Butterworth-Heinemann.

the scruff with one hand and restrain the forelegs with the other.

3. **Action:** The veterinary surgeon will stand in front of the cat and take hold of the ear pinna to be treated, with the finger and thumb of one hand.

    Rationale: In this position the veterinary surgeon can gain maximum access to the ear.

4. **Action:** The veterinary surgeon will gently twist the head so that it faces upwards.

    Rationale: This brings the ear uppermost so that any medication runs down the ear canal by gravity. It also helps to restrain the head.

5. **Action:** Using the other hand, the veterinary surgeon can apply the medication to the ear.

Procedure: Applying eye medication

1. **Action:** Place the cat in a sitting position on a stable examination table with a non-slip surface.

    Rationale: The cat will feel secure and less inclined to escape.

2. **Action:** Place one hand on either side of the cat's rump.

    Rationale: This prevents the cat from trying to go backwards and escape.

3. **Action:** The veterinary surgeon should stand in front of the cat and take the cat's head in one hand, placing the thumb over the cranium and the fingers under the chin. The affected eye should be on the far side of the head away from the palm of the hand.

    Rationale: In this position, the head is held still, reducing the risk of damage to the eye. If the cat struggles, the nozzle of the tube may scratch or penetrate the eye.

4. **Action:** The skin around the affected eye is gently stretched with the forefinger and thumb of this hand.

    Rationale: This will open the eyelids, allowing examination of the eye and conjunctiva.

5. **Action:** Using the other hand, the medication is applied around the edges of the conjunctiva.

    Rationale: If you are too rough you may cause damage to the delicate conjunctiva.

6. **Action:** Relax the stretching around the eyes and eyelids.

    Rationale: This enables the eyelids to close.

7. **Action:** Gently close the eyelids over the medication.

    Rationale: This allows the drops or ointment to spread around the tissues of the eye and eyelids.

8. **Action:** You must maintain control of the forepaws for a short while to prevent the cat from clawing at the eye or rubbing its head on the table.

    Rationale: After a minute or so, the ointment will have dissipated and the cat should not feel any discomfort.

Procedure: Restraint for a subcutaneous injection (Fig. 1.15)

1. **Action:** Place the cat in sternal recumbency on an examination table with a non-slip surface. The cat should face away from you.

    Rationale: In this position, the cat feels secure and cannot slip.

2. **Action:** Grasp the scruff firmly with one hand.

    Rationale: This gives control of the head, as the cat is unable to turn and bite. It also tents the skin ready for injection.

3. **Action:** Using the other hand, introduce the point of the needle with the bevel uppermost, into the raised skin of the scruff.

    Rationale: Be careful to avoid pushing the point of the needle through the skin on the opposite side of the raised scruff.

4. **Action:** Inject the contents into the subcuticular space and withdraw the needle.

    Rationale: If you wish, you may draw back on the syringe, before injecting, to check that you have not penetrated a small blood

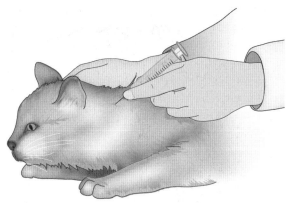

Figure 1.15 Restraint for a subcutaneous injection. Redrawn from Lane and Cooper (1994), Butterworth-Heinemann.

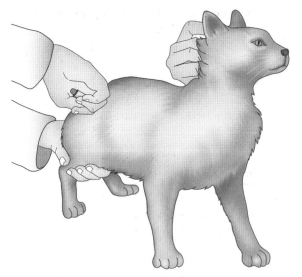

Figure 1.16 Restraint for an intramuscular injection. Redrawn from Lane and Cooper (1994), Butterworth-Heinemann.

capillary, but the blood supply to this area is relatively poor and the risk is low.

5. **Action:** Gently massage the site of injection to disperse the drug.

   Rationale: Absorption from this site takes about 30–45 minutes.

   NB. Most cats will not object to this procedure and it can usually be performed single-handedly provided that you give the injection quickly. However, some cats will need to be restrained by an assistant to prevent struggling.

Procedure: Restraint for an intramuscular injection (Fig. 1.16)

1. **Action:** Place the cat in a standing position on an examination table with a non-slip surface.

   Rationale: In this position, the cat is held firmly but is quite comfortable. It is essential to restrain the cat adequately, as sudden movement may result in damage to the muscle tissues.

2. **Action:** Standing to one side of the cat, restrain the head firmly by grasping the scruff.

   Rationale: The head must be held tightly, as this potentially painful procedure could cause the cat to bite.

3. **Action:** The veterinary surgeon should take the nearest hind leg and locate the quadriceps group of muscles lying on the cranial aspect of the femur. The muscles should be fixed between the thumb and fingers of the hand closest to the caudal end of the cat.

   Rationale: The quadriceps group is a large muscle mass which provides easy access for injection. The hamstring group and the gluteals should not be used as there is a risk of bone and sciatic nerve damage.

4. **Action:** Using the other hand, introduce the needle through the skin and the muscle mass in a direction running towards the femur and almost at right angles to the lateral aspect of the thigh.

   Rationale: At this angle the needle is unlikely to penetrate any major blood vessels or nerves.

5. **Action:** Draw back slightly on the plunger to ensure that a blood vessel has not been penetrated.

   Rationale: Muscle tissue has a good blood supply and there is a risk of vascular penetration.

6. **Action:** If there is no blood present in the needle, inject the contents slowly.

   Rationale: Muscle tissue is very dense and rapid injections of any volume of fluid may be very painful. Avoid giving any more than 2 ml at a time.

7. **Action:** Withdraw the needle and massage the site gently.

   Rationale: Gentle massage will help to disperse the drug into the bloodstream. The effect usually takes about 20–30 minutes.

Procedure: Restraint for an intravenous injection using the cephalic vein (Fig. 1.17)

(Assume that the skin has been clipped and sterilised ready for venepuncture.)

The cephalic vein runs over the dorsal aspect of the lower foreleg.

1. **Action:** Place the cat on a stable examination table with a non-slip surface, in sternal recumbency or in a sitting position.

   Rationale: In this position the cat will feel secure and comfortable and will be less likely to move or try to escape.

2. **Action:** With one hand take a firm grasp of the scruff, facing the cat towards the veterinary surgeon.

   Rationale: It is vital that the cat is held firmly as sudden movement may cause injury to the patient, to yourself or to the vet.

3. **Action:** Use your forearm and elbow to hold the remainder of the body close to you.

   Rationale: Extra control can be achieved by changing the pressure exerted by your elbow.

4. **Action:** Using the other hand, extend a foreleg towards the veterinary surgeon.

5. **Action:** Support the cat's elbow in the palm of your upturned hand and place your thumb across the crook of the elbow.

   Rationale: Your hand can rest on the table ensuring that the foreleg is supported and held firmly.

6. **Action:** Apply gentle pressure with your thumb and rotate your hand slightly outwards.

   Rationale: This pressure acts as a tourniquet, trapping blood passing up the foreleg and resulting in dilation of the vein – referred to as 'raising the vein'.

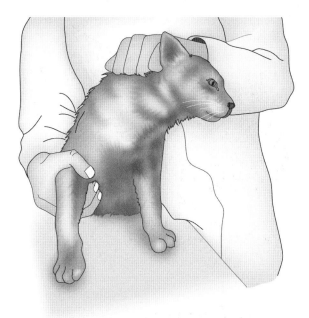

Figure 1.17 Restraint for an intravenous injection using the cephalic vein. Redrawn from Lane and Cooper (1994), Butterworth-Heinemann.

7. **Action:** Maintain this pressure, while the veterinary surgeon inserts the needle through the skin and into the underlying cephalic vein.

   Rationale: The cephalic vein should be clearly visible lying just under the skin.

8. **Action:** The veterinary surgeon should draw back on the syringe to check that the vein has been penetrated.

   Rationale: Perivascular injection may lead to tissue damage and a check must be made that the vein has been penetrated before attempting the injection.

9. **Action:** If blood appears at the hub of the needle, raise your thumb a little and the veterinary surgeon will slowly inject the contents of the syringe into the vein.

   Rationale: Releasing the pressure allows the drug to flow into the vein.

10. **Action:** When the procedure is complete, and the needle has been slowly withdrawn, you should apply gentle pressure to the injection site for about 30 seconds.

Rationale: This prevents haemorrhage into the area around the vein.

NB. If a blood sample is to be collected, maintain pressure on the vein until enough blood is in the syringe.

Procedure: Restraint for an intravenous injection using the lateral saphenous vein

(Assume that the skin has been clipped and sterilised ready for venepuncture.)

The lateral saphenous vein runs over the lateral aspect of the hock.

1. **Action:** Place the cat in lateral recumbency on a stable examination table with a non-slip surface.

    Rationale: The cat will feel secure and comfortable and will be less likely to move or try to escape.

2. **Action:** With one hand grasp the scruff firmly.

    Rationale: The head must be restrained firmly to prevent the cat wriggling or biting.

3. **Action:** With the other hand, extend the uppermost hind leg, at the same time stretching out the body.

    Rationale: If the cat struggles or is aggressive, it may be necessary to exert extra control by wrapping the cat in a towel with the head out. The hind leg can be extended from the towel.

4. **Action:** Position your hand around the lower leg at the level of mid-tibia/fibula and apply gentle pressure.

    Rationale: The lateral saphenous vein collects blood from the hind paw and runs superficially on the caudal aspect of the hock and distal tibia. Pressure applied around the distal tibia acts as a tourniquet, trapping venous blood and causing the vein to dilate – known as 'raising the vein'.

5. **Action:** Maintain this pressure while the veterinary surgeon inserts the needle through the skin and into the underlying saphenous vein.

    Rationale: The saphenous vein should be clearly visible lying just under the skin.

6. **Action:** The veterinary surgeon should draw back on the syringe to check that the vein has been penetrated.

    Rationale: Perivascular injection may lead to tissue damage and a check must be made that the vein has been penetrated before attempting the injection.

7. **Action:** If blood appears at the hub of the needle, release the pressure a little and the veterinary surgeon will slowly inject the contents of the syringe into the vein.

    Rationale: Releasing the pressure allows the drug to flow into the vein.

8. **Action:** When the procedure is complete, and the needle has been slowly withdrawn, you should apply gentle pressure to the injection site for about 30 seconds.

    Rationale: This prevents haemorrhage into the area around the vein.

Procedure: Restraint for an intravenous injection using the jugular vein – method 1 (Fig. 1.18)

(Assume that the skin has been clipped and sterilised ready for venepuncture.)

The jugular veins run in the jugular furrows on either side of the trachea.

1. **Action:** Sit on a chair and place the cat on your lap.

    Rationale: This ensures that you are comfortable and able to support and restrain the cat more easily.

2. **Action:** Turn the cat over into dorsal recumbency.

    Rationale: In this position there is easy access to the ventral part of the neck. If the cat feels secure in your lap it will be more likely to relax.

3. **Action:** Take all four legs in one hand.

    Rationale: Control of the legs prevents the veterinary surgeon from being scratched.

4. **Action:** The veterinary surgeon should gently extend the head with one hand, placing the thumb under the chin and cupping the cranium in the palm of the hand.

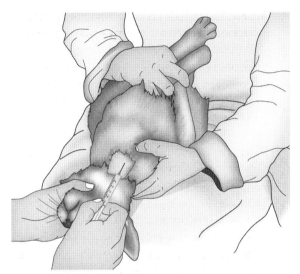

Figure 1.18 Restraint for an intravenous injection using the jugular vein. Redrawn from Anderson and Edney (1991), Pergamon.

Rationale: Extending the head and neck stretches out the jugular as it runs beside the trachea and tenses the overlying skin, making it easier to penetrate the vein with the needle.

5. **Action:** You can now place the thumb of your other hand at the base of the jugular furrow at the point where the trachea enters the thoracic cavity.

   Rationale: The jugular vein on each side of the trachea runs in a groove known as the jugular furrow. It collects venous blood from the head and carries it towards the heart.

6. **Action:** Apply gentle pressure.

   Rationale: Pressure applied at the base of the vein will prevent the flow of blood towards the heart, causing the vein to dilate – known as 'raising the vein'.

7. **Action:** Maintain this pressure while the veterinary surgeon inserts the needle through the skin and into the underlying jugular vein.

   Rationale: The jugular vein should be clearly visible lying just under the skin.

8. **Action:** The veterinary surgeon should draw back on the syringe to check that the vein has been penetrated.

Rationale: Perivascular injection may lead to tissue damage and a check must be made that the vein has been penetrated before attempting the injection.

9. **Action:** If blood appears at the hub of the needle, raise your thumb a little and the veterinary surgeon will slowly inject the contents of the syringe into the vein.

   Rationale: Releasing the pressure allows the drug to flow into the vein.

10. **Action:** When the procedure is complete, and the needle has been slowly withdrawn, you should apply gentle pressure to the injection site for about 30 seconds.

   Rationale: This prevents haemorrhage into the area around the vein.

   NB. The jugular vein is more often used for blood sampling. During this procedure, pressure is maintained until enough blood has collected in the syringe.

Procedure: Restraint for an intravenous injection using the jugular vein – method 2

(Assume that the skin has been clipped and sterilised ready for venepuncture.)

1. **Action:** Place the cat in a sitting position on a stable examination table with a non-slip surface.

   Rationale: The cat will feel secure and comfortable and will be less likely to move or try to escape.

2. **Action:** It may be necessary to ask an assistant to place a hand on either side of the cat's rump to maintain it in this position.

   Rationale: This should prevent the cat from struggling during the procedure. If the cat struggles the assistant should be prepared to use extra force.

3. **Action:** You should bring one hand over the cat's back and restrain the forelegs and paws on the table.

   Rationale: If the cat struggles you may have to use the scruff to restrain and extend the head. However, this leaves the forelegs free and the cat may scratch the veterinary surgeon.

4. **Action:** Place your other hand under the chin and raise the cat's head, so that the neck and chin are in a straight line.

    Rationale: In this position, the jugular vein and overlying skin are tensed, making it easier to penetrate the vein with the needle.

5. **Action:** The veterinary surgeon should apply pressure at the base of the jugular furrow with the fingers of one hand.

    Rationale: The jugular vein on each side of the trachea runs in a groove known as the jugular furrow. It collects venous blood from the head and carries it towards the heart.

6. **Action:** Using the other hand, the veterinary surgeon should insert the needle through the skin into the underlying vein.

    Rationale: The jugular vein should be clearly visible lying just under the skin.

7. **Action:** The veterinary surgeon should draw back on the syringe to check that the vein has been penetrated.

Rationale: Perivascular injection may lead to tissue damage and a check must be made that the vein has been penetrated before attempting the injection.

8. **Action:** If blood appears at the hub of the needle, the veterinary surgeon will release the pressure on the vein and slowly inject the contents of the syringe into the vein.

    Rationale: Releasing the pressure allows the drug to flow into the vein.

9. **Action:** When the procedure is complete, and the needle has been slowly withdrawn, you should apply gentle pressure to the injection site for about 30 seconds.

    Rationale: This prevents haemorrhage into the area around the vein.

NB. The jugular vein is more often used for blood sampling. During this procedure, pressure is maintained until enough blood has collected in the syringe.

REFERENCES AND FURTHER READING

Anderson R S, Edney A T B (eds) 1991 Practical Animal Handling, Pergamon, Oxford

Aspinall V 2006 The Complete Textbook of Veterinary Nursing, Elsevier, Oxford

Dallas S (ed.) 1999 Manual of Veterinary Care, BSAVA, Gloucester

Lane D R, Cooper B (eds) 1994 Veterinary Nursing, Butterworth-Heinemann, Oxford

Lane D R, Cooper B (eds) 2003 Veterinary Nursing, 3rd edn. Butterworth-Heinemann, Oxford

Chapter 2

Measuring clinical parameters

Richard Aspinall

CHAPTER CONTENTS

Introduction 25

To measure the body temperature 26
To measure the pulse rate by palpation of the
femoral artery 27
To measure the pulse rate using a stethoscope 28
To measure the pulse rate by palpation of the
chest 28
To measure the pulse rate using an oesophageal
stethoscope 28
To measure the respiratory rate by direct
observation 29
To measure the respiratory rate using a
stethoscope 29
To measure the respiratory rate using an
oesophageal stethoscope 29
To assess capillary refill time 30
To measure the electrical activity of the heart
using an electrocardiogram 30
To measure the percentage of oxygen (oxygen
saturation) in the blood using a pulse
oximeter 32
To measure central venous pressure 32
To measure arterial blood pressure using a non-
invasive technique 35
To measure carbon dioxide levels using a
mainstream capnograph 36

To measure carbon dioxide levels using a
sidestream capnograph 37
To measure urine production 38
To measure tear production 38
To measure intraocular pressure 39

INTRODUCTION

Diagnosis of a patient's condition is based on a thorough clinical examination followed by a range of diagnostic tests. Part of the clinical examination includes the measurement of certain basic indicators of the body's function known as the clinical parameters. Among the easiest to measure and therefore the most commonly performed are body temperature, pulse or heart rate and respiratory rate. Once these are known, they are compared to normal values for that species and the significance of the result is evaluated in the context of the symptoms. Later, once treatment has started, the parameters can be monitored and used as indicators of the progress of the disease.

Clinical parameters such as the percentage of blood gases or blood pressure require the use of complicated equipment but are essential measurements during anaesthesia and for monitoring the progress of the critically ill and hospitalised patient.

Measurement of clinical parameters and the monitoring of changes in their levels are an essential part of patient care. The veterinary surgeon must be able to rely on the veterinary nurse being able to perform the procedure correctly and accurately, and be confident that the nurse understands that when the results are abnormal, some action must be taken to return them to normal.

This chapter describes the methods of measuring these parameters in detail so that the veterinary nurse can approach the process with a degree of understanding and use the more complicated apparatus without fear.

Procedure: To measure the body temperature (Table 2.1)

Equipment: Mercury or digital thermometer.

1. **Action:** Place the animal in a comfortable standing position on a table.

   Rationale: If the patient feels uncomfortable or insecure it will try to escape.

2. **Action:** Ask an assistant to restrain the dog gently by placing one arm around the neck and the other around the chest. Ensure that the dog is relaxed and quiet. Cats should be held lightly with both hands around the shoulders, or place one hand under the chin and the other around its chest, pulling it close to your body.

   Rationale: In this position, the animal will feel comfortable and unrestricted; however, the assistant will be able to react quickly if it tries to jump off the table.

3. **Action:** Select either a mercury or digital thermometer.

   Rationale: Choice of instrument depends on availability.

4. **Action:** Lubricate the end with KY jelly or a similar lubricant.

   Rationale: Lubrication reduces the discomfort of insertion into the rectum.

5. **Action:** Shake the mercury down to the bulb or check that the digital thermometer is switched on and displaying a reading.

   Rationale: If the mercury is not shaken down the new reading will be inaccurate.

6. **Action:** Gently but firmly, insert the instrument into the rectum through the anus. A slight rotating action may help entrance through the rectal sphincters. Cats,

Table 2.1 Normal clinical parameters in the dog and cat

Clinical parameter	Dog	Cat
Body temperature	38.3–38.7°C	38.0–38.5°C
Pulse rate	60–180 beats/min	110–180 beats/min
Respiratory rate	10–30 breaths/min	20–30 breaths/min
Capillary refill time	1–2 seconds	1–2 seconds
Oxygen saturation	Close to 99%	Close to 99%
Arterial blood pressure: systolic/diastolic	Puppy: 108/60 mmHg Adult: 141/81 mmHg	Kitten: 123/63 mmHg Adult: 129/70 mmHg
Central venous pressure	3–7.5 mm H_2O	3–7.5 mm H_2O
Carbon dioxide concentration	End-tidal: 35–54 mmHg Inspired: less than 8 mmHg	End-tidal: 32–35 mmHg Inspired: less than 8 mmHg
Volume of urine produced	1–2 ml/kg bodyweight/hour	1–2 ml/kg bodyweight/hour
Volume of tears produced	15–25 ml	15–25 ml
Intraocular pressure	25 mmHg	25 mmHg

particularly, may require patient gentle pressure before the sphincters relax.

Rationale: In animals, the oral route is not practical but the rectal route is easy and well tolerated.

7. **Action:** Leave the thermometer in position for at least 30 seconds.

    Rationale: The mercury has to have time to warm up and expand.

8. **Action:** Clean the end of the thermometer by wiping with a paper cloth or cotton wool.

    Rationale: This prevents transmission of disease to another animal the next time the thermometer is used.

9. **Action:** Read the mercury thermometer by looking for the line of mercury against the scale. Read off the figures on the digital thermometer.

    Rationale: The glass of the thermometer magnifies the mercury line and makes it easier to read.

10. **Action:** Record the reading on the hospital record or clinical record.

    Rationale: To monitor rises or falls in the body temperature.

11. **Action:** Shake down the mercury or reset the digital reading.

    Rationale: To prepare the thermometer for use in the future.

12. **Action:** Place the bulb of the instrument in the disinfectant container.

    Rationale: This prevents transmission of disease to another animal the next time the thermometer is used.

Procedure: To measure the pulse rate by palpation of the femoral artery (Table 2.1)

1. **Action:** Place the animal in a comfortable standing position on a table.

    Rationale: If the patient feels uncomfortable or insecure it will try to escape.

2. **Action:** Ask an assistant to restrain the dog gently by placing one arm around the neck and the other around the chest. Ensure that the dog is relaxed and quiet. Cats should be held lightly with both hands around the shoulders, or place one hand under the chin and the other around its chest, pulling it close to your body.

    Rationale: In this position, the animal will feel comfortable and unrestricted; however, the assistant will be able to react quickly if it tries to jump off the table.

3. **Action:** Standing on one side of the animal, place the fingers of one hand on the medial aspect of the thigh. Locate the femoral artery as it runs down the medial aspect of the femur (Fig. 2.1).

    Rationale: The pulse can be palpated at any point where an artery runs over a bone and close to the body surface. The femoral pulse is the easiest to detect.

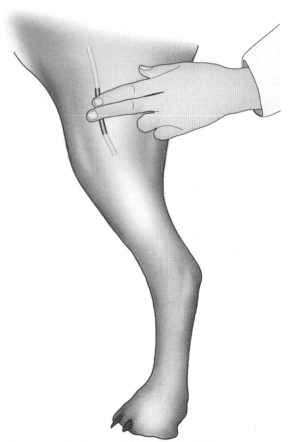

Figure 2.1   Medial view of hind leg of a dog to show position of fingers to measure the pulse rate by palpation of the femoral artery.

4. **Action:** Press gently against the artery with the second and third fingers and feel the pulse.

    Rationale: The tips of the fingers are sensitive to touch. The thumb and the forefinger have a pulse of their own which may be mistaken for the dog's pulse.

5. **Action:** Count the beats of the pulse for 60 seconds.

    Rationale: 60 seconds is enough time in which to detect any abnormalities.

6. **Action:** Record the pulse rate.

    Rationale: If there any irregularities in rate and rhythm, inform the veterinary surgeon.

Procedure: To measure the pulse rate using a stethoscope (Table 2.1)

1. **Action:** Place the animal in a comfortable standing position on a table.

    Rationale: If the animal is quiet and comfortable the heart can be heard more easily.

2. **Action:** Ask an assistant to restrain the dog gently by placing one arm around the neck and the other around the chest. Ensure that the dog is relaxed and quiet. Cats should be held lightly with both hands around the shoulders, or place one hand under the chin and the other around its chest, pulling it close to your body.

    Rationale: In this position, the animal will feel comfortable and unrestricted; however, the assistant will be able to react quickly if it tries to jump off the table.

3. **Action:** Place the earpieces of the stethoscope in your ears and place the stethoscope head on the lower left chest caudal to and just dorsal to the elbow – between the third and sixth ribs.

    Rationale: This is close to the left ventricle where the heartbeat can be best heard.

4. **Action:** Listen to the rhythm of the heart and count the heartbeats for 60 seconds.

    Rationale: 60 seconds is enough time in which to detect any abnormalities.

5. **Action:** Record the pulse rate.

Rationale: If there any irregularities in rate or rhythm, inform the veterinary surgeon.

Procedure: To measure the pulse rate by palpation of the chest (Table 2.1)

1. **Action:** This method is best used for narrow-chested breeds of dog such as whippets, greyhounds or lurchers and most cats.

    Rationale: The hand will reach across the sternum more easily in such animals.

2. **Action:** Place the animal in a comfortable standing position on a table.

    Rationale: If the animal is quiet and comfortable the heart can be heard more easily.

3. **Action:** Ask an assistant to restrain the dog gently by placing one arm around the neck and the other around the chest. Ensure that the dog is relaxed and quiet. Cats should be held lightly with both hands around the shoulders, or place one hand under the chin and the other around its chest, pulling it close to your body.

    Rationale: In this position, the animal will feel comfortable and unrestricted; however, the assistant will be able to react quickly if it tries to jump off the table.

4. **Action:** Either put the flat of the hand on the lower left chest caudal to and just dorsal to the elbow or stretch the hand across to the other side over the sternum and feel the heart beating.

    Rationale: To feel the heart beating within the chest.

5. **Action:** Count the beats over 60 seconds.

    Rationale: 60 seconds is enough time in which to count the rate.

6. **Action:** Record the pulse rate.

    Rationale: If there any irregularities in rate or rhythm, inform the veterinary surgeon.

Procedure: To measure the pulse rate using an oesophageal stethoscope (Table 2.1)

1. **Action:** The patient is anaesthetised with a cuffed endotracheal tube in place.

Rationale: A conscious animal will not tolerate the placing of the tube through the mouth and into the oesophagus.

2. Action: Select the correct diameter of oesophageal stethoscope.

    Rationale: Small dogs require a smaller bore of tube than larger dogs.

3. Action: Lay the stethoscope tube on the outside of the dog or cat and measure the approximate length from the mouth to the heart. Mark the tube with a pen or adhesive bandage at the mouth end.

    Rationale: This ensures that the tube is best placed to hear the heart when inside the oesophagus.

4. Action: Lubricate the end of the stethoscope with KY jelly and introduce it through the patient's mouth and into the oesophagus using gentle pressure. Push it in up to the pre-marked part of the tube.

    Rationale: Gentle pressure enables the tube to enter the oesophagus. Pushing the tube up as far as the mark ensures that the end of the tube lies close to the heart.

5. Action: Insert the earpieces of the stethoscope into your ears and listen to the rhythm of the heart.

    Rationale: If there any irregularities in rate or rhythm, inform the veterinary surgeon.

6. Action: Count the heartbeats for 60 seconds.

    Rationale: 60 seconds is enough time in which to count the rate and detect any abnormalities.

7. Action: Record the pulse rate on the patient's anaesthetic chart.

    Rationale: The use of the oesophageal stethoscope helps to monitor any cardiac changes during the anaesthetic.

Procedure: To measure the respiratory rate by direct observation (Table 2.1)

1. Action: Place the animal in a comfortable standing position on a table.

    Rationale: If the patient feels uncomfortable or insecure it will try to escape.

2. Action: Observe the movement of the rib cage.

    Rationale: The chest expands and contracts once with each breath.

3. Action: Count the number of breaths taken over 60 seconds.

    Rationale: 60 seconds is enough time to obtain an accurate measurement of the rate.

4. Action: Record the respiration rate on the patient's hospital chart or clinical case record.

    Rationale: To produce a permanent record of any changes, which may indicate a need for treatment.

Procedure: To measure the respiratory rate using a stethoscope (Table 2.1)

1. Action: Place the animal in a comfortable standing position on a table.

    Rationale: If the patient feels uncomfortable or insecure it will try to escape.

2. Action: Place the earpieces of the stethoscope in your ears and place the diaphragm of the stethoscope on the upper half of the chest just caudal to the scapula.

    Rationale: This position ensures that the diaphragm of the stethoscope lies over the trachea and bronchi. This is the best place to hear air movement into and out of the lungs.

3. Action: Count the breaths taken over 60 seconds.

    Rationale: 60 seconds is enough time to obtain an accurate measurement of the rate.

4. Action: Record the respiration rate on the patient's hospital chart or clinical case record.

    Rationale: To produce a permanent record of any changes, which may indicate a need for treatment.

Procedure: To measure the respiratory rate using an oesophageal stethoscope (Table 2.1)

1. Action: The patient is anaesthetised with a cuffed endotracheal tube in place.

Rationale: A conscious animal will not tolerate the placing of the tube through the mouth and into the oesophagus.

2. **Action:** Select the correct diameter of oesophageal stethoscope.

    Rationale: Small dogs require a smaller bore of tube than larger dogs.

3. **Action:** Lay the stethoscope tube on the outside of the dog and measure the approximate length from the mouth to the heart. Mark the tube with a pen or adhesive bandage at the mouth end.

    Rationale: This ensures that the tube is best placed to hear the heart when inside the oesophagus.

4. **Action:** Lubricate the end of the stethoscope with KY jelly and introduce it through the patient's mouth and into the oesophagus using gentle pressure. Push it in up to the pre-marked part of the tube.

    Rationale: Gentle pressure enables the tube to enter the oesophagus. Pushing the tube up as far as the mark ensures that the end of the tube lies close to the heart.

5. **Action:** Insert the earpieces of the stethoscope into your ears and listen to the rhythm of the heart.

    Rationale: If there any irregularities in rate or rhythm, inform the veterinary surgeon.

6. **Action:** Record the respiration rate on the anaesthetic chart of the patient.

    Rationale: The use of an oesophageal stethoscope helps to monitor depth of anaesthetic.

Procedure: To assess capillary refill time (CRT) (Table 2.1)

1. **Action:** Ask an assistant to hold, and gently restrain, the animal on the table.

    Rationale: If the animal is held securely it will not try to jump off the table or become stressed.

2. **Action:** Keeping the animal's mouth closed, raise the lip and look at the gum over the upper dental arch.

Rationale: To assess the colour and general appearance of the gum.

3. **Action:** Gently press on the gum with the ball of your thumb.

    Rationale: Pressure will push all the blood out of the squeezed area.

4. **Action:** Lift your thumb and observe the time it takes for the gum to become pink again.

    Rationale: Releasing the pressure allows the blood to flow back into the gum capillaries.

5. **Action:** The gum should take approximately 1 to 2 seconds to return to normal.

6. **Action:** Report any abnormalities to the veterinary surgeon.

    Rationale: So that prompt action can be taken, e.g. a dehydrated dog may have an increased CRT so needs to be given intravenous fluids.

CRT is a quick and useful way of assessing the circulation. Generally a dehydrated animal will have a prolonged CRT because of the reduction in circulating blood volume. The technique also allows assessment of the colour of the mucous membranes – paler gums might indicate anaemia, a blue tinge or cyanosis might indicate respiratory problems, and yellow coloration or jaundice might indicate liver problems or haemolytic anaemia.

Procedure: To measure the electrical activity of the heart using an electrocardiogram (ECG)

An ECG trace (Fig. 2.2) measures the electrical activity of the heart muscle and is produced by attaching electrical contacts to two set points on the outside of the body (Fig. 2.3). One of the leads is the earth wire, which is clipped onto the right hind leg. In animals, the other contacts are on each of the other three limbs and provide three different measurements of the electrical waves produced as the heart muscle contracts.

Equipment: ECG machine and leads, surgical spirit.

1. **Action:** Place the animal in right lateral recumbency. Some cats may resent this

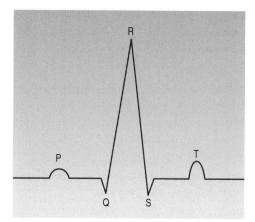

Figure 2.2 A normal lead II ECG trace.

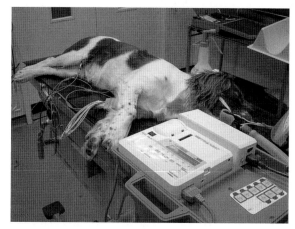

Figure 2.3 Use of an ECG machine to monitor an anaesthetised dog in left lateral recumbency.

position and it may be better to have them in a normal upright sitting position. Do not sedate the animal.

Rationale: This is the standard position for performing ECG recordings. The use of sedatives may affect the ECG trace.

2. **Action:** Ask an assistant to hold the animal's front and back legs so that it lies comfortably on the table.

Rationale: If the patient is comfortable it will not struggle and affect the resulting trace.

3. **Action:** Attach the four leads to the four limbs as follows:

red to the right foreleg
yellow to the left foreleg

black to the right hind leg
green to the left hind leg.

Rationale: The clips should be attached just below the elbows and below the hocks and should be allowed to hang down to minimise movement.

4. **Action:** Soak the crocodile clips with surgical spirit.

Rationale: To ensure good electrical contact.

5. **Action:** Make sure that the room is quiet and stress-free. Set the ECG machine to manual control and switch it on.

Rationale: Any noise or movement will affect the ECG trace.

6. **Action:** Using the markings on the machine, select lead I and do a test trace. Set the electrical filters if required.

Rationale: The filters reduce excessive electrical interference from other electrical circuits in the room, e.g. electric lights or plugged-in appliances, which would affect the trace.

7. **Action:** Record a 1 mV deflection on the test trace

Rationale: This helps to calibrate the measurements of the actual trace.

8. **Action:** Set the paper speed to 2.5 mm per second and record traces from leads I, II, III, AVR, AVL and AVF. Record each lead for 30 seconds.

Rationale: This routine forms a standard initial survey for the detection of any obvious irregularities. Thirty seconds provides enough time for frequent abnormalities to be identified.

9. **Action:** Increase the paper speed to 5 mm per second and record lead II for a further 30 seconds.

Rationale: The most useful and diagnostic measurement is taken across the heart on lead II – from the left foreleg to right hind leg. Faster paper speed will show abnormalities of rhythm or wave form more clearly by stretching the recording over a longer piece of paper.

10. **Action:** Read the trace and look for abnormalities of rhythm and abnormalities in the PQRST waves.

Rationale: Arrhythmias, chamber size irregularities and blocks of the cardiac conduction pathways can be diagnosed by the use of an ECG.

11. **Action:** The veterinary surgeon may require longer traces if an abnormality does not appear in the allocated time.

    Rationale: Some arrhythmias may be intermittent, e.g. in an animal showing signs of fainting. In some cases special small portable ECG units may have to be worn by the animal when exercised. These record digitally and can be used to recall traces from when the dog showed symptoms (e.g. fainting).

12. **Action:** Label the trace by writing on the client's name, date, age and sex of the animal and the case number.

    Rationale: This enables the trace to be identified. If traces are taken at a later date it enables them to be related to the earlier readings.

Procedure: To measure the percentage of oxygen (oxygen saturation) in the blood using a pulse oximeter (Table 2.1)

The pulse oximeter works by transmitting a pulsed infrared light across a thin flap of tissue to a sensor on the other side of a clip. Small pulsing arterioles within this tissue alter the passage of the light and allow the machine to record a pulse rate. Oxygen tension is calculated by using the difference in light absorption by deoxygenated blood compared with that of oxygenated blood. The machine expresses this difference as percentage.

Equipment: Portable pulse oximeter and sensor lead (Fig. 2.4).

1. **Action:** Set up the pulse oximeter near to the patient and either plug it in to the mains or, if battery-operated, ensure that the battery is charged.

    Rationale: The pulse oximeter must be clearly visible to the anaesthetist.

2. **Action:** Set the pulse oximeter to sound its alarm if the pulse rate and oxygen tension go above or below the normal range.

    Rationale: To ensure that action can be taken if the oxygen level falls or the heart rate is too slow or too fast.

3. **Action:** Select the correct sensor for the size of patient.

    Rationale: Smaller animals require smaller clips.

4. **Action:** Select the correct site on which to attach the sensor.

    Rationale: Sites include the tongue, interdigital web, lip, vulva or prepuce.

5. **Action:** Select a site that does not interfere with the surgical procedure.

    Rationale: For instance, using the tongue would interfere with a dental extraction.

6. **Action:** Switch the machine on and monitor the oxygen tension and pulse rate.

    Rationale: In order to identify and correct any reduction in blood oxygen levels or changes in the pulse rate.

7. **Action:** Record the readings on the patient's anaesthetic chart.

    Rationale: Pulse oximetry is used to monitor any changes in anaesthetic level. The heart rate may rise if the depth of anaesthesia is lightening or start to slow if depth is increasing. Oxygen tension may fall if there is a problem with the anaesthetic machine or if the blood in pulmonary circulation is unable to take up the gas, e.g. in cases of pulmonary oedema.

Procedure: To measure central venous pressure (CVP)

Equipment: 1 litre bag of saline, an infusion set, intravenous catheter (14G or smaller), no. 15 scalpel blade, may also need a specially designed 'through the needle' jugular catheter, chlorhexidine solution, swabs, spirit and bandaging materials, three-way tap, 2×0.5 m of sterile drip tubing to connect to the catheter and to the three-way tap, a metric ruler and a stand to hold it vertically.

1. **Action:** Assemble the apparatus required (Fig. 2.5).

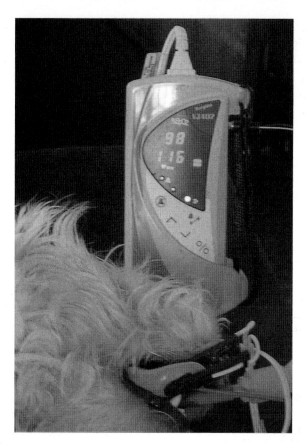

Figure 2.4   A pulse oximeter.

Rationale: CVP can be measured by using simple apparatus usually found in a veterinary practice. Manometers are available but are not a necessity.

2. **Action:** Ask an assistant to restrain the animal for a jugular puncture.

    Rationale: A calm gentle approach will prevent the animal struggling.

3. **Action:** Clip, swab and wipe with spirit an area of the jugular furrow near to the thoracic inlet on the selected side of the neck.

    Rationale: To ensure maximum sterility. The site is at a similar level to the right atrium of the heart, which is where the CVP is measured.

4. **Action:** Put on disposable gloves.

    Rationale: To ensure maximum sterility.

5. **Action:** Ask your assistant to raise the jugular vein by applying digital pressure to the base of the jugular furrow at the thoracic inlet.

Rationale: This will cause the vein to engorge by blocking blood return to the heart – known as 'raising the vein'.

6. **Action:** When the vein is raised, gently push the needle and catheter into the vein with the point towards the head. Check that blood is flowing out of the needle hub and remove the needle while holding the catheter firmly in place.

    Rationale: This will leave the flexible plastic catheter inside the vein. A rigid needle would be likely to dislodge and lacerate the vein if the animal were to move.

7. **Action:** An alternative method is to make a small stab incision through the skin over the vein. If you go too deep you may cut into the vein itself. It can be helpful to mark the spot over the vein and then ask the assistant to release pressure. Move the skin (and spot mark) away from the vein and make the incision.

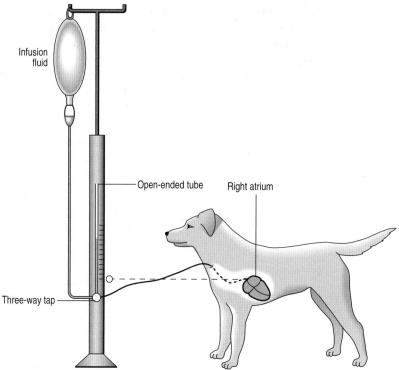

Infusion fluid

Open-ended tube   Right atrium

Three-way tap

Figure 2.5 Method of measuring central venous pressure.

Rationale: Cutting the skin allows the thin through-the-needle catheter to be placed in the vein with minimal resistance. If the skin is not cut first, the catheter may fray or roll back over the needle and may damage the vein.

8. **Action:** Set the three-way tap to allow saline to flow out of the free end of the infusion set, allowing air bubbles in the saline to disperse. Connect the tubing to the end of the catheter once all air bubbles have dispersed.

    Rationale: Air bubbles might cause an air embolism or a block in the circulation and threaten the patient's life. Check that the tube has no blockages or kinks.

9. **Action:** Fix the catheter in place using a bandage or adhesive tape strips.

    Rationale: Under local anaesthetic a butterfly bandage could be placed around the catheter hub or tubing and sutured to the animal's skin.

10. **Action:** Turn the three-way tap to exclude the patient and allow saline to flow up the vertical tubing until halfway up its length (25 cm)

    Rationale: This primes and checks the patency of the tubing and removes any possibility of air entering the patient.

11. **Action:** Check that there are no air bubbles in the pressure tube.

    Rationale: This prevents air inadvertently entering the patient's bloodstream. Bubbles will reduce the accuracy of the measurement.

12. **Action:** Set the three-way tap to exclude the drip bag so that the catheter is now connected, via the tubing and the tap, to the vertical open tubing stretched over the ruler.

    Rationale: Allows the patient's blood pressure to be measured.

13. **Action:** The level in the vertical tube will fall rapidly and settle at a certain mark. Here it will oscillate up and down in time with the patient's breathing.

Rationale: This is the central venous pressure. The pressure of the column of water will equal the pressure in the patient's right atrium.

14. **Action:** Make sure that the zero line on the ruler is level with the right atrium of the heart in the chest.

    Rationale: This is only a rough guide. A spirit level can be used for greater accuracy.

15. **Action:** Read the CVP in centimetres of water against the ruler.

    Rationale: Ask the veterinary surgeon for an interpretation.

16. **Action:** Reconnect the drip to the animal by turning the three-way tap to exclude the pressure arm of the tubing.

17. **Action:** Repeat the readings hourly using the procedure as described from point 10.

    Rationale: This is used to monitor the CVP during the day – usually with an animal on prolonged intravenous therapy.

Central venous pressure is the pressure of the blood entering the right atrium. The jugular catheter must be level with the right atrium of the heart at the time of the measurement. CVP measurement can be useful to determine whether too much fluid is being given to an animal being kept on a drip for a long time.

- A raised CVP may indicate over-perfusion and a raised blood volume.
- A lowered CVP might reflect a failing heart or loss of blood pressure through shock or blood loss. A faster drip rate is required to increase blood volume.

Monitoring such a case might show an increase in CVP as shock improves or blood volume increases. The absolute measurement is less important than the trend shown by the CVP results.

Procedure: To measure arterial blood pressure using a non-invasive technique (Table 2.1)

Invasive (direct) techniques of blood pressure measurement, where arteries are catheterised and linked to a pressure transducer, are more accurate and may be a more common method of blood pressure measurement in university and referral practices. In general veterinary practice non-invasive (indirect) measurement techniques are more likely to be used.

1. **Action:** Place the animal in a comfortable standing position on a table.

   Rationale: If the animal feels uncomfortable or insecure it will try to escape. A distressed animal may have an artificially raised blood pressure. This is particularly important in conscious cats.

2. **Action:** Set up the instrument.

3. **Action:** Choose a cuff of an appropriate size for the animal (Fig. 2.6).

   Rationale: If the cuff is the wrong size the measurement will be inaccurate. Too large a cuff will produce a lower blood pressure reading than is actually shown by the animal and too small a cuff will produce a higher blood pressure reading than the actual pressure.

4. **Action:** Choose a suitable site on a distal limb or the tail (see below).

   Rationale: The cuff is placed over a peripheral artery where a pulse can be palpated. The chosen site must be almost cylindrical for the cuff to sit comfortably and maximise the accuracy of the measurements.

5. **Action:** Shave the transducer site or wet thoroughly with spirit. Lubricate with gel and place transducer over artery while listening for the pulse on the instrument's loudspeaker or earphones. Inflate the cuff

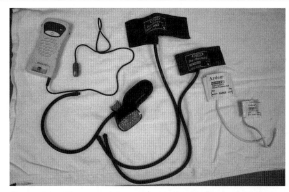

Figure 2.6 Blood pressure monitoring kit with a range of cuff sizes.

until the pulse stops, then, while looking at the pressure dial slowly deflate the cuff until the pulse restarts.

Rationale: Shaving and use of gel reduces air interference between transducer and skin and improves the signal. The cuff pressure at which the pulse restarts is the systolic pressure.

6. **Action:** Take a number of readings over several minutes.

    Rationale: This allows for variations caused by anxiety or movement, which can produce an artificially raised result.

7. **Action:** Record the measurement on the patient's anaesthetic chart or clinical case record.

    Rationale: Blood pressure measurement is used to monitor an anaesthetic or as part of a health check.

    Cuff positioning sites include (Fig. 2.7):

- tail base (coccygeal artery) – best in conscious dogs and cats
- forelimb proximal to carpus (median artery)
- forelimb distal to carpus (common palmar digital artery)
- hindlimb proximal to hock (saphenous artery) – best in anaesthetised dogs
- hindlimb distal to hock (medial plantar artery).

In the dog, blood pressure measurement is usually part of anaesthetic monitoring (Fig. 2.8). Anaesthetic drugs can cause a lowered pressure (hypotension) and fluctuations in the pressure can reflect change in the depth of anaesthesia or blood volume. Monitoring allows necessary treatment to be taken to correct the altered blood pressure. In the cat, raised blood pressure (hypertension) is reasonably common in older animals and is often a consequence of diseases such as renal failure. Routine monitoring of older cats may detect hypertension and allow corrective treatment. Conditions such as retinal haemorrhage and blindness can be directly caused by a raised blood pressure.

Procedure: To measure carbon dioxide levels using a mainstream capnograph (Table 2.1)

A mainstream instrument measures end-tidal CO_2 levels (i.e. it samples the last bit of expired air from each

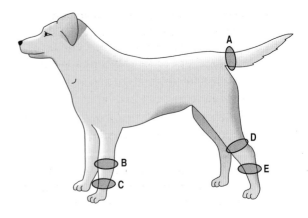

WFF positions
A Tail base (coccygeal artery)
B Proximal to carpus (median artery)
C Distal to carpus (common palmar digital artery)
D Proximal to hock (saphenous artery)
E Distal to hock (median plantar artery)

Figure 2.7 Diagram to show cuff positioning sites for the measurement of blood pressure. A, Tail base – coccygeal artery; B, proximal to carpus – median artery; C, distal to carpus – common palmar digital artery; D, proximal to hock – saphenous artery; E, distal to hock – median plantar artery.

breath). The technique is used during anaesthesia to monitor the inspired and expired carbon dioxide.

1. **Action:** Set up the capnograph.
2. **Action:** After turning off the anaesthetic gas supply, disconnect the endotracheal tube from the gas delivery tube.

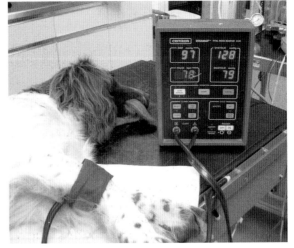

Figure 2.8 Automatic blood pressure monitoring device – purchased from a hospital and adapted for veterinary use.

Rationale: In order to insert mainstream sensor into the gas flow to and from the animal. Turning off the gas first will help prevent spillage of anaesthetic gases into the environment.

3. **Action:** Connect the CO_2 sensor between the endotracheal tube and the gas delivery tube.

   Rationale: Inspired and expired gases pass through the sensor.

4. **Action:** Restart the anaesthetic gases and set the vaporiser to the correct concentration as required by the veterinary surgeon.

   Rationale: To maintain the level of anaesthesia.

5. **Action:** Read the carbon dioxide levels from the digital display.

6. **Action:** Record the levels on the patient's anaesthetic record or print a graph directly from the machine.

   Rationale: To allow monitoring of anaesthesia and early corrective action should the levels start to rise.

7. **Action:** Take readings every 60 seconds throughout the anaesthetic procedure.

   Rationale: To identify any trends and to allow early corrective treatment.

Procedure: To measure carbon dioxide levels using a sidestream capnograph (Fig. 2.9)

A sidestream instrument measures end-tidal CO_2 and inspired CO_2 concentrations.

1. **Action:** Set up the capnograph.

2. **Action:** Without disconnecting the endotracheal tube, attach the small tube leading to the instrument to the special port on the end of the gas delivery tube.

   Rationale: This machine sucks a small sample of gas out of the gas flow rather than being positioned in the midst of the flow.

3. **Action:** Read the levels of inspired and expired CO_2 from the digital display. They are displayed as a scrolling graph showing the changes of CO_2 concentration with each breath.

   Rationale: Both inspired and end-tidal CO_2 levels are measured.

4. **Action:** Record the levels on the patient's anaesthetic record or print a graph directly from the machine.

   Rationale: To allow monitoring of anaesthesia and early corrective action should the levels start to rise.

5. **Action:** Take readings every minute throughout the anaesthetic procedure.

   Rationale: To identify any trends and to allow early corrective treatment.

The sidestream instrument is more accurate and is useful in monitoring both the patient's anaesthetic progress and the efficiency of the anaesthetic equipment. The mainstream type of capnograph has several disadvantages compared with the sidestream type:

- It is more vulnerable to accidental damage as the sensor lies close to the animal during use. The sidestream capnograph can be placed a safe distance away and is less likely to be disturbed.
- It only measures expired end-tidal CO_2 and is useful for identifying a pulmonary problem and a consequent rise in CO_2. However, if the level of CO_2 is high in the inspired gases (e.g. exhausted soda lime in a circuit), the mainstream machine cannot specify whether the cause of the problem is the patient or the apparatus. In a dangerous, life-threatening situation, time may be lost trying to decide the cause of the problem.

Capnographs are available which measure both the CO_2 level and the respiratory rate and may be combined with a pulse oximeter.

Hypercapnia – raised CO_2 levels – may be caused by:

- faulty anaesthetic equipment, e.g. blocked endotracheal tube, excessive dead space, faulty valves, exhausted soda lime
- patient problems, e.g. hypoventilation (reduced respiratory rate, breath holding), any lung condition that prevents the normal exchange of oxygen and carbon dioxide.

Hypocapnia – lowered CO_2 levels – may be caused by:

- patient problems, e.g. hyperventilation caused by panting, or excessive respiratory rate.

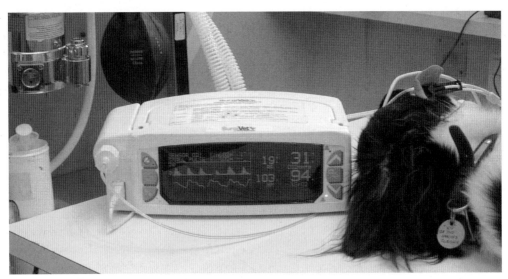

Figure 2.9   A sidestream capnograph combined with a pulse oximeter.

Procedure: To measure urine production (Table 2.1)

Equipment: Sterile urinary catheter, empty used drip bag, infusion set.

1.   **Action:** Catheterise the patient as described in Chapter 3.

2.   **Action:** Drain the bladder with a 50 ml syringe until it is empty.

     Rationale: To get an accurate measure of future urine production.

3.   **Action:** Connect the needle end of the infusion set to the urinary catheter.

4.   **Action:** Make sure that the empty drip bag is level with or, preferably below, the level of the dog's bladder.

     Rationale: This uses gravity to fill the bag and to prevent inadvertent reflux of stale urine back into the bladder.

5.   **Action:** Once an hour **either** weigh the bag on accurate scales **or** empty it with a 50 ml syringe and note the volume.

     Rationale: 1 ml of urine weighs approximately 1 g. Thus the volume can be calculated by the urine weight in grams. This gives the volume of urine produced per hour.

Hourly urinary output is a useful indicator of renal function. Normal kidneys will produce 1–2 ml/kg bodyweight/hour. If urine production is less than 0.5 ml/kg bodyweight/hour then the animal may be severely dehydrated or in renal shutdown.

This procedure is most likely to be performed in hospitalised and recumbent patients. The catheter may be left in place for more than 24 hours and it is very important that a sterile approach is taken to prevent the patient developing cystitis. Bladder infection in a patient that is already ill may cause its condition to deteriorate.

Procedure: To measure tear production (Table 2.1)

Equipment: Schirmer tear measurement strips.

1.   **Action:** Ask an assistant to restrain the animal on the table.

     Rationale: The animal needs to be comfortable to allow the measurement to be made.

2.   **Action:** Remove two Schirmer test strips from their sterile plastic envelope.

     Rationale: These are packaged to keep the strips dry and sterile.

3. **Action:** Fold the end of one strip at the notch near the end. Try not to touch the paper with your fingers.

    Rationale: Touching the strip may cause moisture to be absorbed from your fingers and this may affect the accuracy of the result.

4. **Action:** Gently roll out the lower eyelid and hook the short end of the strip so that it rests against the junction of the cornea and the conjunctiva (Fig. 2.10).

    Rationale: This ensures that the strip makes good contact with the area of tear production.

5. **Action:** Gently close the eyelids.

    Rationale: To hold the strip in place.

6. **Action:** Hold in place for one minute.

    Rationale: This is the standard time of the test.

7. **Action:** Remove the strip and measure the length of the blue-stained area of wet paper.

    Rationale: The longer the length of the stain, the greater the volume of tears produced.

8. **Action:** Repeat the measurement in the other eye using the second strip.

    Rationale: To compare the two eyes.

This simple test is a useful method of assessing tear production. Keratoconjunctivitis sicca (KCS) or 'dry eye' is a distressing problem in certain breeds and the Schirmer test can be used to diagnose and monitor the effectiveness of treatment.

Procedure: To measure intraocular pressure (IOP) (Table 2.1)

Equipment: Either a mechanical IOP instrument (Schiotz) or a digital instrument (Tono-Pen) (Fig. 2.11).

1. **Action:** Ask an assistant to restrain the animal on the table.

    Rationale: The animal needs to be comfortable and firmly restrained to allow the measurement to be taken.

2. **Action:** Put local anaesthetic drops in both eyes. (Proxymetacaine disposable drops are suitable.)

    Rationale: This desensitises the cornea so that it can be touched without the animal blinking or reacting.

3. **Action:** Select the appropriate piece of equipment.

a. Using a Schiotz tonometer

1. **Action:** Calibrate the machine by pressing it gently onto the metal test block. Different weights can be added to the plunger.

    Rationale: This sets the zero pressure level.

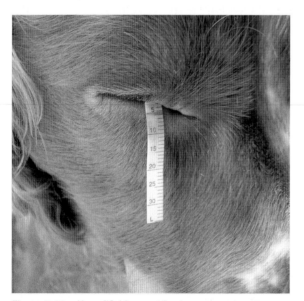

Figure 2.10   Use of Schirmer strips to measure tear production.

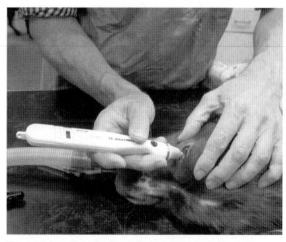

Figure 2.11   Use of a Tono-Pen to measure intraocular pressure.

2. **Action:** Ask the assistant to hold the animal's head up so that the cornea is horizontal.

   Rationale: Readings depend on gravity, so the instrument must be held as vertically as possible.

3. **Action:** Gently rest the instrument on the cornea and take a reading from the needle.

   Rationale: A soft eyeball will only deflect the probe a little, thus producing a reading closer to the zero baseline. Conversely, a harder eyeball will deflect the probe more, thus producing a higher reading.

4. **Action:** Take at least two readings from both eyes.

   Rationale: This allows comparison of the pressure in both eyes and, by repetition, checks the accuracy of the instrument. Each reading should be the same as the previous measurement.

5. **Action:** Record the readings on the clinical case record or hospitalisation chart.

   Rationale: To allow the comparison with later measurements and to monitor the efficacy of treatment.

b. Using a Tono-Pen

1. **Action:** Put a new latex sheath over the end of the Tono-Pen using the cardboard applicator supplied by the manufacturers.

   Rationale: This protects the sensitive end of the instrument and prevents cross-infection.

2. **Action:** Calibrate the machine by pushing the button near the tip with the head of the Tono-Pen held downwards. When it 'beeps', point the head vertically upwards. The machine should read 'good' on the display bar and readings can now be taken. If the display says 'bad' the process has to be repeated until the correct response is obtained.

   Rationale: To calibrate and ensure the accuracy of the actual readings.

3. **Action:** Gently touch the latex covered tip onto the anaesthetised cornea. This should be done several times until a 'beep' is heard.

   Rationale: The machine works by gentle corneal contact not by deforming the surface by pressure.

4. **Action:** Repeat the readings more than once and take them from both eyes.

   Rationale: This allows comparison of the pressure in both eyes and, by repetition, checks the accuracy. Each reading should be the same as the previous measurement.

5. **Action:** Discard the latex sleeve.

   Rationale: To prevent cross-infection.

6. **Action:** Record the readings in the clinical case record or on the hospitalisation chart.

   Rationale: To allow the comparison with later measurements and to monitor the efficacy of treatment.

Intraocular pressure rises if the eye begins to suffer from glaucoma. This increase in pressure can be very destructive to the internal structures of the eye and can cause severe pain, blindness and eventual collapse of the eye. Tonometry readings are a useful method of assessing any rise and allowing time for drugs to be used to reduce the pressure. Serial readings can indicate how effective treatment has been.

The mechanical tonometer is less accurate and is used only as a guide. The Tono-Pen is much more accurate and reliable.

REFERENCES AND FURTHER READING

Chandler E A, Thompson D J, Sutton J B, Price C J 1995 Canine Medicine and Therapeutics. Blackwell Science, Oxford

Hall L W, Clarke K W 1996 Veterinary Anaesthesia, 9th edn. WB Saunders, London

Hotson-Moore A (ed) 1999 Manual of Advanced Veterinary Nursing. BSAVA, Gloucester

Moore M (ed) 1999 Manual of Veterinary Nursing. BSAVA, Gloucester

Peiffer R L, Petersen-Jones S M 1997 Small Animal Ophthalmology. WB Saunders, London

Chapter 3

Medical nursing procedures

Jo Masters

CHAPTER CONTENTS

Introduction   41

General examination of the dog or cat   42
Barrier nursing – avoidance of cross-infection   42
Application of an enema (dogs)   43
Catheterisation of the dog   43
Catheterisation of the bitch   45
Catheterisation of the tomcat   46
Catheterisation of the queen   47
Manual expression of the bladder   48
Cystocentesis   49
Peritoneal dialysis   50
Passive physiotherapy – massage   51
Passive physiotherapy – coupage   51
Passive physiotherapy – supported exercise
   (dogs)   51
Passive physiotherapy – hydrotherapy (dogs)   52
Passive physiotherapy – passive joint therapy   53
Nursing the patient with diarrhoea   53
Nursing the vomiting patient   56
Nursing the paraplegic or recumbent patient   57
Nursing the epileptic patient   58
Nursing the patient with cardiac
   failure – congestive heart failure   59
Nursing the patient with renal disease   60
Nursing the patient with hepatic disease   60
Nursing the patient with pancreatic disease   61
Nursing the patient with diabetes mellitus   62
Nursing the patient with diabetes insipidus   64

INTRODUCTION

Much of the work of the veterinary nurse is concerned with nursing medical patients. These are the patients that are not hospitalised for any type of surgical procedure. Medical conditions can be divided into those that are caused by microorganisms and are infectious, e.g. cat flu or canine parvovirus, and those that develop as a result of an upset in the normal processes of the body, e.g. renal failure, diabetes mellitus or exocrine pancreatic insufficiency. Many patients may not require hospitalisation and may be treated during a consultation or at home, but some will require further diagnostic tests and if critically ill will require observation and skilled nursing care. Those patients that have an infectious disease must be isolated to prevent the spread of infection and barrier nursing procedures must be instigated either at home or within the practice.

The aim of nursing the medical patient is to help the animal to return to a state of normal health as soon as possible. While in the hospital it must be kept warm and comfortable, free from pain and, remembering that this is an animal removed from its normal surroundings, free from fear and apprehension. Veterinary nurses play an extremely important part in the recovery process and the care that they give must be based on an understanding of the disease process and the aims of the treatment regime.

This chapter describes the general techniques used in medical nursing and relates them to some of the more common conditions seen in practice. It is important to understand that most of the techniques can be used in a range of conditions and examples of their use are listed before each procedure.

Procedure: General examination of the dog or cat

1. **Action:** Observe the patient in its kennel and record any abnormalities.

    Rationale: Handling the patient will involve some stress, which may influence clinical signs.

2. **Action:** Remove the patient and place in a comfortable position suited to a full examination.

    Rationale: If the patient feels comfortable it is less likely to try to escape. A cat or small dog should be examined on a table whereas a larger dog may be more suited to an examination on the floor.

3. **Action:** Ask an assistant to reassure and restrain the patient.

    Rationale: Reassuring the patient will help it to relax. An assistant should be ready to restrain the patient if it tries to escape or becomes aggressive during the examination.

4. **Action:** Examine the patient starting at the cranial end, identifying any abnormalities including discharges, wounds, lumps and painful areas.

    Rationale: Examining a patient from head to tail as a routine will limit the likelihood of any area being excluded. Any abnormalities should be noted, however minor or unrelated to the treatment the patient is receiving.

5. **Action:** Temperature, pulse and respiration (TPR) parameters should be taken at this time.

    Rationale: TPR should be noted whenever the patient is examined as a measure of the patient's progress.

6. **Action:** Record all findings on the patient's hospital card.

Rationale: All findings must be recorded on the hospital card to help identify any abnormalities and communicate the patient's progress to all staff. Report any abnormalities to the veterinary surgeon.

Procedure: Barrier nursing – avoidance of cross-infection

1. **Action:** Staff should be allocated solely to the isolation facility and not allowed to nurse patients in the general ward.

    Rationale: Staff could transmit infection from the patient they are nursing to others of the same species or those susceptible to infection such as immunologically challenged patients and paediatric or geriatric patients.

2. **Action:** Personal protective clothing such as disposable gloves, aprons and foot covers should be worn. This should be placed in the clinical waste after use.

    Rationale: Protection from zoonotic disease is a high priority. The wearing of protective clothing will prevent disease being spread via staff clothing.

3. **Action:** Patients who are most likely to spread disease should be cleaned out and treated after all other patients in the isolation facility.

    Rationale: This will prevent disease being spread from the most infectious patient by the nursing staff.

4. **Action:** Each patient in the isolation facility should be allocated its own equipment, i.e. food bowl, water bowl, litter tray, etc. This should be washed and disinfected, or sterilised separately from others. Bedding should all be disposable and should be placed in the clinical waste.

    Rationale: Infection can be spread from fomites such as kennel equipment. Allocation of equipment to specific kennels will limit this as will cleaning the items separately. Keep track of equipment by numbering kennels and their applicable equipment. Most bedding cannot be sterilised satisfactorily and may pass infection on during the cleaning process.

5. **Action:** All findings must be recorded on the patient's hospital sheet. Report all abnormalities to the veterinary surgeon. Barrier nursing notices should be displayed.

   Rationale: The veterinary surgeon should be made aware of the patient's progress. Barrier nursing notices can prevent inadvertent cross-contamination – personnel entering the isolation area should be kept to a minimum.

Procedure: Application of an enema (dogs)

- Examples of uses include emptying the rectum, as a diagnostic aid or to administer drugs.
- Examples of solutions used: water (rectal lavage), soapy water (soap flakes), oily substances (such as liquid paraffin/mineral oil), phosphate enemas (proprietary brands). For cats a proprietary mini enema is usually the product of choice.

1. **Action:** Prepare all equipment – including enema solution at body temperature (and associated tubing, catheters, Higginson's syringe as required), disposable gloves, aprons and absorbent tissue. Lubricant will also be required.

   Rationale: As with all procedures the preparation of the equipment before beginning the procedure is both an efficient and practical method of working. The solution should be warmed to prevent shock and promote tolerance.

2. **Action:** Restrain the patient in a suitable environment – near to an outside door. Two members of staff will be required for this procedure and should wear gloves and aprons to prevent contamination. Place the patient in a standing position.

   Rationale: Giving an enema is a messy procedure and faeces can pass on infection both to the staff and to other patients. The dog will need to evacuate its bowel soon after the application of the enema and will

require an area that can be cleaned and disinfected effectively.

3. **Action:** The end of the tubing to be inserted into the rectum should be lubricated before insertion. The assistant should raise the patient's tail and the anal area should be cleaned with some warm water to remove any faecal material or debris.

   Rationale: Lubricating the tube end will allow easy access and prevent damage to the rectal mucosa. The anal area should be cleaned to prevent infection being introduced from the external area.

4. **Action:** Place the end of the tubing in the patient's anus and gently twist until it is in the rectum. The enema solution should be introduced slowly either by gravity or by pump depending on the method used. The solution may be administered until a back flow is seen.

   Rationale: Gently twisting the tube end will encourage the anal sphincter to relax and allow passage of the tube into the rectum. This is more difficult in cats. A back flow will indicate that the rectum is full of enema solution.

5. **Action:** Once the solution has been delivered, the dog should be allowed free access to a run area to evacuate its bowels.

   Rationale: If the solution has worked as required, bowel evacuation should commence shortly; if not, you may need to repeat the treatment.

6. **Action:** When bowel evacuation is complete, the patient should be cleaned appropriately and a note made of the amount and type of excreta passed.

   Rationale: The patient should be thoroughly clean, dry and comfortable before being put back into its kennel. The type of excreta passed may indicate the reason for a constipation problem, e.g. bones.

Procedure: Catheterisation of the dog

- Two people are required.
- Examples of procedures include short-term catheterisation to obtain a sterile urine sample, or

indwelling catheterisation useful in recumbent patients.

- Examples of catheter types include conventional plastic or Foley silicone dog catheters (Fig. 3.1).

1. **Action:** Prepare all the equipment, including sterile catheter and any application equipment, e.g. stylets to assist with introduction, lubricant, disposable gloves, apron, sterile sample container or collecting vessel such as a kidney dish, syringe, three-way tap or bung. If measurement of urine output and input is required, a urine collection bag will need to be prepared. Absorbent material such as swabs/tissue will be useful and suture material may be required for indwelling catheters.

   Rationale: As with any procedure, the preparation of the equipment before beginning the procedure is both an efficient and practical method of working. Ensure that you understand why the catheter is being introduced and any procedures that will be carried out after its introduction. This will enable all necessary equipment to be prepared. The catheter and collection bag should be sterile to prevent infection being introduced into the urinary tract.

2. **Action:** The assistant should restrain the patient on the examination table. Gloves and aprons should be put on. The preputial area should be cleaned and the penis extruded.

   Rationale: The patient may be standing or in lateral recumbency depending on personal preference. Protective clothing should be worn to prevent the spread of zoonoses and introduction of infection to the patient.

3. **Action:** Remove the catheter from its outer packaging and cut the end from the inner packaging, which is used as a feeder sleeve.

   Rationale: The use of a feeder sleeve allows the catheter to be fed into the urethra without having to touch the sterile tubing.

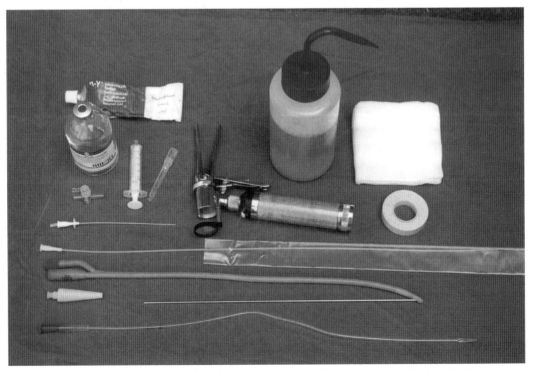

Figure 3.1 Equipment required for general catheterisation. Catheters are from top to bottom: Jackson's cat catheter, conventional dog catheter, latex Foley catheter with stylet correctly placed, Tiemans catheter.

4. **Action:** The catheter tip should be lubricated, introduced into the urethra and then advanced using gentle pressure. Urine will flow back down the catheter when the bladder is reached and may require collection. The bladder may need flushing etc., depending on the procedure to be carried out. Suturing or sticking the catheter to the prepuce will be required if the catheter is to be indwelling.

   Rationale: Gentle pressure should enable the catheter to pass the narrowing of the urethra at the ischial arch or around an enlarged prostate gland. If resistance is met the catheter size may need to be reassessed. The application of zinc oxide tape to the catheter enables it to be sutured to the preputial area.

5. **Action:** Remove the catheter slowly and dispose of correctly. Clean and dry the patient before returning it to its kennel.

   Rationale: Removing the catheter slowly will help prevent tissue damage and urine splashes, which could be a zoonotic risk. All catheters and associated equipment should be disposed of in the clinical waste. Keeping the patient clean will prevent urine scalds.

Procedure: Catheterisation of the bitch

- Two people are required.
- Examples of procedures include short-term catheterisation such as to obtain a sterile urine sample, or indwelling catheterisation useful in recumbent patients.
- Examples of catheter types include Foley indwelling bitch catheters and Tiemans catheters for the bitch. A vaginal speculum (sterile) will be required unless the insertion is to be carried out using the sterile digital method (Fig. 3.1).

1. **Action:** Prepare all the equipment, including sterile catheter and any application equipment (such as vaginal speculum and stylets to assist with introduction if required), lubricant, disposable gloves, apron, sterile sample container/collecting vessel (such as a kidney dish), three-way tap or bung. If measurement of urine output and input is required, a urine collection bag will need to be prepared.

   Rationale: As with all procedures, preparing the equipment before you begin is both an efficient and practical method of working. Ensure that you understand why the catheter is being introduced and any procedures that will be carried out after its introduction. This will enable all necessary equipment to be prepared. The catheter and collection bag should be sterile to prevent infection being introduced to the urinary tract. Foley catheters must not be reused as the balloon weakens after each use.

2. **Action:** Put on gloves and an apron. Ask the assistant to restrain the patient, either in lateral or dorsal recumbency, or in a standing position depending on the insertion method used. If the catheter is to be inserted using the digital method, sterile gloves should be worn by the person carrying out the procedure.

   Rationale: Protective clothing should be worn to prevent the spread of zoonoses and introduction of infection to the patient. For insertion in dorsal recumbency the patient should be in a straight position with the hind legs flexed and drawn cranially. For all methods the tail must be firmly restrained.

3. **Action:** The vulval area should be cleaned and free from debris.

   Rationale: Cleaning the area will prevent introduction of infection to the urogenital tract.

4. **Action:** The catheter should be removed from its outer wrapping, exposing the tip from the inner sleeve, and lubricated. Do not use petroleum-based lubricants on latex catheters. If using a Foley catheter the stylet should be placed and the balloon checked for easy inflation (Fig. 3.1).

   Rationale: Aseptic technique is necessary to prevent introduction of infection. Stylets aid the introduction and placement of the catheter and should be sterile. Most stylets are placed through the tubing but stylets used with Foley catheters should be laid alongside the tubing with the stylet placed in a drainage hole at the catheter's tip.

5. **Action:** Place the speculum blades between the vulval lips. If working with the patient in dorsal recumbency, the blades should be inserted as far caudally as possible, then the speculum should be inserted vertically into the vestibule, turning the handles cranially. If working with the patient standing, the speculum should be inserted at a slight angle towards the spine, then horizontally.

   Rationale: In dorsal recumbency the blades should be inserted to avoid the clitoral fossa.

6. **Action:** Once the speculum is in place, open the blades and identify the urethral orifice.

   Rationale: The urethral orifice should be visible halfway between the vulva and the cervix. If the patient is standing, it will be on the floor of the vestibule; if in dorsal recumbency, it will be on the uppermost side.

7. **Action:** If using the sterile digital method, the first finger of one hand (usually the non-writing hand) should be lubricated and placed into the vestibule, feeling along the ventral surface for a raised area.

   Rationale: The urethral orifice is just cranial to this raised area and can be identified with the finger and the catheter guided in.

8. **Action:** The tip of the catheter should be inserted into the urethral orifice and gradually advanced until it reaches the bladder.

   Rationale: With the patient in dorsal recumbency the hind legs should now be extended caudally to allow straightening of the urethra for easier catheter introduction.

9. **Action:** If a Foley catheter is to be indwelling, the balloon should be inflated, the stylet removed and a collection bag attached. An Elizabethan collar may be used.

   Rationale: The inflated balloon keeps the catheter secure in the bladder without the need for suturing.

10. **Action:** When the appropriate procedure has been completed, remove the catheter slowly, having first deflated the balloon in the Foley catheter, and dispose of it correctly. Ensure that the patient is clean and dry before being returned to its kennel.

    Rationale: Removing the catheter slowly will prevent tissue damage and reduce the risk of urine splashes, which could carry a zoonotic disease. All catheters and associated equipment should be disposed of in the clinical waste. Keeping the patient clean will prevent urine scalds.

Procedure: Catheterisation of the tomcat

This procedure is normally carried out under a general anaesthetic, as it may be painful and struggling may cause penetration of the urethra.

- Two people required.
- Examples of procedures include short-term catheterisation to obtain a sterile urine sample, indwelling catheterisation useful in recumbent patients, or hydropropulsion – using water pressure to dislodge blockages.
- Examples of catheter types include conventional cat catheters, Jackson and silicone catheters for use in the cat.

1. **Action:** Prepare all the equipment, including sterile catheter and any application equipment, e.g. stylets to assist with introduction if required, lubricant, disposable gloves, apron, sterile sample container or collecting vessel (such as a kidney dish), three-way tap or bung. If measurement of urine output is required, a urine collection bag will need to be prepared.

   Rationale: As with all procedures, preparing the equipment before you begin is both an efficient and practical method of working. Ensure that you understand why the catheter is being introduced and any procedures that will be carried out after its introduction. This will enable all necessary equipment to be prepared.

2. **Action:** Put on gloves and apron. Position the cat in lateral or dorsal recumbency, ensuring that the tail is out of the way.

   Rationale: In this position the perineal area and the penis can be easily accessed.

3. **Action:** Remove the catheter from its outer packaging and cut the end from the inner packaging, which is used as a feeder sleeve. Lubricate the tip of the catheter.

   Rationale: The use of a feeder sleeve allows the catheter to be fed into the urethra without touching the sterile tubing. Lubrication of the tip will ensure ease of introduction and will prevent tissue damage.

4. **Action:** Extrude the penis by applying gentle pressure on either side of the prepuce, and introduce the catheter into the urethra (Fig. 3.2). If a Jackson cat catheter is used, remove the metal stylet.

   Rationale: Gentle preputial pressure should result in extrusion of the penis.

5. **Action:** Continue with the procedure – collection of sample, drainage of bladder, hydropropulsion, etc.

   Rationale: If an indwelling Jackson cat catheter is used, suture it to the prepuce. Attach a collection bag and use an Elizabethan collar.

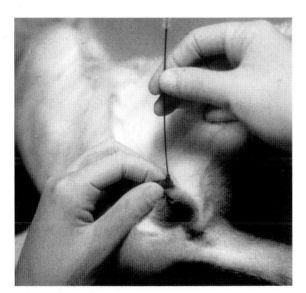

Figure 3.2 Catheterisation of a tomcat.

6. **Action:** Remove the catheter slowly and dispose of it correctly. Return the cat to its kennel when it is clean and dry.

   Rationale: Removing the catheter slowly will prevent tissue damage and urine splashes, which could be a zoonotic risk. All catheters and associated equipment should be disposed of in the clinical waste. Keeping the cat clean and dry will prevent urine scalds.

Procedure: Catheterisation of the queen

- Two people required.
- Examples of procedures include short-term catheterisation to obtain a sterile urine sample, indwelling catheterisation useful in recumbent patients, or hydropropulsion – using water pressure to dislodge blockages.
- Examples of catheter types include conventional cat catheters, Jackson and silicone catheters for use in the cat.

1. **Action:** Prepare all the equipment including sterile catheter and any application equipment, e.g. stylets to assist with introduction, lubricant, disposable gloves, apron, sterile sample container or collecting vessels such as a kidney dish, three-way tap or bung. If measurement of urine output is required, a urine collection bag will need to be prepared.

   Rationale: As with all procedures, preparing the equipment before you begin is both an efficient and practical method of working. Ensure that you understand why the catheter is being introduced and any procedures that will be carried out after its introduction. This will enable all necessary equipment to be prepared.

2. **Action:** Put on gloves and apron. Restrain the cat and ensure that the tail is also restrained.

   Rationale: Restrain the cat either in a standing position or in lateral recumbency.

3. **Action:** Remove the catheter from its outer packaging and cut the end from the inner packaging, which is used as a feeder sleeve. Lubricate the tip of the catheter.

Rationale: The use of a feeder sleeve allows the catheter to be fed into the urethra without touching the sterile tubing. Lubrication of the tip will ensure ease of introduction and will prevent tissue damage.

4. **Action:** Place the catheter between the vulval lips and introduce into the urethra by angling the catheter ventrally, using gentle pressure until the catheter enters the urethral orifice.

   Rationale: The use of a vaginal speculum is not necessary for this procedure. Queen catheterisation is not often performed, as blockages are rare.

5. **Action:** Continue with procedure – collection of sample, drainage of bladder, hydropropulsion, etc.

   Rationale: If an indwelling Jackson cat catheter has been used, suture it in place, attach a collection bag and use an Elizabethan collar.

6. **Action:** Remove the catheter slowly and dispose of it correctly. Return the cat to its kennel when it is clean and dry.

   Rationale: Slowly removing the catheter will prevent tissue damage and urine splashes, which could be a zoonotic risk. All catheters and associated equipment should be disposed of in the clinical waste. Keeping the cat clean and dry will prevent urine scalds.

Procedure: Manual expression of the bladder

• Two people required.

Manual expression of the bladder may be required in recumbent patients or those suffering from bladder paralysis. Natural elimination of the bladder is preferable to urinary catheterisation but it should not be attempted where there is any possibility of urethral obstruction.

1. **Action:** Put on gloves and apron and prepare urinary collection equipment (if required) and absorbent tissue.

   Rationale: Protection of staff from zoonotic diseases transmitted by urine is essential.

Urinary collection equipment, such as a kidney dish, or a sterile sample pot may be required if the urine requires analysing.

2. **Action:** An assistant should restrain the patient in a standing position in a suitable area that is clean and easy to disinfect.

   Rationale: Restraining the patient in the standing position will ensure easy access to the bladder. The area in which the patient urinates should be easy to disinfect to prevent contamination. Dogs will often feel happier urinating outside.

3. **Action:** Isolate the bladder by palpation of the caudal abdomen and place one hand either side of it on the external abdominal wall.

   Rationale: A full bladder should be easy to palpate, as it will feel like a distended sac in the caudal abdomen. If there are difficulties in isolating the bladder, ask a veterinary surgeon to examine the patient for you.

4. **Action:** Apply gentle pressure to the abdominal wall on either side of the bladder to encourage urination. Urine should flow freely and be directed into a collection container (Fig. 3.3). Do not be tempted to squeeze the bladder – if there is any resistance and no urine flow, stop the procedure.

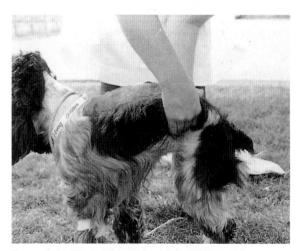

Figure 3.3 Manual expression of the bladder while supporting a recumbent patient. Reproduced, with permission, from Lane and Cooper (2003), Butterworth-Heinemann.

Rationale: Gentle pressure either side of the bladder will mimic the action of the abdominal muscles and should produce a flow of urine. If there is an obstruction in either the bladder or the urethra, no urine will flow. A full bladder may rupture if pressure is put on it. Squeezing a bladder with an obstructed urethra may result in rupture or bruising of the bladder wall.

5. **Action:** When the flow ceases release the pressure. Measure the volume, note its colour, turbidity, smell and the time it was passed. Record your results on the patient's hospital record.

   Rationale: Records should be kept of all procedures. Measuring fluid output is vital in patients on fluid therapy and a comparison of these details will enable accurate assessment of the patient's progress.

6. **Action:** Ensure that the patient is clean and dry before replacing it in its kennel. All areas where urination has occurred should be cleaned and disinfected and disposable clothing placed in the clinical waste.

   Rationale: Ensuring that the patient is clean and dry will prevent urine scalds. Protection of staff and other patients from contamination is vital – disinfection should be a high priority.

Procedure: Cystocentesis

- Two people required – this technique should only be carried out by a veterinary surgeon on a palpable bladder. It may be the only practical method of draining the bladder when obstructed.

1. **Action:** Prepare all the equipment including disposable aprons and gloves, sterile gloves for the veterinary surgeon, a sterile syringe (5–20 ml) and needle of appropriate size (usually 23G × 2.5 cm), three-way tap and sterile urinary collection vessel as required. Clippers and skin preparation solution should be at hand.

   Rationale: As with all procedures, preparing the equipment before you begin is both an efficient and practical method of working. For the welfare of the patient choose a syringe of suitable size and a long needle with a narrow gauge – this should ensure adequate flow. Urine collection may include the preparation of a sterile sample so a suitable pot may be required.

2. **Action:** Put on gloves and apron and restrain the patient in lateral recumbency with the abdomen angled slightly dorsally.

   Rationale: The patient should be restrained to allow easy access to the bladder. Raising of the bladder also reduces the risk of inappropriate puncture of the abdominal organs.

3. **Action:** An area of about 5 cm^2 should be clipped on the midline of the caudal abdomen. Prepare the area in an aseptic fashion using a suitable surgical preparation scrub.

   Rationale: This area needs to be treated as a surgical site and an aseptic technique needs to be maintained.

4. **Action:** The veterinary surgeon will put on the sterile gloves and manually locate and immobilise the bladder through the abdominal wall. Using the syringe with needle attached, the veterinary surgeon will insert the needle through the abdominal wall and into the bladder, Drawing back on the syringe, the urine will be removed.

   Rationale: The aim is to insert the needle into the bladder causing as little trauma as possible and to prevent the introduction of infection by utilising an aseptic technique.

5. **Action:** Gentle pressure should be applied at the injection site when the needle is removed.

   Rationale: Gentle pressure around the injection site will encourage natural tissue recoil around the pierced area and prevent leakage.

6. **Action:** Collect the urine for analysis or dispose of it in the clinical waste. A note should be made of the volume, colour, smell and turbidity for the patient's records.

All equipment used should be disposed of in the clinical waste.

Rationale: Urine should be carefully disposed of in the clinical waste to protect staff and other patients from contamination. A record of urinary output should be noted on the patient's records to enable assessment of its progress.

7.   **Action:** The patient should be thoroughly cleaned and dried before it is placed back in its kennel.

Rationale: Prevention of infection is a high priority.

Procedure: Peritoneal dialysis

- Two people required – this technique should only be carried out by a veterinary surgeon.

Peritoneal dialysis is used to filter waste products from the blood in patients suffering from conditions such as acute renal failure. In these cases, the use of osmotic diuretics may fail to stimulate urine production.

1.   **Action:** Prepare all the equipment including disposable aprons and gloves, sterile gloves for the veterinary surgeon, a small sterile surgical pack, local anaesthetic, peritoneal catheter, trochar, giving set, and dialysis fluid warmed to body temperature. A collection vessel for the waste fluid should be available. Clippers and skin preparation solution should be at hand.

Rationale: As with all procedures, preparing the equipment before you begin is both an efficient and practical method of working. A strict aseptic technique should be used. Dialysis fluid is specific to this procedure and should be warmed to body temperature to prevent shock.

2.   **Action:** Put on gloves and apron and restrain the patient in dorsal recumbency. The hair should be clipped from the ventral abdomen and the site aseptically prepared.

Rationale: Restraining the patient in dorsal recumbency will result in ease of access to the ventral abdomen. The ventral area

needs to be treated as a surgical site and aseptic technique maintained.

3.   **Action:** The veterinary surgeon will inject local anaesthetic into the midline umbilical area.

Rationale: A general anaesthetic would be contraindicated in patients with renal failure.

4.   **Action:** The surgical site should be draped and a small incision made in the skin so that the catheter can be inserted into the abdomen with the aid of a trochar.

Rationale: The site should be draped to aid in asepsis. A trochar is a needle-like instrument which can be used to pierce the abdominal wall.

5.   **Action:** When the catheter is in place, the giving set and the bag containing dialysis fluid should be attached and allowed to flow into the abdominal cavity.

Rationale: The nitrogenous waste flowing through the capillary bed of the peritoneum diffuses into the dialysis fluid.

6.   **Action:** After a specified period of time (usually 30 minutes), the dialysis fluid is removed under gravity. This procedure may be repeated until the blood chemistry improves. Suture placement of the catheter may be required.

Rationale: The dialysis fluid carries the nitrogenous waste out with it, thus benefiting the patient by reducing urea levels. Removing the fluid by gravity can sometimes be difficult and slow but allowing the patient to move around can aid the flow. If necessary repeat the procedure whilst monitoring the blood urea and creatinine levels of the patient.

7.   **Action:** Ensure that the wound is clean and dry before the patient is placed back in its kennel. This patient should be closely monitored as there is a high risk of peritonitis and shock.

Rationale: Ensure that the patient is comfortable and that there is no leakage from the wound before placing it back in its kennel. A patient in acute renal failure may be

immunologically compromised and it is easy for infections such as peritonitis to develop.

Procedure: Passive physiotherapy – massage

Physiotherapy is used to maintain and improve peripheral circulation and is useful in recumbent patients. Massage is especially useful for the limbs.

1. **Action:** Restrain the patient in a comfortable position that enables access to the limbs.

    Rationale: For the procedure to be beneficial, the patient needs to feel relaxed and comfortable. It may be preferable to use the patient's kennel rather than an examination table which it may associate with pain and discomfort.

2. **Action:** Examine each limb in turn to check for wounds and any other abnormalities.

    Rationale: Massage should not be carried out if any abnormalities are present – check with the veterinary surgeon.

3. **Action:** Massage each limb in turn by briskly rubbing from the feet towards the body for at least 5 minutes per limb.

    Rationale: Massaging from the feet towards the trunk of the body encourages venous return.

4. **Action:** Reassure the patient whilst the procedure is being carried out.

    Rationale: Talking to the patient will help it to relax and the massage will become not only beneficial for the circulation but a source of comfort and attention for the animal.

5. **Action:** Regular massage should be part of the patient's daily care.

    Rationale: For full benefit massage should be carried out regularly during the patient's treatment.

Procedure: Passive physiotherapy – coupage

Physiotherapy is used to maintain and improve peripheral circulation and is useful in recumbent patients. Coupage promotes thoracic circulation and helps to prevent hypostatic pneumonia.

1. **Action:** Restrain the patient in sternal recumbency (or standing).

    Rationale: The sternal position allows access to either side of the thorax and facilitates the greatest possible lung expansion.

2. **Action:** Examine the patient for signs of abnormality – such as wounds, tumours, fractures, etc.

    Rationale: Coupage may be contraindicated with some conditions such as fractured ribs, where further damage could be caused. If in doubt consult the veterinary surgeon.

3. **Action:** Cup your hands and slap either side of the thorax from the most caudal part of the area to the cranial part. Repeat for up to 5 minutes.

    Rationale: This slapping promotes coughing and improves the thoracic circulation. It also assists in the removal of bronchial secretions.

4. **Action:** This procedure should be carried out up to 4–5 times daily or as recommended by the veterinary surgeon.

    Rationale: Coupage must be carried out regularly to maintain thoracic circulation in a recumbent patient.

Procedure: Passive physiotherapy – supported exercise (dogs)

Physiotherapy is used to maintain and improve peripheral circulation and is useful in recumbent patients. Supported exercise can be carried out using proprietary frames, but 'towel walking' is the most common method used for paraplegic patients in a practice (Fig. 3.4).

1. **Action:** Depending on the size of dog, 'towel walking' can be carried out by one or two people. A strong towel and dog lead will be required – the size is dependent on the size of the patient.

    Rationale: For large dogs one person will be needed to support the hindquarters and one to support and control the front of the patient. In giant breeds two people may be required to support the hindquarters alone.

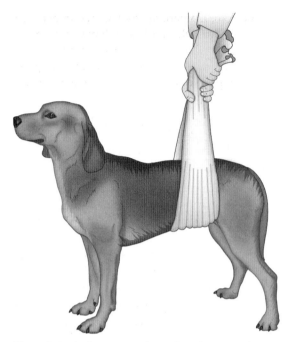

Figure 3.4   Active supported exercise using a towel.

Health and safety should always be taken into consideration and the procedure should not be attempted without sufficient staff available.

2.   **Action:** Restrain the dog and attach a lead. Roll the towel into a 'sausage' shape and pass under the caudal abdomen. Hold the towel at each end supporting the body so that the feet are on the ground (Fig. 3.4).

  Rationale: The towel is used to support the hindquarters of the patient and mimic its usual stance (Fig. 3.4). In a small dog, one person may be able to hold the ends of the towel with one hand and the patient's lead with the other.

3.   **Action:** Encourage the dog to walk while supporting the hindquarters.

  Rationale: Supported walking encourages the circulation and gives the patient confidence to try and use its limbs whilst they are being supported.

4.   **Action:** Encourage urination and defecation and improve the patient's mental attitude by carrying out this procedure in an outside environment.

  Rationale: The opportunity to be outside is often invaluable in changing the patient's mental attitude and will encourage normal behaviour such as urination and defecation.

5.   **Action:** The opportunity for a supported walk should be offered to the patient at least three times a day as part of a physiotherapy technique.

  Rationale: This procedure needs to be carried out regularly to promote improvement in the patient's condition.

Procedure: Passive physiotherapy – hydrotherapy (dogs)

Physiotherapy is used to maintain and improve peripheral circulation and is useful in recumbent patients. Hydrotherapy can be carried out for small dogs in sinks or baths available in the practice. For larger patients, referral to specialised facilities may be necessary. Hydrotherapy causes more stress than benefit in most cats!

1.   **Action:** Fill a sink or bath of suitable size with warm water – ideally slightly above body temperature.

  Rationale: The water should be deep enough to force the patient to move or swim and should be warm enough to be inviting and not chill the patient.

2.   **Action:** Gradually lower the patient into the water supporting the patient's body. Ideally the patient should start to move the limbs in a swimming action. Do not leave the patient – it will require constant support and reassurance.

  Rationale: Support the patient's body at all times to prevent panic or drowning. The swimming action provides excellent physiotherapy to the limbs without weight bearing and will help build muscle tissue and increase its strength.

3.   **Action:** The length of time required will vary from patient to patient but as a general rule start with approximately 5 minutes, building up the time as the patient becomes more confident.

Rationale: Initially the patient will tire quickly, but as its strength builds it will tolerate a longer session in the water.

4. **Action:** The patient should be dried properly and placed in a warm kennel when each session is over.

   Rationale: Do not allow the patient to become chilled as it goes back into an environment in which it cannot move.

5. **Action:** As with all physiotherapy techniques, hydrotherapy sessions need to be regular to have a beneficial effect on the patient.

   Rationale: Regular exercise of the limbs will build up muscle mass.

Procedure: Passive physiotherapy – passive joint movement

Physiotherapy is used to maintain and improve peripheral circulation and is useful in recumbent patients. Passive joint movement will improve limb circulation and helps prevent stiffness of the joints.

1. **Action:** Ensure the patient is comfortable and relaxed – you may wish to carry out this procedure with the patient in its kennel rather than on an examination table.

   Rationale: A relaxed patient will benefit more from the procedure than a patient that is anxious and tense.

2. **Action:** An assistant may be required to restrain the patient's head until the patient becomes familiar with the process. It may be possible to carry out the procedure single-handed if the patient is in lateral recumbency in its kennel.

   Rationale: The patient may be supported in a standing position or in lateral recumbency in its kennel. This will depend on its condition. The help of an assistant may be required in some cases.

3. **Action:** Slowly flex and extend the joints, one limb at a time, starting with the carpal/tarsal joints and then moving upwards to the next joint.

   Rationale: Slowly flexing and extending the joints will enable them to become more

flexible. If a patient has been recumbent for a few days, the joints may have become very stiff. Be careful to keep within the normal range of movement to prevent joint damage. Working up the limb encourages venous return.

4. **Action:** The amount of time spent working on each joint should be related to the patient's condition and the degree of joint degeneration. It is usual for the duration of the sessions to increase as the patient's condition improves.

   Rationale: Seek advice from the veterinary surgeon.

5. **Action:** As with all physiotherapy techniques, joint movement sessions need to be regular to have a beneficial effect on the patient.

   Rationale: Regular movement of the joints will improve circulation and prevent stiffness.

Procedure: Nursing the patient with diarrhoea

A patient with diarrhoea of unknown aetiology should always be treated as a possible source of infection. Infectious diseases that may have diarrhoea as a clinical sign include canine parvovirus and feline infectious enteritis. Diseases that are also zoonotic include campylobacteriosis and salmonellosis. If an infectious disease is suspected, barrier nursing should be maintained throughout the patient's stay.

1. **Action:** If no definite diagnosis has been made, provide isolation facilities, or choose a kennel that is easy to clean and disinfect.

   Rationale: Always suspect an infectious disease if no diagnosis has been made or whilst diagnostic tests are being carried out. It is likely that the kennel occupied by a diarrhoeic patient will require regular cleaning and disinfection so management of this should be taken into account.

2. **Action:** If an infectious disease is suspected, instigate barrier nursing techniques.

   Rationale: Barrier nursing should be employed to protect both staff and other patients from the spread of infection.

3. **Action:** Provide a comfortable environment for the patient including absorbent bedding and warmth. For cats ensure that a clean litter tray is available at all times.

   Rationale: These patients will be feeling uncomfortable and insecure. They may defecate frequently and therefore will require bedding that is absorbent and disposable. Most cats will prefer to use a clean litter tray so make sure it is cleaned every time it is used.

4. **Action:** Ensure that the medical treatment prescribed by the veterinary surgeon is carried out and recorded on the patient's record (Fig. 3.5).

   Rationale: The veterinary surgeon may have prescribed drugs which must be given at the advised times to have maximum effect. The administration of any drug should be noted on the patient's records, to ensure that all members of staff are aware that the treatment has been given.

5. **Action:** Monitor any fluid therapy that is being given. This is likely to be administered intravenously. An example of a fluid commonly used for diarrhoeic patients is Hartmann's solution.

   Rationale: Patients with diarrhoea lose water and electrolytes, which need to be replaced by the appropriate fluid. In cases of chronic diarrhoea, a metabolic acidosis may occur and sodium bicarbonate may be required.

6. **Action:** Monitor and record the usual patient parameters, i.e. temperature, pulse and respiration. An assessment of the patient's hydration status should be made and recorded.

   Rationale: Patient parameters are required to assess progress. Clinical signs of dehydration include slightly sunken eyes, dry mucous membranes and a loss of skin elasticity.

7. **Action:** Monitor and record the patient fluid intake and output, i.e. the rate and volume of fluid the patient is given as well as the amount and type of urine and faeces it produces.

   Rationale: Monitoring fluid intake and output gives us the information to gauge the hydration status and progress. The amount, colour and type of faeces passed should be recorded to assess the recovery process.

8. **Action:** A soiled patient should be bathed immediately with warm water and dried with disposable absorbent towel before being placed back in the clean kennel. Disposable aprons and gloves should be worn throughout the procedure and should be disposed of in the clinical waste after use.

   Rationale: Clip away heavily soiled hair, ensuring that it is easy to clean the area if further diarrhoea occurs. The patient may be sore in places; check this with the veterinary surgeon. Thoroughly drying the patient before returning it to its kennel will prevent further soreness and the patient will not become chilled. All contaminated equipment should be regarded as a possible source of infection and be disinfected or placed in the clinical waste. Faecal material should be disposed of in the clinical waste unless required for analysis.

9. **Action:** Diagnostic tests may be planned for this patient. Blood samples may be taken to measure the patient's hydration status. Faecal material may be required to aid in the diagnosis of the condition and may require collection at regular intervals. Check with the veterinary surgeon before disposing of any faecal material from the patient.

   Rationale: Packed cell volume (PCV) and blood electrolyte levels will help monitor the hydration status of the patient. Analysis of the components of the faecal material may include bacteriology.

10. **Action:** The nutritional requirements of the patient will depend on the severity of the condition. Initially 'nil by mouth' is likely to be advised, with feeding starting gradually once the veterinary surgeon has approved this. A bland diet is then offered with a gradual reintroduction of the patient's usual food.

Kennel Chart							
Animal		Owner			Case Number		
Species		Clinician			Student		
Breed		Clinical Summary					
Colour							
Sex							
Age							

Date		Day No.		Date		Day No.	
Weight		Diet		Weight		Diet	

	AM	PM			AM	PM	
Temp				Temp			
Pulse				Pulse			
Resp				Resp			
Fed				Fed			
Ate				Ate			
Drank				Drank			
Taken Out					Taken Out			
Urine					Urine			
Faeces					Faeces			

MEDICATION		MEDICATION	
PROCEDURES		PROCEDURES	
COMMENTS		COMMENTS	

Figure 3.5   Example of a hospitalisation kennel chart. Adapted, with permission, from Masters and Bowden (2001), Butterworth-Heinemann.

Rationale: Nil by mouth is instigated to rest the gastrointestinal tract. Once the inflammatory reaction has begun to subside food may gradually be reintroduced. The use of a bland diet is less likely to inflame the gastrointestinal tract – a proprietary diet may be used in the practice. Once this diet is being tolerated without causing diarrhoea, the patient's usual diet can be reintroduced.

11. **Action:** If you have any concern over the condition of the patient, notify the veterinary surgeon immediately.

    Rationale: These patients can develop problems very rapidly and require constant veterinary care.

Procedure: Nursing the vomiting patient

A patient with vomiting of unknown aetiology should always be treated as a possible source of infection. Infectious diseases that have vomiting as a clinical sign include canine parvovirus and feline infectious enteritis. Zoonotic diseases include leptospirosis. If an infectious disease is suspected, barrier nursing should be maintained throughout the patient's stay. Vomiting can range from a minor episode such as that resulting from scavenging to a major attack as occurs with some forms of poisoning. Each type will require different degrees of nursing.

1. **Action:** If no definite diagnosis has been made, provide isolation facilities, or choose a kennel that is easy to clean and disinfect.

   Rationale: Always suspect an infectious disease if no diagnosis has been made or whilst diagnostic tests are being carried out. It is likely that the kennel occupied by a vomiting patient will require regular cleaning and disinfection so management of this should be taken into account.

2. **Action:** If an infectious disease is suspected, use barrier nursing techniques.

   Rationale: Barrier nursing should be employed to protect both staff and other patients from infection.

3. **Action:** Provide a comfortable environment for the patient including absorbent bedding and warmth.

   Rationale: These patients will be feeling uncomfortable and insecure. Vomiting may occur frequently and will require efficient cleaning. The patient may be shocked and will need to be kept warm.

4. **Action:** Ensure that the medical treatment prescribed by the veterinary surgeon is carried out and recorded on the patient's record (Fig. 3.5).

   Rationale: The veterinary surgeon may have prescribed drugs for this patient which must be given at the advised times to have maximum effect. The administration of any drug should be noted on the patient's records, to ensure that all members of staff are aware that the treatment has been given.

5. **Action:** Monitor any fluid therapy that is being given. This is likely to be administered intravenously. An example of a fluid commonly used for vomiting patients is 0.9% sodium chloride solution. Oral electrolyte replacement may be used in minor cases.

   Rationale: Patients that are persistently vomiting will lose water and electrolytes, which need to be replaced by an appropriate fluid.

6. **Action:** Monitor and record the usual patient parameters, i.e. temperature, pulse and respiration. An assessment of the patient's hydration status should be made and recorded.

   Rationale: Patient parameters are required to assess progress. Clinical signs of dehydration include slightly sunken eyes, dry mucous membranes and a loss of skin elasticity.

7. **Action:** Monitor and record the patient fluid intake and output, i.e. the rate and volume of fluid the patient is given as well as the amount and type of vomit, urine and faeces it produces.

   Rationale: Monitoring fluid intake and output gives us the information to gauge its hydration status and progress. The amount, colour and type of vomit should be recorded to make an assessment of progress.

8. **Action:** Diagnostic tests may be planned for this patient. Blood samples may be taken to measure the patient's hydration status. Prepare equipment as required.

    Rationale: Packed cell volume (PCV) and blood electrolyte levels will help monitor the hydration status of the patient.

9. **Action:** Nutritional requirements of the patient will depend on the severity of the condition. Initially, 'nil by mouth' is likely to be advised with feeding starting gradually once the veterinary surgeon has approved this. A bland diet is then offered with gradual reintroduction of the patient's usual food. Oral fluids may require monitoring initially, being given 'little and often' until the vomiting has ceased.

    Rationale: 'Nil by mouth' is instigated to rest the gastrointestinal tract. Once the inflammatory reaction has begun to subside, food may gradually be reintroduced. This may begin as a bland diet, which is less likely to inflame the gastrointestinal tract – a proprietary diet may be used in the practice. Once this diet is being tolerated without causing vomiting, the patient's usual diet is gradually reintroduced.

10. **Action:** If you have any concern over the condition of the patient, notify the veterinary surgeon immediately.

    Rationale: These patients can develop problems very rapidly and require constant veterinary care.

Procedure: Nursing the paraplegic or recumbent patient

Examples of conditions that may result in paraplegia include spinal trauma, spinal neoplasia, head injuries, pelvic fractures, and medical diseases such as cardiac disease.

1. **Action:** Choose a kennel of a size in which the patient can lie comfortably on its side. Waterproof bedding such as a foam mattress is ideal, with absorbent bedding material placed on top. Try to prop the patient in sternal recumbency with foam pads or sandbags. Remember that these patients may be lying in the same kennel for some time so try to place them in an area where they can see some activity to keep them stimulated.

    Rationale: The patient needs to be able to lie comfortably but the kennel should not be so large that the patient could move around and damage itself. Sternal recumbency will help to prevent hypostatic pneumonia. Foam mattresses are comfortable for the patient and help to prevent the formation of decubitus ulcers. Absorbent bedding is required, as these patients are often incontinent.

2. **Action:** Monitor and record the usual patient parameters, i.e. temperature, pulse and respiration. Urinary and faecal outputs should be recorded as well as any progress. Any abnormalities should be recorded and the veterinary surgeon notified.

    Rationale: Patient parameters are required to assess progress. Recumbent patients will lose heat quickly and may require covering with blankets, or use an infrared lamp or other heating device. Heat pads are not recommended for patients that are unable to move as they may be burnt.

3. **Action:** Provide a concentrated, highly digestible diet. Ensure that food and water are placed within reach of the patient. Some of these patients may refuse to eat and tempting them with their usual favourite foods may stimulate the appetite. Water must be available at all times – intake should be measured.

    Rationale: Energy requirements are low but recumbent patients require a diet that will supply enough energy for tissue repair and the stress of being kennelled over a long period. Some of these patients may be overweight and a reducing diet may be introduced if advised by the veterinary surgeon. It is important to keep the appetite stimulated.

4. **Action:** Even if the patient is incontinent, dogs should be taken outside for a change in environment on a regular basis using 'towel walking' techniques (Fig. 3.4).

   Rationale: A change in the patient's environment will be stimulating. Supported exercise techniques promote good circulation and enable the patient to gain confidence.

5. **Action:** Turn the patient in its kennel every 4 hours to prevent hypostatic pneumonia and decubitus ulcers. Apply padding to bony prominences to prevent decubitus ulcers. Make sure that the patient is clean and dry every time it is turned to prevent urine scalding – the patient may have an indwelling catheter and this should be cared for accordingly.

   Rationale: Hypostatic pneumonia occurs when there is pooling of the blood in the lungs and is seen in patients left in lateral recumbency for long periods without turning. Decubitus ulcers occur on the bony prominences and are extremely slow in healing. Urine scalds are easily prevented with good nursing. The patient must be kept clean and dry at all times – barrier creams can be applied to the most susceptible areas.

6. **Action:** Carry out physiotherapy techniques.

   Rationale: Simple physiotherapy such as supported exercise, passive joint movement and massage should be carried out. If equipment is available, hydrotherapy may be used.

Procedure: Nursing the epileptic patient

Epilepsy is a condition of the central nervous system in which the brain sends out confused electrical messages, which result in convulsions. The convulsions consist of three phases – pre-ictal, ictal and post-ictal, with collapse occurring during the ictal phase. These convulsions, or 'fits', will often take place at home and advice will initially be given to the owner (often over the telephone). Personal safety must be taken in account – an animal that is fitting may inadvertently bite.

1. **Action:** Advise the owner not to touch the animal and to ask all people to leave the room. Move all furniture away from the animal to prevent injury. Reduce noise and darken the environment. Observe the animal until the fit is over and then reassure the animal.

   Rationale: A fitting animal should not be brought down to the surgery as this stimulation could prolong the fit. Transporting a fitting animal in the car could cause an accident. All stimulation should be removed from the animal, i.e. people, noise, light – a quiet environment will help the animal recover more quickly. The animal will be confused after the fit and will require comfort.

2. **Action:** If the fit becomes continuous or repeated fits occur one after the other, the animal must be brought to the surgery. A padded kennel should be prepared.

   Rationale: Prolonged fitting is known as status epilepticus – these patients will require anticonvulsant therapies and constant observation. Padding in the kennel will prevent the animal damaging itself during convulsions.

3. **Action:** The veterinary surgeon may wish to give intravenous anticonvulsants. The patient's pulse, respiration and mucous membrane colour should be monitored frequently. An oxygen supply should be readily available in case of respiratory difficulties. Do not touch the patient until the fitting has subsided. The temperature should be taken regularly to monitor for hypothermia.

   Rationale: Anticonvulsants will depress the central nervous system and control the fit. However, they may also cause respiratory problems so constant observation is required. These patients will essentially be sedated and lying still for long periods, which could lead to a situation where hypothermia develops.

4. **Action:** The progress and continuing nursing care of these patients depends on the aetiology of the fit. Some patients (i.e. those

with idiopathic epilepsy) can be stabilised and may be discharged with anticonvulsive therapies. Other patients may have signs of an underlying disease of which the fit is one of the symptoms – diagnostic tests may be required to confirm this.

Rationale: Idiopathic epilepsy can be treated with oral anticonvulsants, but other disease conditions such as renal disease or poisoning may cause fitting and will be treated differently.

Procedure: Nursing the patient with cardiac failure – congestive heart failure

Congestive heart failure occurs when the heart fails to function effectively – it compensates by changing its rate, leading to clinical signs which will indicate the side of the heart that is affected. Right-sided heart failure will result in poor venous return to the heart, congestion of organs such as the liver and spleen, and possibly the development of ascites. Left-sided heart failure will result in poor venous return from the lungs, causing pulmonary congestion and oedema, tachypnoea and coughing.

1. Action: Choose a kennel of a size in which the patient can lie comfortably. Bedding should be comfortable and absorbent. The kennel needs to be in a quiet area.

    Rationale: The patient needs to be able to lie comfortably. It may be on drug therapy that results in an increase in urination so acrylic bedding or incontinence pads may be useful in case of leakage. These patients require a stress-free environment.

2. Action: Monitor and record the usual patient parameters, i.e. temperature, pulse and respiration. Urinary and faecal output should be recorded. Note any progress. Any abnormalities should be recorded (Fig. 3.5) and the veterinary surgeon notified. Take the patient out to urinate frequently.

    Rationale: Patient parameters are required to assess progress. Geriatric patients will lose heat quickly and may require covering with blankets or the use of an infrared lamp or

other heating device. Heat pads are not recommended for patients that are unable to move away from the heat as they may be burnt. The patient may be under treatment with diuretics and therefore need to urinate more frequently.

3. Action: Cardiac patients need a diet that is low in salt, contains protein of high biological value and is highly digestible. However, it is important to stimulate the patient's appetite, which may mean that salt is added to improve the taste. Cardiac patients are often overweight and a diet with reducing capabilities may be utilised at the discretion of the veterinary surgeon. Potassium supplementation may be required. Water must be available at all times – intake should be measured.

    Rationale: A diet that is low in salt will help to reduce pulmonary oedema and ascites, which occur as a result of hypertension and venous congestion. However, salt does increase the palatability of the diet and these patients must be prevented from becoming anorexic. Potassium levels may drop in patients on diuretic therapy as it is being lost in the urine.

4. Action: Ensure that the medical treatment prescribed by the veterinary surgeon is carried out and recorded on the patient's record. Cardiac drug therapy includes diuretics, bronchodilators, vasodilators and glycosides.

    Rationale: The veterinary surgeon may have prescribed drugs for this patient which must be given at the advised times to have the maximum effect. The administration of any drug should be noted on the patient's records, to ensure that all members of staff are aware that the treatment has been given.

5. Action: Canine patients must be taken outside on a lead to urinate or defecate. Cats must have access to a clean litter tray at all times.

    Rationale: The patient must be rested as much as possible and not exercised.

Procedure: Nursing the patient with renal disease

Renal diseases include acute renal failure – complete/almost complete lack of renal function, chronic renal failure – progressive loss of renal function, and nephrotic syndrome – associated with the development of glomerulonephritis. Leptospirosis – a zoonotic disease – can be a differential in acute renal failure and barrier nursing may be instigated until a diagnosis is made.

1. **Action:** Choose a kennel that is of a size in which the patient can lie comfortably. Bedding should be comfortable and absorbent.

    Rationale: The patient needs to be able to lie comfortably. Acrylic bedding or incontinence pads may be useful in cases of incontinence. White bedding is useful in identifying the colour of the urine absorbed – the presence of blood will be especially noticeable.

2. **Action:** Monitor and record the usual patient parameters, i.e. temperature, pulse and respiration. Urinary and faecal output should be recorded. Note any progress. Any abnormalities should be recorded (Fig. 3.5) and the veterinary surgeon notified.

    Rationale: Patient parameters are required to assess progress. Measure urinary output and fluid intake. This will be vital in assessing the progress of treatment.

3. **Action:** Renal patients require a diet that is low in protein and phosphorus. The protein used must be of high biological value. Patients may have oral ulceration and may require much encouragement to eat. Hand feeding or tube feeding may be considered.

    Rationale: Low protein levels will help to reduce levels of nitrogenous waste. The protein must be of a high biological value to enable it to be utilised for maintenance and repair. Phosphorus levels will be elevated in uraemic patients so the diet must contain low phosphorus levels.

4. **Action:** Ensure that the medical treatment prescribed by the veterinary surgeon is carried out and recorded on the patient's record. Drugs that may be used include anti-emetics, antibiotics, anabolic steroids and diuretics.

    Rationale: Drugs prescribed for this patient by the veterinary surgeon must be given at the advised times to have maximum effect. The administration of any drug should be noted on the patient's records, to ensure that all members of staff are aware that the treatment has been given.

5. **Action:** The continuing nursing care will be dependent on the disease condition. Patients with renal failure will require intravenous fluid therapy and this must be carefully monitored. Treatment for patients with acute renal failure may include peritoneal dialysis.

    Rationale: Fluid therapy will be given to correct electrolyte loss and maintain hydration.

6. **Action:** It is likely that the veterinary surgeon will require samples for diagnostic assessment of the patient's progress.

    Rationale: Blood and urine may be utilised to monitor the patient's progress.

7. **Action:** Canine patients must be taken outside to urinate or defecate. Cats should have access to a clean litter tray at all times.

    Rationale: Urine may require collection – check with the veterinary surgeon.

Procedure: Nursing the patient with hepatic disease

Hepatic disease is usually caused by a bacterial or viral infection. Examples include adenovirus, which causes infectious canine hepatitis, and *Leptospira icterohaemorrhagiae*, which causes leptospirosis. Both of these are infectious diseases and if they are suspected, barrier nursing should be instigated until a definitive diagnosis is made. Leptospirosis is a zoonosis, so extra care should be taken to protect all personnel involved. Toxic damage caused by poisoning or prolonged drug therapy can sometimes result in hepatitis.

1. **Action:** Choose a kennel that is of a size in which the patient can lie comfortably. Bedding should be comfortable and absorbent.

Rationale: The patient needs to be able to lie comfortably. Acrylic bedding or incontinence pads may be useful in cases of incontinence.

2. **Action:** Monitor and record the usual patient parameters, i.e. temperature, pulse and respiration. The mucous membranes may be jaundiced and ascites may develop. Urinary and faecal output should be recorded. Note any progress. Any abnormalities should be recorded (Fig. 3.5) and the veterinary surgeon notified.

   Rationale: Patient parameters are required to assess progress. Jaundice occurs where there are excessive levels of bilirubin in the blood – a result of the hepatitis affecting the biliary system. Ascites is the result of fluid accumulation (due to portal hypertension) in the abdomen – this could include blood, urine, transudates and exudates.

3. **Action:** Most hepatic patients need an energy-dense diet with moderate amounts of protein with a high biological value and increased levels of water-soluble vitamins. These patients are often anorexic and good nutritional support is essential. Hand feeding or tube feeding may be required.

   Rationale: Protein is required to supply the patient's basic needs and support regeneration of damaged tissue.

4. **Action:** Ensure that the medical treatment prescribed by the veterinary surgeon is carried out and recorded on the patient's record. Drugs that may be used are of a supportive nature.

   Rationale: Drugs prescribed for this patient by the veterinary surgeon must be given at the advised times to have maximum effect. The administration of any drug should be noted on the patient's records, to ensure that all members of staff are aware that the treatment has been given.

5. **Action:** The continuing nursing care will depend on the cause of the disease. Patients are likely to require intravenous fluid therapy and this must be carefully monitored.

Rationale: Fluid therapy will be given to correct electrolyte loss and maintain hydration.

6. **Action:** It is likely that the veterinary surgeon will require samples to confirm the diagnosis and assess the patient's progress. Diagnostic imaging techniques may be used. If a liver biopsy is required, the patient will have to be prepared for surgery.

   Rationale: Blood biochemistry will be monitored to assess the patient's progress.

7. **Action:** Canine patients must be taken outside to urinate or defecate. Cats must have access to a clean litter tray at all times.

   Rationale: Supportive therapies must include good nursing techniques.

Procedure: Nursing the patient with pancreatic disease

Disease conditions of the exocrine part of the pancreas include pancreatitis and exocrine pancreatic insufficiency.

1. **Action:** Choose a kennel that is of a size in which the patient can lie comfortably. Bedding should be comfortable and absorbent.

   Rationale: The patient needs to be able to lie comfortably. Acrylic bedding or incontinence pads may be useful in cases of incontinence.

2. **Action:** Monitor and record the usual patient parameters, i.e. temperature, pulse and respiration. Any abnormalities should be recorded (Fig. 3.5) and the veterinary surgeon notified.

   Rationale: Patient parameters are required to assess progress. Care should be taken when handling the patient as there is likely to be pain in the cranial abdomen.

3. **Action:** Patients with pancreatitis vomit persistently and quickly become dehydrated. Intravenous fluid therapy is required and should be monitored closely – use Hartmann's solution.

Rationale: The fluid and electrolytes that have been lost must be replaced with a suitable fluid such as Hartmann's.

4. **Action:** Initially patients should be kept on 'nil by mouth'. After 3 to 5 days gradually introduce a low fat diet with additional replacement enzymes. This diet may be required for a long period.

   Rationale: Pancreatic patients are unable to digest fat, so a low fat diet is required. Added enzyme supplementation will aid the digestive process.

5. **Action:** Pancreatitis is an extremely painful condition and peritonitis may develop as a complication. Ensure that the medical treatment prescribed by the veterinary surgeon is carried out and recorded on the patient's record. Drugs that may be used include analgesics and antibiotics.

   Rationale: Drugs prescribed for this patient by the veterinary surgeon must be given at the advised times to have maximum effect. The monitoring of the analgesic regime is vital as these patients will be in extreme pain if the dose of analgesic is insufficient. The administration of any drug should be noted on the patient's records, to ensure that all members of staff are aware that the treatment has been given.

6. **Action:** Tests will be carried out to confirm the diagnosis and to assess the patient's progress. Blood and faecal samples may be required.

   Rationale: Diagnostic tests for pancreatitis include haematology (a leucocytosis may be present), biochemistry (to assess serum amylase and lipase) and abdominal radiography (to assess the degree of peritonitis). For patients with suspected exocrine pancreatic insufficiency, a serum raised trypsin-like immunoreactivity test (TLI) may be carried out.

7. **Action:** Once hospital treatment has finished, the patient will require strict dietary management and may need the provision of proprietary enzymes to aid digestion for the remainder of its life.

Rationale: Once the pancreas has been damaged it is unlikely to return to normal function.

Procedure: Nursing the patient with diabetes mellitus

Diabetes mellitus is caused by degeneration of the endocrine part of the pancreas. This normally secretes the hormone insulin, which stimulates glucose uptake by the cells and storage of excess glucose in the liver as glycogen. In patients with diabetes mellitus, insufficient amounts of insulin are released, resulting in hyperglycaemia (raised blood glucose) and excretion of glucose in the urine.

1. **Action:** The patient may be admitted with ketoacidosis and will require immediate intravenous fluid therapy. Initially Hartmann's solution is used, followed by 0.9% saline to maintain the patient once it is stable. The veterinary surgeon will also administer a short-acting soluble insulin intravenously.

   Rationale: Ketoacidosis occurs when the patient starts to break down proteins to use as a source of energy. The cells are unable to use the more normal glucose as a source of energy as this requires the presence of insulin. A metabolic acidosis occurs and ketones build up in the circulation. Hartmann's solution will correct the metabolic acidosis, whilst saline is used for maintenance. Soluble insulin begins working rapidly and the utilisation of glucose can begin.

2. **Action:** Choose a kennel that is of a size in which the patient can lie comfortably. Bedding should be comfortable and absorbent.

   Rationale: The patient needs to be able to lie comfortably.

3. **Action:** Monitor and record the usual patient parameters, i.e. temperature, pulse and respiration. Any abnormalities should be recorded and the veterinary surgeon notified.

Rationale: Patient parameters are required to assess the progress.

4. **Action:** Maintenance of a patient with diabetes mellitus requires a strict routine. First thing each morning, a urine sample should be collected and its glucose level tested using a simple dipstick test. A blood sample may also be collected to test for blood glucose levels.

   Rationale: Testing the urine glucose gives a level on which to base the dose of insulin. Urine may also be tested for ketones but these should not be present unless the condition of the patient has become unstable. Blood glucose levels can be monitored to give baseline levels but are not usually used except in a practice, as owners find it difficult to collect a blood sample.

5. **Action:** Use the level of the glucose in the urine to calculate the dose of insulin to be given to the patient.

   Rationale: Calculations are based on an initial dose of 0.5 IU (international units) per kg of bodyweight. If the morning urine glucose is more than 1%, give the previous day's dose plus 2 IU. If the urine glucose is 0%, give the previous day's dose less 2 IU. If the glucose is 0.1%, give the previous day's dose. Check all dosages with the veterinary surgeon before administering the insulin.

6. **Action:** Before administering the insulin, give the patient one-quarter of its daily food ration. If the patient eats this, inject the prepared dose of insulin. Insulin is usually given subcutaneously in proprietary insulin syringes. Ensure that the subcutaneous injection has been given correctly to enable the insulin to work efficiently. If the patient does not eat its food, seek advice from the veterinary surgeon.

   Rationale: The insulin will require some glucose in the blood to metabolise so food is given before the insulin to provide this. The dose of the insulin must be calculated and administered accurately. Proprietary syringes which are calibrated in international units ensure this.

7. **Action:** All treatments must be noted on the patient's record.

   Rationale: If the patient does not respond or there is an excessive response to the insulin injection, the record can be checked and used to adjust the dose.

8. **Action:** The remainder of the patient's food ration should be given 8 hours after the insulin injection. A blood sample may be taken at this time to monitor levels of glucose.

   Rationale: The maximum effect of the insulin will coincide with the peak of blood glucose levels from the digested food.

9. **Action:** Nutritional support of the diabetic patient includes a high fibre diet. It is vital that the patient is kept to a strict regime and that no extra food or titbits are offered.

   Rationale: High fibre diets reduce the speed and prolong the time of glucose absorption from the small intestine. This helps the insulin control the blood glucose by preventing the glucose surges that can occur after a meal.

10. **Action:** Hypoglycaemia can be a complication and may occur around the time of the peak of insulin activity. Clinical signs include tremors, weakness, ataxia, collapse and coma. A conscious patient should be given oral glucose in the form of glucose powder, sugar, honey, etc. An unconscious patient will require intravenous glucose as soon as possible.

    Rationale: Hypoglycaemia (low blood glucose) can occur when too much insulin has been given, if the patient has failed to eat, or if the peak effect of the insulin has occurred before the patient has received the major part of its daily food ration.

11. **Action:** Diabetic patients must continue with a strict regime in order to keep their condition stable. This includes a constant amount of food and of a constant constituency. Exercise must be monitored and should be the same amount at the same time each day. Some cases of diabetes mellitus are transient

while other patients may require insulin for the remainder of their life.

Rationale: High levels of blood glucose or high levels of insulin may cause the condition of the patient to become unstable. Unusual energy demands, such as a very long walk, can also result in instability. Some patients may have diabetes as a secondary condition, e.g. a bitch may develop diabetes after her 'season'. If she is spayed she may not require insulin in the future.

Procedure: Nursing the patient with diabetes insipidus

Diabetes insipidus results from either a failure of the pituitary gland to produce antidiuretic hormone (ADH) or of the kidneys to respond to ADH. Either type leads to an inability to control the concentration of urine and so to conserve body fluid.

1. **Action:** The patient will present with a marked polydipsia and polyuria.

   Rationale: The patient is unable to concentrate the urine so will pass dilute urine frequently.

2. **Action:** Choose a kennel that is of a size in which the patient can lie comfortably. Bedding should be comfortable and absorbent. Water must be available and canine patients must be frequently taken outside to urinate.

   Rationale: The patient needs to be able to lie comfortably. If the patient is not offered water it will dehydrate quickly as it will still exhibit polyuria.

3. **Action:** Monitor and record the usual patient parameters, i.e. temperature, pulse and respiration. Fluid intake and output should be noted. Any abnormalities should be recorded and the veterinary surgeon notified.

   Rationale: Patient parameters are required to assess progress. Fluid intake and output will indicate the degree of the problem.

4. **Action:** Diagnosis of diabetes insipidus involves the use of the water deprivation test. The patient must be well hydrated and have good renal function.

   Rationale: The water deprivation test assesses the ability of the patient to concentrate its urine. The patient can become dehydrated quickly and this test should only be carried out by a veterinary surgeon. Assessment of the patient's hydration status should be made throughout the test. The renal function of the patient should be taken into consideration as further complications could occur.

5. **Action:** Empty the patient's bladder and measure the specific gravity using a refractometer. Record the results.

   Rationale: The specific gravity measurement will assess the concentration of the urine before water deprivation.

6. **Action:** The patient should be weighed and 5% of its bodyweight calculated. It should then be placed in a kennel without food and water for 1 hour.

   Rationale: This provides a measurement on which to base the subsequent results.

7. **Action:** After an hour its bladder should be emptied, the patient weighed and the urine specific gravity measured. Repeat this process until 5% of the patient's bodyweight is lost.

   Rationale: When a normal patient loses 5% of its bodyweight it will concentrate its urine to a specific gravity of more than 1.020. If the patient has diabetes insipidus it will still produce dilute urine of a specific gravity of less than 1.007 and a diagnosis can be made.

8. **Action:** When the testing is finished the patient should be allowed free access to water.

   Rationale: The patient may become severely dehydrated if water is withheld for too long.

9. **Action:** Ensure that the medical treatment prescribed by the veterinary surgeon is carried out and recorded on the patient's record.

   Rationale: The veterinary surgeon may have prescribed drugs for this patient which must be given at the advised times to have maximum effect. The administration of any drug should be noted on the patient's records, to ensure that all members of staff are aware that the treatment has been given.

REFERENCES AND FURTHER READING

Agar S 2001 Small Animal Nutrition. Butterworth-Heinemann, Oxford

Aspinall V 2006 The Complete Textbook in Veterinary Nursing. Elsevier, Oxford

Blood D C, Studdert V P 2000 Comprehensive Veterinary Dictionary. WB Saunders, London

Cooper B, Lane D R (eds) 1999 Veterinary Nursing, 2nd edn. Butterworth-Heinemann, Oxford

Lane D R, Cooper B (eds) 2003 Veterinary Nursing, 3rd edn. Butterworth-Heinemann, Oxford

Masters J, Bowden C 2001 Pre-Veterinary Nursing Textbook. Butterworth-Heinemann, Oxford

Chapter **4**

Administration of fluid therapy

Carole Martin

CHAPTER CONTENTS

Introduction 67

Appreciation of water content in the body 68
Appreciation of water balance in the body 68
Assessing level of dehydration of the patient 69
Selection of fluids in relation to their action in the body 69
Selection of fluid for specific needs 69
Oral fluid therapy 70
Subcutaneous fluid therapy 70
Intraperitoneal fluid therapy 72
Preparation of equipment for intravenous fluid administration 72
Intravenous access to the cephalic vein and administration of fluid therapy 74
Intravenous access to the saphenous vein and administration of fluid therapy 75
Intravenous access to the jugular vein and administration of fluid therapy 76
Calculation of fluid deficit and maintenance requirements 77
Calculation of drip rate 77
Maintenance of intravenous fluid therapy – general maintenance 78
Maintenance of fluid therapy – replacement/changing of intravenous fluid bags 78
Maintenance of fluid therapy – removal of intravenous fluid therapy equipment from patient 79

Monitoring of fluid therapy – general guidelines 80
Monitoring of fluid therapy – essential parameters 80
Blood collection for transfusion 80
Blood transfusion 83
Monitoring for blood transfusion reactions 85

INTRODUCTION

The healthy body contains between 60% and 70% water, which is found inside and surrounding all the cells. This fluid maintains a balanced state within the body so that the normal metabolic processes can function efficiently – a process known as homeostasis. Dissolved in the body fluids are chemical materials that are essential for the body's metabolism and which play a part in controlling the movement of fluid around the body. Many medical conditions and surgical procedures cause an upset in fluid balance and if nothing is done to correct this the animal may become severely dehydrated or go into shock and die. The purpose of fluid therapy is to replace any deficit so that the circulating fluid volume is restored and renal function is improved.

There are many types of fluid used in fluid therapy and the fluid replaced must be as close as possible, in terms of the chemical constituents and volume, to that lost from the general circulation. This chapter explains the theory that underpins the selection of fluids and describes in detail the procedures involved in supplying the fluid to the patient.

Procedure: Appreciation of water content in the body (Fig. 4.1)

1. **Action:** 100% total bodyweight.
   Rationale: 60% water + 40% other body structures.
2. **Action:** Intracellular fluid (ICF) = 2/3 of body fluid.
   Rationale: ICF is located within the cells.
3. **Action:** Extracellular fluid (ECF) = 1/3 of body fluid.
   Rationale: ECF is located outside the cells; plasma – water contained within blood, interstitial fluid bathing cells, transcellular fluid within specialised areas.
4. **Action:** Body fluids contain electrolytes, which yield ions.
   Rationale: It is important to know the electrolyte and ion composition of body fluids to ensure the correct fluid is administered.

5. **Action:** Ions are small water-soluble particles carrying one or more negative or positive charges. Sodium chloride (NaCl) is an electrolyte which dissociates into sodium ions and chloride ions when dissolved in water.
   Rationale: It is important to know which ions are in ICF and ECF to ensure that the correct fluid therapy is administered. Cations are ions that are positively charged; the main cations in ICF are potassium and magnesium and the main one in ECF is sodium. Anions are ions that are negatively charged; the main anions in ECF are chloride and bicarbonate.
6. **Action:** Water balance and concentration need to be maintained equally within the body.
   Rationale: Osmosis is the process by which water moves from a low concentration to a high concentration through a semi-permeable membrane. Osmotic pressure is the pressure needed to prevent osmosis from happening. Osmotic pressure is maintained in the healthy animal by various homeostatic mechanisms.

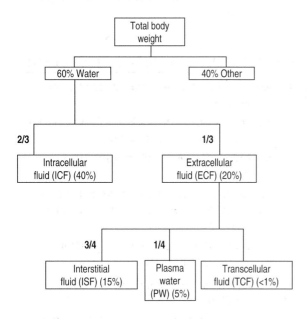

Figure 4.1 The distribution of body water into its principal compartments. Adapted, with permission, from Lane and Cooper (2003), Butterworth-Heinemann.

Procedure: Appreciation of water balance in the body

1. **Action:** Water intake – ingestion.
   Rationale: Ingestion of fluids and foods.
2. **Action:** Water intake – metabolism.
   Rationale: Metabolism of fats and carbohydrates.
3. **Action:** Water loss – 50 ml/kg bodyweight/24 h.
   Rationale: This is the amount that needs to be replaced daily to ensure water balance.
4. **Action:** Sensible water loss – 25 ml/kg bodyweight/24 h.
   Rationale: Sensible loss via urine.
5. **Action:** Insensible water loss – 25 ml/kg bodyweight/24 h.
   Rationale: Insensible losses – respiratory, cutaneous and faeces.
6. **Action:** Water replacement = 50 ml/kg/24 h.
   Rationale: To balance water loss.

7. **Action:** Electrolyte replacement:
sodium 1 mmol/kg/24 h
potassium 2 mmol/kg/24 h.
Rationale: To balance electrolyte loss.

8. **Action:** Metabolic acidosis = loss of alkaline ions.
Rationale: Replace loss with fluid containing alkaline ions to correct acid/base imbalance.

9. **Action:** Metabolic alkalosis = loss of acidic ions.
Rationale: Replace loss with fluid containing acidic ions to correct acid/base imbalance.

Procedure: Assessing level of dehydration of the patient

1. **Action:** Normal physical appearance despite a history of fluid loss.
Level (degree of dehydration as a percentage of bodyweight): Slight >5%.

2. **Action:** Mild to dry mucous membranes, slight decrease in skin turgor.
Level: Mild 5–6%.

3. **Action:** Decrease in skin turgor; dry mucous membranes; mild tachycardia; sunken eyes; slight increase in capillary refill time.
Level: Mild 6–8%.

4. **Action:** Marked decrease in skin turgor; dry mucous membranes; sunken eyes; weak pulse; increased capillary refill time; oliguria; cold extremities.
Level: Moderate 10–12%.

5. **Action:** Very marked decrease in skin turgor; pale and dry mucous membranes; sunken eyes; tachycardia; cold extremities; muscle weakness; collapse; depression; anuria.
Level: Severe 12–15%.

Procedure: Selection of fluids in relation to their action in the body

1. **Action:** Isotonic fluid.
Rationale: Equal osmotic pressure to blood – no fluid movement thereby maintaining equilibrium.

2. **Action:** Hypertonic fluid.
Rationale: Greater osmotic pressure than blood – thereby encouraging movement of fluid from cells into circulation.

3. **Action:** Hypotonic fluid.
Rationale: Lower osmotic pressure than blood – thereby encouraging movement of fluids into cells.

4. **Action:** Crystalloids.
Rationale: These fluids contain small molecules that enter and temporarily increase the blood volume before passing into the cells and equilibrating with the ICF.

5. **Action:** Colloids.
Rationale: These fluids contain large molecules that remain within the circulation, thereby increasing osmotic pressure and expanding plasma volume.

6. **Action:** Blood product – plasma.
Rationale: This helps to expand plasma volume and treat hypoproteinaemia.

7. **Action:** Whole blood.
Rationale: Used in cases where replacement of red blood cells and plasma volume expansion are required.

Procedure: Selection of fluid for specific needs

1. **Action:** 0.9% NaCl – normal saline (isotonic crystalloid).
Rationale: Replace ECF. Gastric losses or loss of acidic ions from vomiting.

2. **Action:** 0.18% NaCl + 4% dextrose (isotonic crystalloid).
Rationale: Maintenance requirements; primary water deficit replacement; neonatal ECF replacement.

3. **Action:** 5% dextrose (isotonic crystalloid).
Rationale: Primary water deficit replacement.

4. **Action:** Hartmann's solution (isotonic crystalloid).
Rationale: Replace ECF. Diarrhoea and postgastric losses/alkaline ions.

5. **Action:** Ringer's solution (isotonic crystalloid).

Rationale: Replace ECF; gastric losses from vomiting.

6. Action: Haemaccel/Gelofusine (isotonic colloids).

   Rationale: Expand plasma volume; moderate to severe fluid loss and blood loss where no blood products are available.

7. Action: Plasma (blood product – isotonic).

   Rationale: Replace plasma proteins; expand plasma volume as above; clotting defects.

8. Action: Whole blood (isotonic).

   Rationale: Replace blood loss; meet any ongoing or anticipated blood loss; anaemia; circulatory insufficiency.

Procedure: Oral fluid therapy

Indications: Animal willing to drink, not vomiting, absence of intestinal obstruction.

Fluid choice: Hypotonic electrolyte solution or water.

1. Action: Select equipment – dosing syringe with catheter tip, towel, assistant, fluid.

   Rationale: A dosing syringe is the most suitable method of accurate administration. It is important to select all equipment prior to the procedure to ensure efficient method of administration.

2. Action: Measure correct volume of fluid in syringe.

   Rationale: Important to accurately measure fluid replacement to avoid excess or insufficient fluid.

3. Action: Request assistance to hold patient.

   Rationale: Ensure that the patient is kept at ease and feels safe.

4. Action: Support patient's nose and mouth with left hand in normal position.

   Rationale: Firm but sympathetic handling will ensure fluid is delivered safely and effectively. Head must be in normal position to prevent aspiration pneumonia.

5. Action: Introduce the catheter tip syringe into the mouth between upper and lower premolars above the tongue surface.

Rationale: This area is the most suitable to administer fluid safely and accurately.

6. Action: Slowly introduce 5–10 ml of fluid into the mouth and allow the patient to swallow. Stroke the ventral aspect of the pharynx to encourage swallowing.

   Rationale: Avoid giving too much fluid at any one time as this may induce choking. Allow patient to swallow and breathe between administrations.

7. Action: Continue until required volume has been delivered or the patient becomes agitated.

   Rationale: Only continue if patient is taking fluid well and swallowing between doses. At any time if the patient gets distressed or fails to swallow stop the procedure immediately.

8. Action: Dry the patient's mouth and surrounding area and replace in ready prepared clean kennel.

   Rationale: Always dry the area to help prevent heat loss and make the patient comfortable.

9. Action: Record total fluid volume given and the frequency on the hospital record.

   Rationale: Ensure record keeping is accurate to prevent over- or under-administration.

10. Action: Dispose of equipment safely and appropriately.

   Rationale: It is essential to dispose of equipment correctly to avoid contamination and accidents.

Procedure: Subcutaneous fluid therapy

Indications: Mild dehydration with adequate peripheral circulation.

Fluid choice: Any crystalloid isotonic solution such as 0.9% NaCl, 0.18% NaCl + 4% dextrose or Hartmann's solution.

1. Action: Select and prepare equipment – prewarmed fluid, measured volume in sterile syringe with new sterile needle attached (maximum 10–20 ml/kg/site), clippers, surgical skin scrub, gloves, swabs (Fig. 4.2).

Rationale: Fluid must be prewarmed to prevent shock and discomfort and aid absorption. Isotonic or hypotonic fluid is used to promote absorption. Ensure all equipment is prepared in advance to allow for efficient procedure.

2. **Action:** Request assistant to restrain patient in lateral recumbency.

   Rationale: Firm, effective handling ensures that the patient remains comfortable throughout procedure.

3. **Action:** Clip an area of approximately 3 cm × 3 cm on either side of the thorax over the ninth rib, midway between ventral and dorsal borders.

   Rationale: Area must be free of hair to reduce the risk of infection. This area allows effective movement and absorption of fluid.

4. **Action:** Prepare skin aseptically with surgical scrub solution. Wear gloves.

   Rationale: Skin must be cleaned aseptically to reduce risk of infection.

5. **Action:** Infiltrate local anaesthetic into the prepared site as per veterinary surgeon instructions. Drape the area.

   Rationale: Local anaesthetic will desensitise the area, preventing pain and discomfort. Draping the area will help to maintain asepsis.

6. **Action:** Tent the skin and introduce the needle, attached to the fluid-filled syringe, subcutaneously.

   Rationale: Administration must be subcutaneous, avoiding any puncture of thoracic cavity.

7. **Action:** Withdraw the plunger of the syringe.

   Rationale: To check that a vein has not been punctured by accident.

8. **Action:** Administer the volume of fluid slowly and withdraw the needle (maximum 10–20 ml/kg/site).

   Rationale: Fast infusion of fluid can cause considerable discomfort.

9. **Action:** Massage the area.

   Rationale: To ensure even and effective distribution.

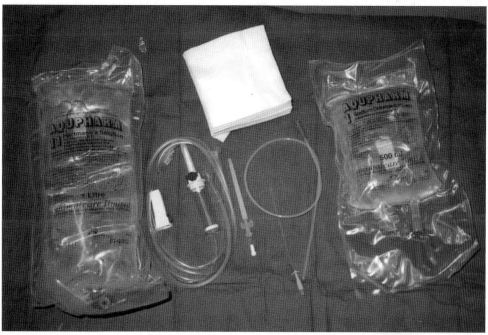

Figure 4.2   Fluids and equipment used in fluid therapy and catheterisation. From left to right: Hartmann's solution, infusion set, intravenous catheter, Jackson's cat catheter, dog urinary catheter, normal saline.

10. **Action:** Repeat the procedure on the other side of the thorax.

    Rationale: To ensure equal distribution in the body.

11. **Action:** Remove the drapes and dry the area. Allow the patient to resume sternal recumbency and place back in the kennel.

    Rationale: Ensure patient is comfortable in kennel.

12. **Action:** Dispose of equipment safely and appropriately.

    Rationale: It is essential to dispose of equipment correctly to avoid contamination and accidents.

Procedure: Intraperitoneal fluid therapy

Indications: Mild dehydration where fluids cannot be administered orally; where larger volumes need to be infused rapidly; neonates and exotics.

Fluid Choice: Any isotonic crystalloid fluid such as 0.9% NaCl; 0.18% NaCl + 4% dextrose; Hartmann's solution.

1. **Action:** Select and prepare equipment – prewarmed fluid, measured volume in sterile syringe with sterile new needle attached, clippers, surgical skin scrub solution, swabs, gloves.

    Rationale: Avoid shock and drop in body temperature by prewarming fluid. Prepare all equipment in advance of procedure to ensure efficient administration.

2. **Action:** Assistant to restrain patient in dorsal recumbency and reassure patient throughout procedure.

    Rationale: To present the correct area for administration and encourage the viscera to gravitate away from site, thereby avoiding puncture during procedure.

3. **Action:** Clip area surrounding umbilicus.

    Rationale: Reduce risk of infection by clipping hair, allowing a wide margin around umbilicus.

4. **Action:** Prepare skin aseptically and drape area.

    Rationale: To reduce risk of infection.

5. **Action:** Infiltrate local anaesthetic into prepared site – region of umbilicus – as per veterinary surgeon instructions.

    Rationale: To desensitise area prior to administration of fluid.

6. **Action:** Introduce sterile needle attached to fluid syringe through the skin and central line (linea alba) into the peritoneal cavity.

    Rationale: Ensure asepsis maintained and introduction efficient and smooth.

7. **Action:** Withdraw plunger of syringe.

    Rationale: Accident – if blood appears in hub of syringe, withdraw and start again. If urine or gut contents appear in the syringe, the bladder or intestine may have been punctured – withdraw and start again.

8. **Action:** Introduce prewarmed fluid into the peritoneal cavity.

    Rationale: If any resistance is felt, stop and restart procedure from point 6.

9. **Action:** Withdraw needle and syringe, putting gentle pressure over injection site.

    Rationale: Clean, swift removal of needle to prevent any discomfort. Pressure to prevent leakage of body fluid.

10. **Action:** Remove drapes and dry area. Allow patient to regain sternal recumbency, reassure and replace in kennel.

    Rationale: Resume normal position as soon as possible to restore equilibrium. It is important to ensure patient is comfortable before placing back in kennel.

11. **Action:** Record fluid administration details.

    Rationale: To ensure accurate monitoring.

12. **Action:** Dispose of equipment safely and appropriately.

    Rationale: It is essential to dispose of equipment correctly to avoid contamination and accidents.

Procedure: Preparation of equipment for intravenous fluid administration

1. **Action:** Wash hands and wear disposable gloves.

Rationale: It is essential to maintain levels of asepsis to avoid contamination and infection.

2. **Action:** Select correct equipment for intravenous fluid administration – clippers, surgical scrub solution, swabs, tapes, blade, intravenous catheter, heparinised saline, three-way tap or bung, fluid bag, infusion set, kick bowl, drip stand (Fig. 4.3).

   Rationale: All equipment must be selected prior to patient restraint to ensure that the procedure is performed efficiently and thoroughly.

3. **Action:** Check the expiry date on the fluid bag, look for any damage to the outside of the bag or for any artefacts within the fluid.

   Rationale: Any sign of damage, abnormality or expiry date passed indicates that sterility of the product cannot be guaranteed; therefore it would be unsafe to use.

4. **Action:** Remove the fluid bag from its outer covering and identify the correct outlet port. Prewarm fluid to body temperature and hang fluid bag on drip stand.

Rationale: Careful handling to reduce risk of contamination. Use of a drip stand facilitates handling. Warming of fluid to just below body temperature will prevent shock.

5. **Action:** Remove infusion set from its outer coverings and switch off the flow control.

   Rationale: Switching off the flow control will prevent loss of fluid prior to connection to bag.

6. **Action:** Remove the cover from the infusion spike and introduce into the fluid bag carefully.

   Rationale: Careful handling will avoid puncture of fluid bag with the spike, thereby avoiding contamination and fluid loss.

7. **Action:** Squeeze fluid chamber so that it fills by one-third.

   Rationale: To aid control of fluid during infusion and prevent air bubbles.

8. **Action:** Remove the cap from the end of infusion line, taking care not to touch a non-sterile surface.

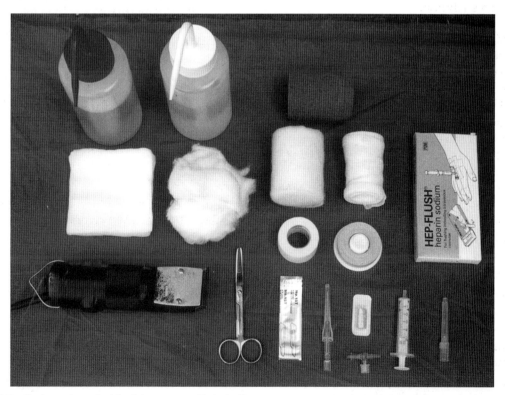

Figure 4.3 Equipment required for intravenous catheterisation.

Rationale: It is important to maintain sterility at all times.

9. **Action:** Open flow control and allow fluid to travel down infusion set in a controlled manner, removing all air bubbles.

    Rationale: No air bubbles should enter the circulation and excess fluid loss should be avoided from fluid bag.

10. **Action:** Switch off flow control and replace cap. Hang giving set on drip stand.

    Rationale: To prevent leakage and maintain sterility.

11. **Action:** Dispose of equipment safely and appropriately.

    Rationale: It is essential to dispose of equipment correctly to avoid any clutter of equipment and reduce risk of contamination and accidents.

Procedure: Intravenous access to the cephalic vein and administration of fluid therapy

1. **Action:** Select equipment and prepare fluid infusion. Prewarm fluid to body temperature.

    Rationale: Prepare equipment in advance of restraining the patient. Maintain body temperature and minimise discomfort by prewarming the fluid.

2. **Action:** Assistant to restrain the patient in sternal recumbency, in the correct manner to allow access to the cephalic vein.

    Rationale: Firm handling will keep the patient at ease and reduce the risk of any accident.

3. **Action:** Wearing gloves, clip and prepare the site aseptically using surgical scrub or surgical spirit.

    Rationale: This will help to prevent infection.

4. **Action:** Ask the assistant to raise the vein.

    Rationale: This dilates the vein, making it easier to see.

5. **Action:** With gloved hands, insert the catheter tip into the vein. A cut down technique with a scalpel blade may be employed for venous access. Once blood appears within the catheter, remove the needle and advance the catheter fully (Fig. 4.4).

    Rationale: Cut down technique reduces risk of blunting catheter tip. The needle is removed to prevent accidental puncture of vein further along lumen.

6. **Action:** Ask the assistant to release the pressure over the vein. Place a bung or three-way tap to close over end of catheter.

    Rationale: To avoid excess blood loss.

7. **Action:** Dry the area and secure the catheter to the leg with tapes.

    Rationale: It is important to dry the area to ensure that any tape adheres to the leg and holds the catheter in place, thus preventing movement and blood leakage.

8. **Action:** Flush the catheter with a small amount of heparinised saline.

    Rationale: This is to ensure patency of the catheter and prevent blood clot formation in the catheter.

9. **Action:** Remove the cap from the infusion set and attach the infusion tube to the intravenous catheter. Secure the infusion tube to the patient's leg with tapes. Bandage if necessary.

    Rationale: To ensure that the fluid infusion tube remains in place if the patient moves. Movement could cause it to become dislodged, resulting in blood loss.

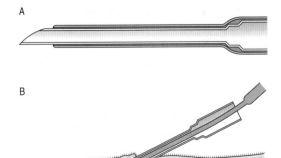

Figure 4.4 Types of intravenous catheter. A, 'over the needle' cannula; B, 'through the needle' cannula.

10. **Action:** Open fluid flow control.

   Rationale: To assess if the fluid is flowing freely. If the drip is not flowing, assess the reason and deal with it appropriately.

11. **Action:** Adjust the fluid control to the drip rate required for the patient. Syringe drivers and infusion pumps may be used to facilitate the delivery of the calculated drip rate.

   Rationale: It is essential to control rate of delivery of the fluid replacement, to avoid over- or under-infusion.

12. **Action:** Record fluid type and drip rate on hospital card.

   Rationale: This is to ensure accurate monitoring and clear communication between all veterinary personnel.

13. **Action:** To prevent self-mutilation by the patient, bandage the area and apply an Elizabethan collar as necessary.

   Rationale: If patient mutilates area there is a risk of blood loss, sepsis and thrombosis.

14. **Action:** Dispose of equipment safely and appropriately.

   Rationale: It is essential that all items are disposed of correctly to avoid contamination and accidents.

Procedure: Intravenous access to the saphenous vein and administration of fluid therapy

1. **Action:** Select equipment and prepared fluid infusion. Prewarm fluid to body temperature.

   Rationale: Prepare all equipment in advance of restraining the patient. Maintain body temperature and minimise discomfort by prewarming fluids.

2. **Action:** Ask the assistant to restrain the patient in lateral recumbency to allow intravenous access to the saphenous vein. Two assistants may be required to maintain patient in required position.

   Rationale: Firm handling will keep the patient at ease and reduce the risk of any accident. As the patient will need to be in lateral

recumbency, a second assistant would be required to extend the hindlimb.

3. **Action:** Wearing gloves, clip and prepare site aseptically using surgical scrub or surgical spirit.

   Rationale: This will help to prevent infection.

4. **Action:** Ask the assistant to raise vein.

   Rationale: This dilates the vein, making it easier to see.

5. **Action:** With gloved hands insert the catheter tip into the vein. Once blood appears in the catheter, remove the needle and advance catheter fully.

   Rationale: The needle is removed to prevent accidental puncture of the vein further along lumen.

6. **Action:** Ask the assistant to release the pressure on the vein. Place a bung or three-way tap to close over the end of catheter.

   Rationale: To avoid excess blood loss.

7. **Action:** Dry the area and secure the catheter to the leg with tapes.

   Rationale: It is important to dry the area to ensure any tape adheres to the leg and holds the catheter in place. Tapes are used to secure the catheter, preventing movement and blood leakage.

8. **Action:** Flush the catheter with a small amount of heparinised saline.

   Rationale: This is to ensure patency of the catheter and prevent blood clot formation in the catheter.

9. **Action:** Remove the cap from the infusion set and attach the infusion tube to the intravenous catheter. Secure the infusion tube to the patient's leg with tapes. Bandage if necessary.

   Rationale: To ensure that the fluid infusion tube remains in place if the patient moves. Movement could cause it to become dislodged, resulting in blood loss.

10. **Action:** Open fluid flow control.

   Rationale: To assess if the fluid is flowing freely. If the drip is not flowing, assess the reason and deal with it appropriately.

11. **Action:** Adjust the fluid control to the drip rate required for the patient. Syringe drivers and infusion pumps may be used to facilitate the delivery of the calculated drip rate.

    Rationale: It is essential to control the rate of delivery of the fluid replacement to avoid over- or under-infusion.

12. **Action:** Record fluid type and drip rate on the hospital card.

    Rationale: This is to ensure accurate monitoring.

13. **Action:** To prevent self-mutilation by the patient, bandage the area and apply an Elizabethan collar as necessary.

    Rationale: If the patient mutilates the area there is a risk of blood loss, sepsis and thrombosis.

14. **Action:** Dispose of equipment safely and appropriately.

    Rationale: It is essential that all items are disposed of correctly to avoid contamination and accidents.

Procedure: Intravenous access to the jugular vein and administration of fluid therapy

1. **Action:** Select equipment and prepared fluid infusion. Prewarm fluid to body temperature.

    Rationale: Prepare all equipment in advance of restraining the patient. Maintain body temperature and minimise discomfort by prewarming fluid.

2. **Action:** Ask the assistant to restrain the patient in the correct manner to provide access to the jugular vein (see Chapter 1). Two assistants may be required maintain the patient in the required position.

    Rationale: Firm handling will keep the patient at ease and reduce risk of any accident.

3. **Action:** Wearing gloves, clip and prepare site aseptically using surgical scrub or surgical spirit.

    Rationale: This will help to prevent infection.

4. **Action:** The vein will be raised by the operator by applying pressure at the base of the neck (see Chapter 1).

    Rationale: This dilates the vein making it easier to see.

5. **Action:** With gloved hands insert the catheter tip into the vein. Once blood appears in the catheter, remove the needle and advance the catheter fully.

    Rationale: The needle is removed to prevent accidental puncture of the vein further along lumen.

6. **Action:** Ask the assistant to release the pressure on the vein. Place a bung or three-way tap to close over the end of catheter.

    Rationale: To avoid excess blood loss.

7. **Action:** Dry the area and secure the catheter to the skin with the aid of adhesive tapes and bandage or suture in place.

    Rationale: It is important to dry the area to ensure that any tape adheres to the skin holding the catheter in place. Accidental movement or displacement of the catheter must be avoided from the jugular vein, as blood loss could be considerable.

8. **Action:** Flush the catheter with a small amount of heparinised saline.

    Rationale: This maintains the patency of the catheter and prevents blood clot formation in catheter.

9. **Action:** Remove the cap from the infusion set and attach the infusion tube to the intravenous catheter. Secure the infusion tube to the neck region. Bandage if necessary.

    Rationale: To ensure fluid infusion remains in place if patient moves, thereby preventing dislodgement and blood loss.

10. **Action:** Open fluid flow control.

    Rationale: To assess if the fluid is flowing freely. If the drip is not flowing, assess the reason and deal with it appropriately.

11. **Action:** Adjust the fluid control to the drip rate required for the patient. Syringe drivers and infusion pumps may be used to facilitate the delivery of the calculated drip rate.

    Rationale: It is essential to control the delivery of the fluid replacement rate to avoid over- or under-infusion.

12. **Action:** Record fluid type and drip rate on the hospital card.

    Rationale: This is to ensure accurate monitoring and clear communication between all veterinary personnel.

13. **Action:** To prevent self-mutilation by the patient, bandage the area and apply an Elizabethan collar as necessary.

    Rationale: If the patient mutilates the area, there is a risk of blood loss, sepsis and thrombosis.

14. **Action:** Dispose of equipment safely and appropriately.

    Rationale: It is essential that all items are disposed of correctly to avoid contamination and accidents.

Procedure: Calculation of fluid deficit and maintenance requirements

Example: 20 kg dog that has been off food and water for 3 days and has been vomiting four times a day for the last 2 days.

Fluid choice: Colloid to replace or expand plasma volume, e.g. Haemaccel or Gelofusine, followed by a crystalloid to replace remainder of deficit, e.g. 0.9% NaCl or Hartmann's solution, and crystalloid to meet maintenance requirements, e.g. 0.18% NaCl + 4% dextrose.

1. **Action:** Calculate insensible losses × 3 days (25 ml/kg/24 h × 20 kg) = 1500 ml.

   Rationale: Insensible losses (respiratory; cutaneous; faecal) will initially continue in spite of the lack of fluid intake.

2. **Action:** Calculate sensible losses × 3 days (25 ml/kg/24 h × 20 kg × 1) = 500 ml.

   Rationale: Sensible losses (urine) will be reduced by the lack of fluid intake, therefore calculation based on 1 day instead of 3 days.

3. **Action:** Calculate loss from vomiting four times a day for 2 days (4 ml/kg/vomit × 20 × 4 × 2) = 640 ml.

   Rationale: Fluid loss from vomit can only be estimated but does need to be taken into account when calculating the total deficit.

4. **Action:** Calculate total fluid deficit = all of the above factors added together = 2640 ml, of which ECF deficit is 880 ml and 220 ml represents plasma volume.

   Rationale: This amount has been calculated by adding all of the above factors and represents the deficit only.

5. **Action:** This volume should be replaced over 24 hours, with half of the replacement being administered over 6–8 hours.

   Rationale: One-twelfth of the total deficit should be replaced with a plasma substitute as one-twelfth of the body fluid represents plasma volume (Fig. 4.1).

6. **Action:** Meet ongoing losses/maintenance requirements at 50 ml/kg/24 h × 20 kg = 1250 ml/24 h.

   Rationale: While the deficit needs to be replaced, water loss will continue due to body metabolism so it is essential to meet the ongoing maintenance requirements until the patient has recovered.

7. **Action:** Alternatively calculate deficit from packed cell volume/haematocrit measurement: for every 1% rise in PCV allow for fluid deficit of 10 ml/kg.

   Rationale: This can only be assessed if compared with PCV reading for normal, healthy patient.

Procedure: Calculation of drip rate

Example: Daily maintenance for 20 kg dog to be administered over an 8-hour period.

1. **Action:** Calculate the daily maintenance fluid requirements for a 25 kg dog at 50 ml/kg bodyweight/24 h = 1250 ml/24 h.

   Rationale: Daily fluid requirement is a total of 50 ml/kg bodyweight to allow for 25 ml/kg bodyweight/24 h sensible losses and 25 ml/kg bodyweight/24 h insensible losses. The weight of the patient is multiplied by the millilitres of fluid for a 24-hour period.

2. **Action:** The above fluid is to be given over 8 hours. Calculate the volume of fluid to be given per hour = 156 ml/hour.

Rationale: The calculation in step 1 is based on a 24-hour period. This is to be administered over an 8-hour period. Divide 1250 ml by 8.

3. **Action:** Calculate the volume of fluid to be given per minute = 2.60 ml/minute.

   Rationale: The hourly rate is 156 ml. There are 60 minutes in one hour, therefore divide 156 by 60.

4. **Action:** The infusion set delivers 20 drops/ml. Calculate the drips per minute = 52 drops per minute.

   Rationale: The volume in millilitres per minute is 2.60 and the infusion set delivers 20 drops/ml; therefore multiply 2.6 by 20.

5. **Action:** Calculate the drops per second = 0.8 drop per second or approximately 1 drop per second.

   Rationale: 52 drops are to be delivered over one minute; there are 60 seconds in one minute, therefore divide 52 by 60 = 0.8.

6. **Action:** Once the drip rate is calculated, an infusion pump or syringe driver may be employed.

   Rationale: An infusion pump or syringe driver accurately delivers the calculated fluid rate and will alarm if problems arise.

Procedure: Maintenance of intravenous fluid therapy – general maintenance

1. **Action:** Ensure the infusion site is kept clean. Avoid touching the barrel of the catheter or the site of insertion.

   Rationale: It is essential that the area is kept clean to avoid infection. Bandage the area where possible.

2. **Action:** Replace dressings if they become soiled.

   Rationale: Any soiled dressings near to the infusion site dressing could introduce infection so the dressings must be checked and changed regularly. Antibiotic or antiseptic cream can be applied to the site of catheter insertion to reduce risk of infection.

3. **Action:** Check catheter placement for any abnormalities such as redness, heat or swelling of the area.

Rationale: The signs of infection include perivascular leakage and thrombus. A new catheter may have to be placed.

4. **Action:** Take the patient's temperature 3–4 times daily.

   Rationale: An increasing body temperature could indicate infection.

5. **Action:** Flush the catheter at least twice daily with a small amount of heparinised saline.

   Rationale: This is to ensure patency of the catheter. If resistance is experienced, assess the viability of the catheter and replace with a new catheter if necessary.

6. **Action:** Check that fluid is kept warm, is flowing freely and at the correct drip rate.

   Rationale: Warm fluids will prevent infusion shock. Failure of the fluid to flow could mean that the catheter has moved or become blocked or there are problems with the infusion set or pump – all of which require immediate attention. Flush the catheter and assess the patency of the infusion set. If patency is not achieved, replace faulty or damaged equipment as necessary.

7. **Action:** Check the patient's demeanour.

   Rationale: If the patient shows any change in its behaviour pattern and appears to be in discomfort, examine the infusion site for any problems. Stop infusion and consult the veterinary surgeon.

8. **Action:** Allow the patient to urinate either by catheterisation, taking a dog for walks, providing litter trays for cats, and providing absorbent bedding.

   Rationale: To ensure the patient remains comfortable it must be allowed to urinate while receiving fluids. The method will depend on each individual case. Remember to measure urine voided.

Procedure: Maintenance of fluid therapy – replacement/changing of intravenous fluid bags

1. **Action:** Select and prepare equipment – correct fluid prewarmed, check expiry date, wash hands, wear gloves and apron.

Rationale: It is essential to make sure that all equipment is ready prior to the procedure to ensure efficient changing of fluid bags.

2. **Action:** Remove the new fluid bag from its outer wrapping. Identify the correct fluid outlet port and remove the cover, maintaining asepsis. Hang the new fluid bag on patient's drip stand.

   Rationale: It is essential to identify the correct site to insert the infusion set to prevent damage or contamination. Placing the fluid bag on the drip stand will facilitate easy and efficient handling.

3. **Action:** Ask assistant to restrain the patient.

   Rationale: This is essential to avoid movement of the patient and risk of removal or contamination of equipment.

4. **Action:** Switch off flow control on infusion set connected to patient.

   Rationale: The infusion must be switched off before changing the bags to prevent any air entering the infusion tube.

5. **Action:** Holding the empty fluid bag at the base, carefully remove the infusion set and immediately insert spike into new fluid bag, taking care not to puncture bag or contaminate the infusion.

   Rationale: Removal and reintroduction of the infusion set to a new bag needs to be swift to reduce the likelihood of contamination. Any contamination could result in infection entering the circulatory system.

6. **Action:** Switch on flow control to ensure that the fluid is flowing freely, and adjust to required drip rate.

   Rationale: It may be necessary to flush the patient's catheter after a fluid change as some backflow of blood into catheter and infusion line may occur.

7. **Action:** Record all details of fluid replacement.

   Rationale: It is essential to keep accurate records to prevent under- or over-infusion of the patient.

8. **Action:** Dispose of all equipment safely and appropriately and disinfect area.

Rationale: It is essential for all areas to remain hygienic and for equipment to be disposed of correctly to prevent infection and accidents.

Procedure: Maintenance of fluid therapy – removal of intravenous fluid therapy equipment from patient

1. **Action:** Select and prepare equipment – tapes, swab, scissors; wash hands, assistant, wear gloves and apron.

   Rationale: It is essential to ensure all equipment is ready prior to starting the procedure to ensure efficient and safe removal of the catheter from the vein.

2. **Action:** Ask assistant to restrain patient.

   Rationale: It is essential that the patient is made to feel safe and any movement minimised to prevent discomfort or unnecessary haemorrhage during the procedure.

3. **Action:** Remove all tapes and sutures and terminate flow by switching off flow control.

   Rationale: The infusion must be switched off before removal to prevent fluid leakage and contamination.

4. **Action:** Gently and quickly remove catheter while assistant applies pressure over the vein.

   Rationale: Removal of the catheter should be quick and efficient to ensure minimal discomfort to the patient.

5. **Action:** Maintain pressure on the site of catheter removal while placing a swab over the area. Secure with adhesive tape or bandage.

   Rationale: Pressure must be exerted to prevent haemorrhage and haematoma formation. It may be necessary to apply sutures if a cut down technique has been used for jugular access.

6. **Action:** Dispose of all equipment safely and appropriately and disinfect area.

   Rationale: It is essential for all areas to remain hygienic and for equipment to be disposed of correctly to prevent infection.

Procedure: Monitoring of fluid therapy – general guidelines

1. **Action:** Baseline parameters must be recorded prior to any fluid administration.

   Rationale: It is essential to know the results of baseline tests in order to compare and assess the effectiveness of fluid administration.

2. **Action:** Monitoring must be performed at regular intervals and recorded on a fluid administration chart.

   Rationale: Regular results will indicate a trend, which is more useful than a one-off measurement. Accuracy and regularity are essential requirements for effective monitoring. Everything must be recorded in writing to avoid error.

3. **Action:** All deviations or abnormalities must be noted immediately.

   Rationale: It is essential that any abnormalities are reported immediately to the veterinary surgeon and acted upon to avoid further deterioration or complications to the patient.

Procedure: Monitoring of fluid therapy – essential parameters

Indications: All patients receiving fluids (Figs 4.5 and 4.6).

1. **Action:** Pulse rate, rhythm and quality including core and peripheral pulses.

   Rationale: To check circulatory volume is adequate for tissue perfusion and to ensure circulation is the same throughout body.

2. **Action:** Mucous membrane colour and feel.

   Rationale: Check oxygenation levels are adequate – membranes will change colour. Check level of hydration by feel – membranes may feel moist, tacky or dry. Excess moisture and lacrimation may indicate over-infusion – contact the veterinary surgeon.

3. **Action:** Capillary refill time.

   Rationale: To assess effectiveness of circulating fluid volume – should be 1–2 seconds.

4. **Action:** Chest auscultation/respiratory rate and depth.

   Rationale: Should be clear lung sounds. Laboured, rapid or noisy respiratory patterns may indicate over-infusion or cardiac problems.

5. **Action:** Peripheral oedema.

   Rationale: This could indicate over-infusion of fluid.

6. **Action:** Body temperature – core and peripheral.

   Rationale: To assess vasoconstriction/vasodilation, and to check if patient is suffering from a systemic infection.

7. **Action:** Urine output.

   Rationale: Minimum output per hour = 1 ml/kg/h. To assess renal function and associated circulatory volume. Less than 1 ml/kg/h could indicate renal problems due to insufficient circulatory volume.

8. **Action:** Skin turgor.

   Rationale: To assess pliability of skin. Tenting can indicate dehydration.

9. **Action:** Bodyweight.

   Rationale: To assess any change over a period of hours/days. Marked increase could indicate over-infusion.

10. **Action:** General demeanour/clinical observation.

    Rationale: Any sign of distress or discomfort could indicate a problem, e.g. infection, over-infusion, medical condition deteriorating.

Procedure: Blood collection for transfusion

Indication: Blood required for storage or by a recipient to replace acute or chronic haemorrhage, anaemia, clotting problems.

1. **Action:** Select an appropriate donor.

   Rationale: Correct species and blood group.

2. **Action:** Select equipment for blood collection – acid citrate/citrate dextrose blood collection bag, local anaesthetic, syringe, needle,

Patient I.D.	Clinical history
Species and breed	
Age Sex Weight	
Veterinary surgeon	
Veterinary nurse	

Monitor and record every.................. daily

Date and time	T	P	R	MM CRT	Demeanour	Fluid type	Drip rate	Fluid input	Fluid/urine output	Weight	Medication	Comments

Figure 4.5   Example of a chart for monitoring patients receiving fluid therapy.

Name _____

Case number _____

Date and time	Fluid offered	Fluid intake	IV fluid	Drip rate

Figure 4.6   Example of a chart for monitoring fluid balance.

clippers, surgical skin scrub solution, gloves, swabs, assistant.

Rationale: Anticipation and preparation is essential for effective collection.

3. **Action:** An assistant is needed to restrain the patient in a suitable position allowing access to the jugular vein. The patient is reassured throughout the procedure.

   Rationale: Firm restraint is required to make the donor feel safe and comfortable.

4. **Action:** Clip small area over jugular vein and prepare skin aseptically.

   Rationale: To reduce risk of infection.

5. **Action:** Local anaesthetic is infiltrated into the prepared site as per veterinary surgeon's instructions. Massage the area.

   Rationale: Local anaesthetic desensitises the area. The area is massaged to help absorption.

6. **Action:** The needle attached to the donor blood bag is introduced by the veterinary surgeon into the jugular vein. Once blood flows into the donor bag the needle is advanced and held in place manually.

   Rationale: As collection is via a needle rather than a catheter, it needs to be held securely to prevent further puncture of the jugular vein resulting in considerable blood loss.

7. **Action:** Hold blood bag below the patient and roll it continually and gently.

   Rationale: Blood is collected by the action of gravity. The bag is rolled to ensure mixing of the acid citrate/citrate dextrose anticoagulant thus preventing clotting.

8. **Action:** Once the required volume of blood has been collected, the veterinary surgeon removes the needle and the assistant exerts pressure on the jugular puncture site.

   Rationale: To prevent further blood loss by providing back pressure, thereby arresting haemorrhage from venepuncture site.

9. **Action:** Fold over the blood collection tube to occlude it.

   Rationale: To avoid excess wastage within the tube.

10. **Action:** If the blood is not to be administered immediately, store at 4–8°C for a maximum of 3 weeks. Label bag clearly with the species and date of collection.

    Rationale: It is essential that blood products are stored correctly to avoid deterioration.

11. **Action:** Dispose of equipment safely and appropriately.

    Rationale: It is essential to dispose of equipment correctly to avoid contamination and accidents.

Procedure: Blood transfusion

Indications: Acute or chronic haemorrhage, acute or chronic anaemia, platelet and clotting problems.

1. **Action:** Select and prepare equipment (Fig. 4.7) – blood warmed to body temperature (if from storage), blood infusion set, adhesive tape, bandage, patient with intravenous catheter in place.

   Rationale: Blood must be prewarmed prior to administration to maintain body temperature and cause minimal discomfort to the patient. All equipment must be prepared in advance of beginning the procedure to ensure efficient administration.

2. **Action:** Remove the cover from the spike of the blood infusion set. Switch off flow control and insert the spike into the correct port of the blood bag, taking care not to puncture the bag.

   Rationale: Puncturing the blood bag would result in a waste of blood and contamination of the blood bag, making it unsafe to use for transfusion.

3. **Action:** Squeeze both chambers of blood infusion set to fill with blood to one-third in each of them.

   Rationale: The extra chamber within the blood infusion set provides a fibrin filter to collect any fibrin clots, preventing them entering the circulation.

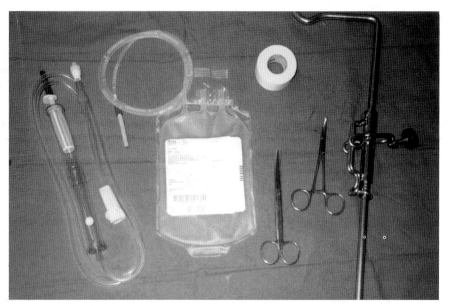

Figure 4.7   Blood transfusion kit (blood collection bag, blood infusion set, scissors, clamps, tape and drip stand). Reproduced, with permission, from Masters and Bowden (2003), Butterworth-Heinemann.

4. **Action:** Remove cap from the end of infusion line and hold over kick bowl, taking care not to contaminate the tip.

    Rationale: It is essential to keep all items sterile.

5. **Action:** Turn on flow control switch to allow blood to travel down infusion line to the tip in a controlled manner to remove all air bubbles.

    Rationale: To avoid risk of air embolism, all air bubbles must be removed from the infusion line prior to connection to patient.

6. **Action:** Replace cap on infusion line and hang infusion on drip stand prior to connection to the patient.

    Rationale: Ensure equipment remains aseptic.

7. **Action:** Restrain patient, and ensure the patency of the catheter by flushing with a small amount of heparinised saline.

    Rationale: It is essential to check the patency of the catheter before attachment to the blood infusion line to avoid unnecessary contamination or wastage of blood.

8. **Action:** Remove cap from infusion line and attach to the intravenous catheter. Switch on flow control to allow blood to flow into the patient.

    Rationale: Connect and access patency. If not flowing freely, check equipment and reflush.

9. **Action:** When flowing freely, adjust flow control to required rate of transfusion.

    Rationale: Rapid transfusion of blood should be avoided to prevent circulatory overload or reaction.

10. **Action:** Attach infusion line securely to the patient by means of tapes, bandages or sutures (depending on which intravenous route has been chosen).

    Rationale: It is essential that the infusion line is secure to avoid displacement or leakage.

11. **Action:** Monitor constantly for any signs of blood transfusion reaction and record details of transfusion rate and time.

    Rationale: It is essential to keep accurate records and monitor constantly as any reaction to a blood transfusion is undesirable and requires immediate attention.

12. **Action:** Dispose of equipment safely and appropriately.

    Rationale: It is essential to dispose of all equipment correctly to avoid contamination and accidents.

Procedure: Monitoring for blood transfusion reactions

Indications: All patients receiving blood transfusions.

1. **Action:** Assess baseline parameters prior to transfusion – temperature, pulse, respiration, mucous membrane colour, packed cell volume.

    Rationale: It is essential to obtain baseline parameters in order to notice any deviations from normal during the transfusion.

2. **Action:** Continue to monitor patient parameters as above and record results.

    Rationale: Immediate action is required if any signs of a reaction become apparent.

3. **Action:** Monitor the patient for any of the following signs: pyrexia, salivation, vomiting, diarrhoea, tachycardia, muscle tremors, facial oedema.

    Rationale: Any of these signs could indicate a transfusion reaction due to incompatibility or over-administration and requires immediate attention.

4. **Action:** If any of the above signs are apparent, stop the infusion and inform the veterinary surgeon immediately.

    Rationale: It is essential to stop the infusion if these signs are apparent to prevent further deterioration.

5. **Action:** Reassure the patient and make it comfortable.

    Rationale: Patients can become disorientated and confused during a blood transfusion reaction and require reassurance to avoid undue stress.

REFERENCES AND FURTHER READING

Aspinall V 2006 The Complete Textbook of Veterinary Nursing. Elsevier, Oxford

Houlton J E F, Taylor P M 1987 Trauma Management. Wright, Bristol

Lane D R, Cooper B (eds) 2003 Veterinary Nursing, 3rd edn. Butterworth-Heinemann, Oxford

Masters J, Bowden C 2003 Quick Reference Guide to Veterinary Medical Kits. Butterworth-Heinemann, Oxford

Taylor R A, McGehee R 1995 Manual of Small Animal Postoperative Care. Williams and Wilkins, Baltimore

Chapter 5

Provision of nutritional support

Carole Martin

CHAPTER CONTENTS

Introduction 87

Enteral feeding 88
Calculation of energy needs 88
Calculation of food quantities to be
    administered 88
Selection of food for enteral feeding 89
Forced feeding – placing food in mouth 89
Forced feeding by syringe 90
Naso-oesophageal and nasogastric tube
    placement and tube feeding 90
Pharyngostomy tube placement and tube
    feeding 92
Gastrostomy tube placement and tube
    feeding 94
Maintenance of feeding tubes 97
Monitoring techniques for enteral feeding 97
Monitoring enteral feeding – essential
    parameters 98

Parenteral feeding 98
Calculation of nutrition requirements
    and suggested feeding regime 98
Intravenous access to jugular vein
    and administration of parenteral feeding 101
Monitoring techniques for parenteral
    feeding 102
Monitoring parenteral feeding – essential
    parameters 102

INTRODUCTION

All animals must receive a balanced diet to maintain optimum levels of health. When an animal is ill, it may not want to eat or may not be able to eat, leading to deficiencies of certain vital nutrients and energy. These deficiencies will seriously slow down the rate of recovery and impair the healing process. Failure to consider some method of nutritional support may compromise the patient's chances of recovery.

When nursing the sick animal consideration must be given to certain factors which differ from those in the healthy animal:

1. Energy requirement – a healthy animal needs energy for basic metabolism and for exercise. A sick animal will use much less energy in exercise but disease and stress increase the normal energy requirements.
2. Type of food – sick animals often have a reduced desire to eat and thought must be given to palatability and how to tempt them to eat. If the animal does eat it may only eat small quantities, giving rise to the need to supply energy-dense food. In addition, the consistency must be considered in relation to the route of administration.
3. Route of administration: nutritional support can be given by the enteral route – making use of the gastrointestinal tract – or by the parenteral route – providing nutrients intravenously.

In some cases a patient may not be able to use part of the gastrointestinal tract, e.g. the oral cavity, and steps must be taken to bypass it using some form of feeding tube.

This chapter considers all these factors and describes in detail the techniques involved in placing feeding tubes and the nursing care needed to maintain them.

ENTERAL FEEDING

(Administration of nutritional support using the gastrointestinal tract.)

Procedure: Calculation of energy needs

1. **Action:** Calculate basic energy requirement (BER) for over 5 kg bodyweight.

   Formula: BER = (30 × kg bodyweight) + 70 kcal.
   For example, to find the BER for a 10 kg dog:
   BER = (30 × 10) + 70
   $$= 300 + 70$$
   $$= 370 \,\text{kcal/day.}$$

   Rationale: The energy required to meet the metabolic needs of patients is measured in kilocalories (kcal). The BER is based on the metabolic energy needs of a patient at rest including processes such as respiration, circulation and kidney function. Age, bodyweight and composition, and activity may affect it.

2. **Action:** Calculate daily BER for 5 kg bodyweight and under.

   Formula: BER = (60 × kg bodyweight) + 70 kcal.
   For example, to find BER for a 3 kg cat:
   BER = (60 × 3) + 70
   $$= 180 + 70$$
   $$= 250 \,\text{kcal/day.}$$

   Rationale: Animals under 5 kg have a faster metabolic rate, so require more energy per kg bodyweight than do animals over 5 kg. This also applies to neonates, where the metabolic rate is greater than that of adults.

3. **Action:** Calculate illness energy requirement (IER) in relation to daily BER:

   hospitalised/cage rest = 1.2 × BER
   surgery/trauma = 1.3–1.5 × BER
   cancer/sepsis = 1.7 × BER
   burns = 2 × BER.

   Rationale: Illness and disease factors must be taken into account when artificially feeding patients. Stress and disease processes require an increase in energy to meet metabolic needs and counteract weight loss. The factors shown should be multiplied by the RER to give the kcal/day requirements.

Procedure: Calculation of food quantities to be administered

1. **Action:** Calculate quantity of kcal to be fed to a hospitalised 10 kg dog.

   For example, 10 kg dog requires 370 kcal/day at rest:
   = 370 (BER) × 1.2 (IER) for hospitalised patient
   = 444 kcal/day.

   Rationale: It is essential to ascertain the energy requirement in kcal before calculating the quantity of food in millilitres (ml).

2. **Action:** Calculate the quantity of food in ml to be fed to a 10 kg hospitalised dog. Food value 1.5 kcal/ml.

   For example, dog requires 444 kcal/day:
   = 444 kcal ÷ 1.5 kcal
   = 296 ml/day.

   Rationale: For artificial feeding it is important to choose a food that is energy dense, i.e. a small volume contains a large number of kcal. This will reduce the volume given, providing easier and more efficient administration.

3. **Action:** Divide quantity in ml into equal feeds to be administered throughout the day:

   296 ÷ 6 = 50 ml per feed
   296 ÷ 8 = 37 ml per feed
   296 ÷ 10 = 29 ml per feed.

   Rationale: Always divide the food quantity into equal workable amounts depending on the method of artificial feeding. Consider the time available for feeding and each patient's needs. Avoid excessive quantities in single feeds to prevent discomfort, regurgitation or vomiting. Avoid small quantities that necessitate excessive handling and discomfort to the patient.

NB. Larger tubes, such as gastrostomy tubes, allow for larger quantities to be administered at each feed – calculations can be adjusted accordingly.

Procedure: Selection of food for enteral feeding

Indications: Aim to select a food with high calorie density (at least 1 kcal/ml).

1. **Action:** Concentrated tinned food, e.g. recovery and convalescent diets.

    Rationale: Forced feeding by hand, or for syringe and gastrostomy tube feeding. Not always easily liquidised, therefore unsuitable for smaller bore tubes.

2. **Action:** Semi-solid foods.

    Rationale: Syringe and all tube feeding. May require further liquidising for smaller bore tubes to prevent blockage by food particles.

3. **Action:** Liquid complete foods.

    Rationale: Suitable for syringe feeding, naso-oesophageal tube feeding, nasogastric and pharyngostomy tubes.

Procedure: Forced feeding – placing food in mouth

Indications: General inappetence due to change in environment, stress, underlying disease.

Food choice: Any proprietary, complete, balanced tinned food or energy-dense food; food of a high aroma is desirable.

1. **Action:** Select and prepare equipment – check expiry date of food; prewarm food; wash hands; wear gloves and apron; damp swabs, towel.

    Rationale: Ensure all equipment is selected and prepared prior to beginning the procedure to allow for efficient administration.

2. **Action:** Reassure patient and ask the assistant to restrain the patient, holding the head in a normal position.

    Rationale: Kind but firm handling will ensure the animal feels secure. Keeping the head in a normal position will reduce the risk of aspiration pneumonia.

3. **Action:** With gloved hands, take a small quantity of food. Open the patient's mouth and place some food on the back of the tongue (Fig. 5.1).

    Rationale: Wear gloves to ensure hygiene is maintained. If the patient resents the procedure in any way, stop and offer reassurance before recommencing.

4. **Action:** Allow the patient to swallow and lick its lips, reassuring it throughout the procedure.

    Rationale: Encourage patient to swallow by externally massaging the ventral pharynx.

5. **Action:** Repeat until required amount of food has been administered.

    Rationale: If the patient becomes distressed before all of the food has been administered, stop the procedure and allow the patient to calm down fully before commencing again.

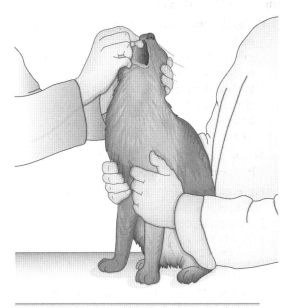

Figure 5.1   Placing food by hand directly into the oral cavity may encourage animals to begin eating after a period of illness or major surgery.

6. **Action:** Once all food has been administered, clean the patient's mouth with damp swabs and dry the area.

   Rationale: The mouth must free of any food debris to discourage bacterial growth.

7. **Action:** Record food administration and repeat at required intervals.

   Rationale: It is essential to keep accurate records of food administration to prevent any error.

8. **Action:** Dispose of equipment safely and appropriately.

   Rationale: This is essential to avoid contamination.

9. **Action:** Any food in tins must be covered and stored at 4–8 °C between feeds.

   Rationale: Food must be stored according to the manufacturer's instructions to avoid any loss of nutrients and subsequent deterioration of food quality.

Procedure: Forced feeding by syringe

Indications: General inappetence due to underlying disease.

Food choice: Food of high calorific value, liquid consistency or easy to liquidise and feed with a syringe, e.g. proprietary convalescent foods.

1. **Action:** Select and prepare equipment – calculate energy requirements and food quantity. Prewarmed food, catheter tip syringe, towel, assistant; wash hands, wear gloves and apron.

   Rationale: It is essential to select and prepare all equipment prior to beginning the procedure to ensure efficient administration.

2. **Action:** Measure correct volume of food into syringe.

   Rationale: Accurately measure volume required based on calculation of energy/kcal needed.

3. **Action:** Request assistance to hold patient.

   Rationale: Ensure patient feels safe.

4. **Action:** Support patient's nose and mouth, keeping the head in a normal position.

Rationale: Firm but effective handling will ensure food is delivered safely. Keeping the head in a normal position will reduce the risk of aspiration pneumonia.

5. **Action:** Introduce the syringe into the mouth between the upper and lower premolars above the surface of the tongue.

   Rationale: This area is the most suitable to aid administration and control food intake.

6. **Action:** Applying gentle pressure to the syringe, introduce approximately 10 ml of food into the mouth and allow patient to swallow. Stroke ventral aspect of pharynx to encourage swallowing.

   Rationale: Avoid giving food quickly or in one bolus as this may cause choking. Allow the patient to swallow and breathe between administrations.

7. **Action:** Continue with administration until the required volume has been delivered.

   Rationale: Only continue if patient is taking the food well and swallowing between administrations. If the patient gets distressed or fails to swallow, stop immediately.

8. **Action:** Clean and dry the patient's mouth thoroughly and replace in kennel.

   Rationale: Always ensure mouth is free of any food debris and is dry, to discourage bacterial growth.

9. **Action:** Record food administered.

   Rationale: Accurate record keeping is essential to avoid error.

10. **Action:** Dispose of equipment safely and appropriately. Clean and disinfect surface areas.

   Rationale: It is essential to dispose of equipment correctly to avoid contamination.

Procedure: Naso–oesophageal and nasogastric tube placement and tube feeding

Indications: Generally short-term tube feeding where there is failure to stimulate voluntary eating or a physical inability to eat. Use liquid foods only.

1. **Action:** Select and prepare equipment – naso-oesophageal or nasogastric tubes, water-soluble lubricant, speculum, pen torch, gloves, tissue glue or suture equipment, swabs, syringe and water, prewarmed food to room temperature; wash hands, wear gloves and apron.

   Rationale: It is essential to prepare equipment prior to beginning the procedure to ensure efficient administration. Always prewarm food to at least room temperature as cold food can induce vomiting.

2. **Action:** Request an assistant to restrain the patient, supporting its head in a normal position. The patient will be conscious or be mildly sedated.

   Rationale: Firm handling makes the patient feel safe and facilitates the procedure. General anaesthesia is not normally used for placement of these tubes.

3. **Action:** Measure the distance from the external nares to the seventh rib space for naso-oesophageal tube and from external nares to the tenth rib space for nasogastric tube (Fig. 5.2). Mark position on the tube.

   Rationale: It is important to measure the distance prior to the procedure to check placement is correct.

4. **Action:** Local anaesthetic gel or spray can be applied to the internal aspect of nares. (No need to use local anaesthetic if patient is anaesthetised.)

   Rationale: Local anaesthetic agents can be used to desensitise the nasal mucous membrane, reducing any discomfort.

5. **Action:** Lubricate the tip of the tube with water-soluble lubricant (avoid the use of petroleum jelly on silicone tubes).

   Rationale: This will allow for easy passage of the tube and minimal discomfort for the patient. Petroleum jelly reacts with silicone.

6. **Action:** The tube is introduced into the nasal cavity and advanced down the pharynx and oesophagus. In the case of a nasogastric tube, the tube is advanced to the caudal oesophagus.

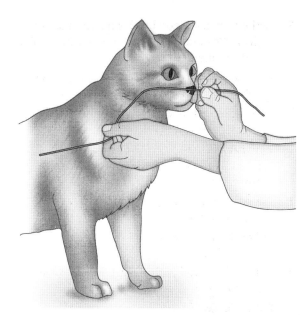

Figure 5.2 Naso-oesophageal tube placement. Before inserting the tube, determine the correct tubing length by measuring and marking the tube distance from the cat's mouth to the seventh or eighth rib space (eighth or ninth rib space for dogs).

   Rationale: Nasogastric tube placement is preferred in some cases. The placement is more caudal than that of a naso-oesophageal tube, which reduces the risk of gastric reflux.

7. **Action:** Check for correct positioning by observing any coughing and by the introduction of up to 5 ml of water followed by auscultation for borborygmi. Once in place, occlude end of tube with suitable bung.

   Rationale: It is essential to ensure that the tube is placed correctly to prevent inhalation of food. Coughing and lack of borborygmi could indicate that the tube is in the trachea – the tube should be repositioned. The end of the tube must be occluded once in place to prevent excessive air being swallowed.

8. **Action:** Secure the exterior part of the tube to the patient's head with the aid of tissue glue or sutures over the nose and between the eyes.

   Rationale: The remainder of the tube must be secured to prevent displacement.

9. **Action:** Food may now be administered to the conscious patient (Fig. 5.3). If feeding is not to take place immediately, occlude the end of the tube with a bung and apply an Elizabethan collar.

    Rationale: It is essential to prevent patient interference, tube displacement and swallowing of air, if the patient is not to be fed immediately.

10. **Action:** Measure the correct volume of prewarmed food into a syringe, as calculated previously.

    Rationale: It is important that the food quantity/energy requirements are calculated prior to procedure, facilitating easy measurement at this point.

11. **Action:** Remove bung from the feeding tube and flush the tube with 3–10 ml of water.

    Rationale: Flushing the tube will ensure it is patent. If resistance is experienced, repeat the procedure (carbonated water may be used in cases where food and mucus may be blocking the tube).

12. **Action:** Administer the food slowly (do not exceed 50 ml/kg/feed).

    Rationale: Rapid administration can lead to discomfort, regurgitation and vomiting and should therefore be avoided.

13. **Action:** Flush tube with a further 5–10 ml water.

    Rationale: Water must be flushed after the food to ensure tube is clear of any particles.

14. **Action:** Replace bung in feeding tube.

    Rationale: The bung must be replaced to prevent any leakage of fluid or food and prevent air being ingested.

15. **Action:** Clean around tube site.

    Rationale: It is essential to keep the tube insertion site clean. An antibiotic or antiseptic cream may be applied to the area to help moisturise and to prevent infection.

16. **Action:** Apply an Elizabethan collar to the patient and return patient to the kennel.

    Rationale: Patient interference must be avoided to prevent displacement of the tube.

17. **Action:** Follow same feeding regime for repeat feeds. Record all administration details.

    Rationale: It is essential to keep accurate records to avoid any error in administration.

18. **Action:** Store any remaining food according to the manufacturer's instructions and dispose of all other equipment safely and appropriately.

    Rationale: It is essential that any food is stored hygienically and equipment is disposed of correctly to avoid contamination.

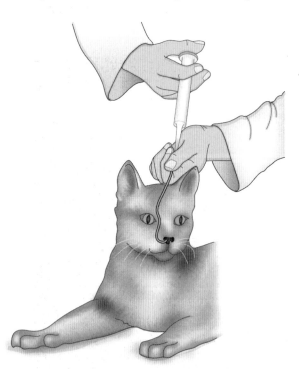

Figure 5.3 Naso-oesophageal tube feeding. Attach a syringe and instil 3 ml of water. Slowly administer food. After administration, flush with water to prevent blockage. Cap or cover tube opening. Redrawn from Lane and Cooper (1994), Butterworth-Heinemann.

Procedure: Pharyngostomy tube placement and tube feeding

Indications: Short-term feeding where there is underlying disease or injuries cranial to the pharynx. Use liquid diets or liquidised tinned foods.

1. **Action:** Select and prepare equipment (Fig. 5.4) – pharyngostomy tube, clippers, surgical skin scrub solution, forceps, gloves, minor surgical kit and suture equipment, swabs, syringe and water, prewarmed food; wash hands, wear gloves and apron.

   Rationale: It is essential to prepare equipment prior to beginning the procedure to ensure efficient administration. Food should be warmed to at least room temperature as cold food can induce vomiting.

2. **Action:** The patient will be anaesthetised or sedated. Position in right lateral recumbency with pharynx slightly elevated.

   Rationale: Correct positioning is essential in aiding correct placement of the tube.

3. **Action:** Measure the distance from the external nares to approximately the tenth rib space and mark the position on the tube.

   Rationale: It is important to measure the distance prior to the procedure to check that the placement is correct.

4. **Action:** Clip an area of approximately 6 cm × 6 cm lateral to and caudal to the angle of the jaw and prepare the skin surgically. Drape the area.

   Rationale: It is essential to provide asepsis for the surgical procedure.

5. **Action:** The veterinary surgeon then places the pharyngostomy tube surgically (this may be aided by a specially designed introducer).

   Rationale: This will allow for easy passage of the tube and minimal discomfort for patient.

6. **Action:** Correct positioning of the tube is checked by the introduction of 2–3 ml of water. Respiratory and gastric sounds are monitored. Once confirmed, occlude end of tube.

   Rationale: It is essential to ensure that the tube is placed correctly to prevent inhalation of food. The end of the tube must be occluded once in place, to prevent excessive air travelling down tube.

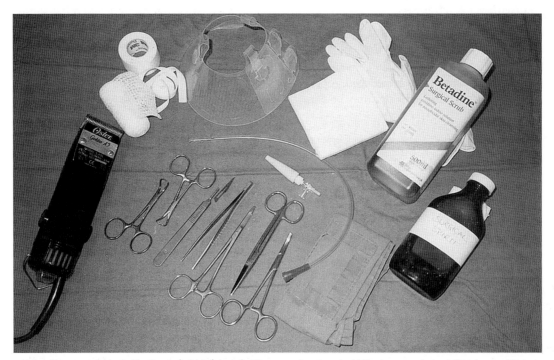

Figure 5.4 Pharyngostomy tube placement kit (electric clippers, minor surgical kit, pharyngostomy tube, drape, skin preparation solutions, swab, gloves, Elizabethan collar, tapes). Reproduced, with permission, from Masters and Bowden (2003), Butterworth-Heinemann.

7. **Action:** The tube is then sutured to the skin at the insertion site. Remove drapes and cover the tube with sterile dressing and bandage (Fig. 5.5).

   Rationale: The remainder of the tube must be secured to prevent displacement and a bandage placed over it to prevent patient interference.

8. **Action:** As placement is performed under general anaesthetic, do not administer food until the patient is fully conscious. Once it is conscious, request an assistant to restrain the patient in sternal recumbency, reassuring it throughout the procedure.

   Rationale: Food must not be administered in the unconscious patient due to the absence of or reduced swallow and cough reflexes.

9. **Action:** Measure the correct volume of prewarmed food into a syringe as calculated previously.

   Rationale: It is important that the food quantity/energy requirements are calculated prior to procedure, facilitating easy measurement at this point.

10. **Action:** Remove the bung from the feeding tube and flush tube with 3–10 ml of water.

    Rationale: Flushing the tube will ensure it is patent. If resistance is experienced, repeat procedure (carbonated water may be used in cases where food and mucus may be blocking the tube).

11. **Action:** Administer the food slowly – do not exceed 50 ml/kg/feed.

    Rationale: Rapid administration can lead to discomfort, regurgitation and vomiting and should therefore be avoided.

12. **Action:** Flush tube with a further 5–10 ml of water.

    Rationale: Water must be flushed after the food to ensure tube is clear of any particles.

13. **Action:** Replace bung in feeding tube.

    Rationale: The bung must be replaced to prevent any leakage of fluid or food and prevent air being ingested.

14. **Action:** Clean around tube site.

    Rationale: It is essential to keep tube insertion site clean. An antibiotic or antiseptic cream may be applied to the area to help moisturise and prevent infection as directed by the veterinary surgeon.

15. **Action:** Apply a dressing and light bandage to the area, being careful not to occlude the airways by excessive pressure. An Elizabethan collar may be used in some cases.

    Rationale: Patient interference must be avoided to prevent displacement of the tube.

16. **Action:** Repeat the procedure as required and record all food administration details.

    Rationale: It is essential to record accurately to prevent an error in administration.

17. **Action:** Store any remaining food according to the manufacturer's instructions and dispose of all other equipment safely and appropriately.

    Rationale: It is essential that any food is stored hygienically and equipment is disposed of correctly to avoid contamination.

Procedure: Gastrostomy tube placement and tube feeding

Indications: Preferred method for longer-term feeding, underlying disease, surgery or trauma to the oesophagus. The tube can be left in place for several months; use liquidised foods.

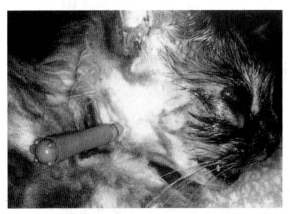

Figure 5.5 A pharyngostomy tube (placed under general anaesthesia) in a cat with a fractured jaw. Reproduced, with permission, from Lane and Cooper (1994), Butterworth-Heinemann.

1. **Action:** Select equipment (Fig. 5.6) – gastrostomy (mushroom tipped) catheter, stilette and introducing equipment, clippers, surgical skin scrub solution, forceps, gloves, minor surgical kit and suture equipment, swabs, prewarmed food; wash hands, wear gloves and apron.

    Rationale: It is essential to prepare equipment prior to beginning the procedure to ensure efficient administration. Food should be warmed to at least room temperature as cold food can induce vomiting.

2. **Action:** The patient will be anaesthetised. Position in right lateral recumbency. The tube may also be placed during a midline laparotomy – if so the patient will be in dorsal recumbency.

    Rationale: As the placement of this tube requires surgical intervention, a general anaesthetic is required. Correct positioning of the patient is essential to facilitate efficient preparation and tube placement.

3. **Action:** Clip an area of approximately 15 cm × 15 cm on the lateral aspect of the patient, midway between dorsal and ventral body surfaces and caudal to the costal arch. Prepare skin aseptically and drape area.

    Rationale: It is essential to provide asepsis for surgical procedures, thereby reducing the risk of infection.

4. **Action:** The veterinary surgeon places the gastrostomy tube surgically. This can be facilitated by a specially designed introducer or with the aid of an endoscope (percutaneous endoscopic gastrostomy – PEG).

    Rationale: This will allow for easy passage of the tube and minimal discomfort for the patient.

5. **Action:** Correct placing of the tube is checked by the introduction of 2–3 ml of water. Gastric sounds are monitored. Once confirmed, occlude the end of tube.

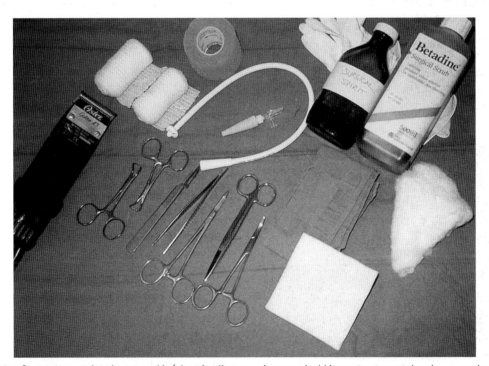

Figure 5.6 Gastrostomy tube placement kit (electric clippers, minor surgical kit, gastrostomy tube, drape, swabs, surgical skin preparation solutions, bandages, gloves). Reproduced, with permission, from Masters and Bowden (2003), Butterworth-Heinemann.

Rationale: It is essential to ensure that the tube is placed correctly in the stomach and not between the visceral and parietal layers of the peritoneum. The end of the tube must be occluded, once in place, to prevent excessive air being ingested.

6. **Action:** The exterior part of the tube is secured to the patient's body wall by means of a suture or tissue glue. Remove drapes (Fig. 5.7).

   Rationale: The remainder of the tube must be secured to prevent displacement.

7. **Action:** As placement is performed under general anaesthetic, it is not advisable to administer food until the patient has regained consciousness. Once fully conscious, request an assistant to restrain the patient in sternal recumbency reassuring it throughout the procedure. Apply a dressing and an abdominal bandage to cover the tube until food is administered.

   Rationale: Food must not be administered in the unconscious patient due to an inability to swallow or cough if gastric reflux occurs.

8. **Action:** When ready to feed the patient, measure the correct volume of prewarmed food into a syringe as calculated previously.

   Rationale: It is important that the food quantity/energy requirements are calculated prior to the procedure, facilitating easy measurement at this point.

9. **Action:** Remove bung from the feeding tube and flush the tube with 3–10 ml of water.

   Rationale: Flushing the tube will ensure it is patent. If resistance is experienced, repeat the procedure (carbonated water may be used in cases where food and mucus may be blocking the tube).

10. **Action:** Administer the food slowly as calculated previously. Larger quantities of food can be administered by this route – do not exceed 50 ml/kg/feed.

    Rationale: Rapid administration can lead to discomfort and vomiting and should therefore be avoided.

11. **Action:** Flush tube with a further 5–10 ml water.

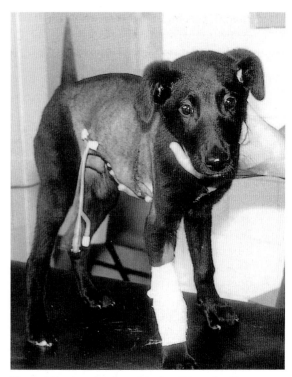

Figure 5.7 A gastrostomy tube in a 12-week-old puppy after removal of an oesophageal foreign body. Partial thickness oesophageal damage necessitated tube placement. Tube feeding (including all water requirements) was maintained for 5 days. Antibiotics were also given. Reproduced, with permission, from Lane and Cooper (1994), Butterworth-Heinemann.

   Rationale: Water must be flushed after the food to ensure tube is clear of any particles.

12. **Action:** Replace bung in feeding tube.

    Rationale: The bung must be replaced to prevent any leakage of fluid or food and prevent air being ingested.

13. **Action:** Clean around tube site.

    Rationale: It is essential to keep tube insertion site clean. An antibiotic or antiseptic cream may be applied to the area to help moisturise and to prevent infection, as directed by the veterinary surgeon.

14. **Action:** Apply a dressing and an abdominal bandage to the area. Also apply an Elizabethan collar.

    Rationale: Patient interference must be avoided to prevent displacement of the tube.

15. **Action:** Repeat feeding regime as required and record administration details.

    Rationale: It is essential to record accurately to prevent any error in administration.

16. **Action:** Store any remaining food according to the manufacturer's instructions and dispose of all other equipment safely and appropriately.

    Rationale: It is essential that any food is stored hygienically and equipment is disposed of correctly to avoid contamination.

Procedure: Maintenance of feeding tubes

1. **Action:** Ensure tube and insertion site is clean and dry at all times.

    Rationale: As the food being administered contains the ideal constituents for the growth of microorganisms it is essential to remove any food leakage from the tube and surrounding area and to keep the area dry to prevent infection. Antiseptic and antibiotic creams may be applied to the skin at the tube insertion site under the direction of the veterinary surgeon.

2. **Action:** Check the position and condition of the tubes at least twice daily.

    Rationale: It is important to check tube position and check for signs of movement or displacement. The tubes should also be checked for cracks or damage.

3. **Action:** Flush tube before and after administration of fluids.

    Rationale: Always flush the tube with water prior to the administration of food, to ensure that the tube is not blocked. Always listen for any coughing or lack of borborygmi indicating that the tube has moved. If in doubt, do not continue and inform the veterinary surgeon. Always flush after feeding to ensure no food particles remain within the tube and cause a blockage later.

4. **Action:** Ensure tube remains occluded when not in use.

    Rationale: It is essential to occlude the tube when not in use to prevent unnecessary

ingestion of air leading to discomfort and distension of the abdomen.

5. **Action:** Keep tube area covered and free from patient interference.

    Rationale: It is essential to prevent patient interference, which may cause tube displacement. In the case of pharyngostomy and gastrostomy tubes it is advisable to cover with dressings and bandages.

6. **Action:** Flush mouth regularly with water and dry afterwards.

    Rationale: As any form of tube feeding excludes the mouth, it is essential to flush the mouth with water regularly to improve the patient's comfort.

7. **Action:** When tube is to be removed, remove all tapes and sutures. Pull the tube out gently but quickly while an assistant exerts pressure on the exit site. Sutures may be placed if necessary.

    Rationale: Tube removal is indicated if there are problems or if the animal begins to eat sufficient food voluntarily. Gastrostomy tubes should be left in place for at least 5 days to ensure adhesion of the stomach to the body wall. The procedure needs to be quick and efficient to produce minimal discomfort and reduce risk of aspiration of air or stomach contents.

8. **Action:** Dispose of all equipment and disinfect the area.

    Rationale: It is essential to maintain a clean environment at all times, thereby reducing risk of infection.

Procedure: Monitoring techniques for enteral feeding

1. **Action:** Baseline parameters must be recorded prior to any enteral feeding.

    Rationale: It is essential to know the results of baseline tests in order to compare and assess the effectiveness of enteral feeding.

2. **Action:** Monitoring must be performed at regular intervals and recorded on the feeding chart.

Rationale: Regular results will indicate a trend, which is more useful than a one-off measurement. Accuracy and regularity are essential requirements for effective monitoring. Everything must be recorded in writing to avoid error.

3. **Action:** All deviations or abnormalities must be noted immediately.

   Rationale: It is essential that any abnormalities are reported immediately to the veterinary surgeon and acted upon to avoid further deterioration or complications in the patient.

Procedure: Monitoring enteral feeding – essential parameters

Indications: All patients receiving enteral nutrition (Fig. 5.8A and B).

1. **Action:** Temperature, pulse and respiration.
   Rationale: To identify infection or inflammation.
2. **Action:** Bodyweight – measure daily.
   Rationale: To identify any large fluctuations that may indicate fluid imbalance.
3. **Action:** Plasma glucose concentration – daily until stable.
   Rationale: To monitor blood glucose levels.
4. **Action:** Urine output.
   Rationale: Minimum output per hour = 1 ml/kg. To assess renal function and associated circulatory volume. Less than 1 ml/kg/h could indicate renal problems due to insufficient circulatory volume.
5. **Action:** Urine glucose – every 6 hours until stable.
   Rationale: To identify hyperglycaemia.
6. **Action:** General demeanour/clinical observation.
   Rationale: Any sign of distress or discomfort could indicate a problem.
7. **Action:** Check tube insertion site for any signs of heat, redness or swelling.
   Rationale: It is essential to monitor the insertion site to check for any signs of discomfort or infection.

8. **Action:** Continue to feed until the patient eats ⅔ to ¾ of nutritional requirements voluntarily.

   Rationale: This would indicate a need to reduce or cease tube feeding due to patient progress.

9. **Action:** Record all results accurately.

   Rationale: It is essential to record all results accurately in order to measure the patient's progress or deterioration.

PARENTERAL FEEDING

(Administration of nutritional support by the intravenous route.)

Procedure: Calculation of nutrition requirements and suggested feeding regime

1. **Action:** 10 kg patient with a septic condition requires 630 kcal/day.

   Rationale: Bodyweight × BER × IER.

2. **Action:** 4 g of protein are required per 100 kcal/day = 25 g protein/day.

   Rationale: 630 kcal/day × 4 g protein/100 kcal.

3. **Action:** 8.5% amino acid solution (AAS) available = 294 ml/day of 8.5% AAS.

   Rationale: 8.5% solution = 8.5 g in 100 ml
   25 g protein/day × 100 ÷ 8.5 = 294 ml.

4. **Action:** 100% Glucose provides 3.4 metabolisable kcal/g, therefore 50% solution = 1.7 kcal/g.

   Rationale: 100% solution = 100 g in 100 ml
   50% solution = 50 g/100 ml (half of 100)
   3.4 kcal/g in 100%
   1.7 kcal/g in 50%.

5. **Action:** 630 kcal energy are required = 370 ml/day of 50% glucose.

   Rationale: 630 kcal ÷ 1.7 kcal of 50% glucose solution = 370 ml.

6. **Action:** The patient's energy needs can be met by feeding 370 ml of a glucose solution and 294 ml of an amino acid solution daily.

   Rationale: This will meet the patient's maintenance and illness requirements.

Patient I.D.

Species and breed

Age   Sex   Weight

Veterinary surgeon

Veterinary nurse

Clinical history

Monitor and record every .... intervals daily

Date and time	T	P	R	MM CRT	Demeanour	Food administration	Type and rate	Food input	Fluid/urine output	Weight	Medication	Comments

Figure 5.8A,B Examples of charts used for monitoring patients undergoing enteral feeding.

Small animal nutrition sheet

Client name   Admission date   Veterinary surgeon

Patient name   Age

Sex   Weight   Veterinary nurse

Condition

emaciated ☐   ....

underweight ☐   ....

correct for breed ☐   Medical/surgical problems

overweight ☐   1.   3.

grossly obese ☐   2.   4.

Resting energy requirement (RER)

RER kcal/day: **Dogs**   >5 kg = 30 × kg + 70
                Cats/dogs   5 kg and under = 60 × kg + 70

Illness energy requirement (IER)

Cage rest/hospitalisation	1.2	× RER	☐	**RER =** kcal/day
Post surgery/trauma	1.3–1.5	× RER	☐	
Sepsis/cancer	1.7	× RER	☐	
Head trauma/major burn	2	× RER	☐	**IER =** kcal/day

IER = RER × ....

Dietary recommendations

Protein ☐   Fat ☐

Fibre ☐   Other ☐

Selected food ....

Calorific density ....

Amount to feed daily = $\dfrac{\text{IER}}{\text{Calorific density}}$ **OR**

Amount =	**ml/day**
Amount =	**g/day**

Food dosage and route

DAY 1

DAY 2

DAY 3

Plan

Continue diet for: 2 weeks   Post surgery
                   2–4 weeks   Trauma
                   4–12 weeks   Head trauma/burns
                   months   Chronic disease/neoplasia

Continue ....diet for .... weeks

Figure 5.8A,B   Examples of charts used for monitoring patients undergoing enteral feeding.

7. **Action:** Electrolyte requirements are supplied by the amino acid solution.

   Rationale: Further electrolyte solutions are unnecessary unless otherwise indicated by plasma electrolyte concentrations.

8. **Action:** Vitamin B complex should be given daily.

   Rationale: To meet maintenance requirements.

9. **Action:** Continuous feeding may be achieved at an approximate rate of 30 ml/h.

   Rationale: To meet total energy requirement over 24 hours.

10. **Action:** The rate should start at 10 ml in the first hour, 20 ml in second hour; 30 ml in third and subsequent hours. At completion of feeding, the rate should decrease in a similar manner.

    Rationale: It is essential to avoid rapid increases or decreases during parenteral feeding as this may cause hyperglycaemia, uraemia and shock.

Procedure: Intravenous access to jugular vein and administration of parenteral feeding

Indications: Where a patient cannot be fed enterally due to gastrointestinal disease, hepatitis, pancreatitis or intestinal obstruction. Such conditions require complete bowel rest.

Food choice: Proprietary solutions containing amino acids, glucose and lipids.

1. **Action:** Select and prepare equipment – intravenous jugular catheter, clippers, surgical skin scrub solution, prewarmed parenteral feeding solution and infusion set, suture equipment, local anaesthetic, bandage; wash hands, wear gloves and apron.

   Rationale: It is essential that equipment is prepared prior to beginning the procedure to ensure efficient administration.

2. **Action:** Ask an assistant to hold the patient in the correct manner, allowing intravenous access to the jugular vein. Two assistants may be required to maintain the patient in the required position.

   Rationale: Prewarm food for parenteral administration to prevent discomfort during administration and a subsequent drop in body temperature. Firm handling will keep the patient at ease and reduce risk of any accident.

3. **Action:** Wearing gloves, clip and prepare site aseptically using surgical scrub and surgical spirit.

   Rationale: This will help to prevent infection.

4. **Action:** The assistant will raise the vein.

   Rationale: To visualise the site.

5. **Action:** With gloved hands insert the catheter tip into the vein. Once blood appears in the catheter, remove the needle and advance the catheter fully.

   Rationale: The needle is removed to prevent accidental puncture of vein further along lumen.

6. **Action:** Ask the assistant to release the pressure on the vein and place a bung or three-way tap to occlude end of catheter.

   Rationale: To avoid excessive blood loss.

7. **Action:** Dry the area and secure the catheter to the skin with the aid of adhesive tapes, or suture in place.

   Rationale: It is important to dry the area to ensure any tape adhesive sticks to the skin and holds the catheter in place. It is essential to avoid accidental movement or displacement of the catheter from the jugular vein, as blood loss could be considerable.

8. **Action:** Flush the catheter with a small amount of heparinised saline.

   Rationale: This is to ensure patency of the catheter and prevent blood clot formation.

9. **Action:** Remove the cap from the parenteral infusion set and attach the infusion line to the intravenous catheter. Secure the infusion tube to the neck region and bandage if necessary.

   Rationale: To ensure parenteral food infusion line remains in place if patient moves, thereby preventing dislodgement and blood loss.

10. **Action:** Provide correct infusion of parenteral fluid in relation to the calculation of fluid and calorie requirements. Check that the fluid is flowing freely.

    Rationale: If the infusion is not flowing freely, look for the reason and deal with it appropriately.

11. **Action:** Adjust the fluid control to the drip rate required for the patient. Syringe drivers and infusion pumps may be used to facilitate the delivery of the calculated flow rate.

    Rationale: It is essential to control the delivery of fluid replacement rate to avoid over- or under-infusion.

12. **Action:** If the administration is not continuous, remove the parenteral infusion line and occlude the jugular catheter with a three-way tap. Flush the catheter with heparinised saline every 4 hours.

    Rationale: It is not always necessary to provide continuous parenteral fluids. Where feeding is intermittent the catheter must be sealed and maintained aseptically.

13. **Action:** Keep catheter site clean and dry at all times.

    Rationale: As parenteral feeding solutions are composed of amino acids and glucose they provide the perfect environment for the growth of microorganisms, so strict aseptic technique is essential.

14. **Action:** Record parenteral fluid administration rate on hospital card. Repeat administration at required intervals.

    Rationale: This is to ensure accurate monitoring and clear communication to all veterinary personnel.

15. **Action:** Prevent self-mutilation by the patient, bandage the area and apply an Elizabethan collar as necessary.

    Rationale: If the patient mutilates the area there is a risk of blood loss, sepsis and thrombosis.

16. **Action:** Dispose of equipment safely and appropriately.

    Rationale: It is essential that all items are disposed of correctly to avoid contamination and accidents.

Procedure: Monitoring techniques for parenteral feeding

1. **Action:** Baseline parameters must be recorded prior to any parenteral feeding.

   Rationale: It is essential to know the results of baseline tests in order to compare and assess the effectiveness of parenteral feeding.

2. **Action:** Monitoring must be performed at regular intervals and recorded on feeding chart.

   Rationale: Regular results will indicate a trend, which is more useful than a one-off measurement. Accuracy and regularity are essential requirements for effective monitoring. Everything must be recorded in writing to avoid error.

3. **Action:** All deviations or abnormalities must be noted immediately.

   Rationale: It is essential that any abnormalities are reported immediately to the veterinary surgeon and acted upon to avoid further deterioration or complications in the patient.

Procedure: Monitoring parenteral feeding – essential parameters

Indications: All patients receiving parenteral nutrition. Administration of amino acids and glucose via the intravenous route requires strict monitoring and aseptic technique due to an increased risk of infection (Fig. 5.8A,B).

1. **Action:** Temperature, pulse and respiration.

   Rationale: To identify infection or inflammation.

2. **Action:** Bodyweight – measured daily.

   Rationale: To identify any large fluctuations that may indicate food and fluid imbalance.

3. **Action:** White blood cell count (twice weekly).

   Rationale: To identify infection or inflammation.

4. **Action:** Plasma glucose concentration – taken daily until stable.

   Rationale: To control blood glucose levels and feeding regimes.

5. **Action:** Plasma electrolytes.

Rationale: To identify any deviations.

6. **Action:** Urine output.

   Rationale: Less than 1 ml/kg/hour would indicate inadequate renal perfusion due to insufficient circulatory volume.

7. **Action:** Urine glucose – every 6 hours until stable.

   Rationale: To identify hyperglycaemia.

8. **Action:** Blood urea – as needed, particularly if it becomes elevated.

   Rationale: Large increases suggest too rapid administration of amino acids.

9. **Action:** General demeanour/clinical observation.

   Rationale: Any sign of distress or discomfort could indicate a problem.

REFERENCES AND FURTHER READING

Agar S 2001 Small Animal Nutrition. Butterworth-Heinemann, Oxford

Aspinall V 2006 The Complete Textbook of Veterinary Nursing. Elsevier, Oxford

Houlton J E F, Taylor P M 1987 Trauma Management in the Dog and Cat. Wright, Bristol

Lane D R, Cooper B (eds) 1994 Veterinary Nursing. Butterworth-Heinemann, Oxford

Lane D R, Cooper B (eds) 2003 Veterinary Nursing, 3rd edn. Butterworth-Heinemann, Oxford

Lewis L D, Morris M, Hand M S 2000 Small Animal Clinical Nutrition, 4th edn. Morris Marks Associates, Topeka, Kansas

Masters J, Bowden C 2003 Quick Reference Guide to Veterinary Medical Kits. Butterworth-Heinemann, Oxford

Taylor R A, McGehee R 1995 Manual of Small Animal Postoperative Care. Williams and Wilkins, Baltimore

Chapter 6

Anaesthetic procedures

Pip Millard

CHAPTER CONTENTS

Introduction   105

The anaesthetic machine   106
Checking the anaesthetic machine before
   use   106
Shutting down the anaesthetic machine   106

Patient preparation   107
Pre-anaesthetic instructions   107
Admitting the patient   109
Pre-anaesthetic check – carried out by the
   veterinary surgeon   110

Stages of anaesthesia   112
To intubate a patient   112
To remove the endotracheal tube –
   extubation   119
Care of endotracheal tubes   119

Anaesthetic masks   119

Anaesthetic circuits   120
Jackson Rees modified T-piece
   (non-rebreathing)   120
Magill (non-rebreathing)   120
Lack and parallel Lack (non-rebreathing)   120
Modified Bain (non-rebreathing)   121
To and fro (rebreathing)   121
Circle system (rebreathing)   122
Humphrey ADE system (rebreathing
   and non-rebreathing)   122

Replacing soda lime   123

Calculating anaesthetic gas flow rates   123

Patient recovery   127
Care of the patient during recovery   128
Discharging a patient   128

Anaesthetic emergencies   128
Intermittent positive pressure
   ventilation (IPPV)   129

Specialised techniques   130
Local anaesthesia   130
Muscle relaxation   131

Control of pollution – scavenging   132

INTRODUCTION

Anaesthesia may be defined as the production of a reversible state of insensitivity. By using certain drugs designed to have an effect on the nervous system, anaesthesia may be general, i.e. the animal is unconscious and the entire nervous system is rendered insensitive to stimuli, or local, i.e. a small area is rendered insensitive to stimuli. Anaesthesia is used for the welfare of the animal, as it is obviously unpleasant for painful procedures to be performed on a fully sentient animal. It may also be used as a means of restraint, e.g. when using X-rays or if examining an aggressive animal, and when properly managed anaesthesia may significantly increase the chances of an animal's survival of an operation.

Local anaesthesia is most commonly used in large animal practice. However, it may be used in small animal practice for superficial surgery such as stitching a small skin wound, to aid diagnosis and in some cases to reduce the depth of general anaesthesia by desensitising a particular small area under treatment.

General anaesthesia is now a routine procedure in small animal practice and its use is becoming more common in exotic species (see Chapter 12). It can be achieved by the use of injectable agents for which very little specific equipment is needed or by the use of inhalational agents, i.e. gases or volatile liquids. The administration of inhalational agents requires the use of some expensive and complicated equipment and it is usually the job of the veterinary nurse to set up and maintain this equipment and to monitor the level of anaesthesia in the patient. It is vital that the veterinary nurse has a thorough understanding of the anaesthetic process if the patient is to survive the procedure and make a complete recovery.

This chapter describes all the procedures involved in preparing the anaesthetic equipment, and in caring for the patient preoperatively, during the operation and postoperatively. It also describes the different types of circuits in common veterinary usage.

THE ANAESTHETIC MACHINE

Anaesthetic machines are designed to deliver accurate amounts of carrier gases and volatile liquids in a vapour form to the patient to produce anaesthesia (Fig. 6.1). Table 6.1 describes the parts of the anaesthetic machine.

Procedure: Checking the anaesthetic machine before use

1. **Action:** Turn on the **spare** oxygen cylinder and check that it is full. It should read 137 bar.

   Rationale: The contents of the spare cylinder must be noted to ensure a constant supply of oxygen throughout the anaesthetic.

2. **Action:** Turn the cylinder off and label it as full.

   Rationale: If the current cylinder and the spare cylinder are both on, they will empty at the same time.

3. **Action:** Turn on the **in-use** cylinder, check the contents and replace if necessary. Label it as in-use.

   Rationale: If the pressure reading is in the red area of the scale, the cylinder should be changed.

4. **Action:** Repeat the process for the nitrous oxide cylinders. The spare, full cylinder should read 44 bar.

5. **Action:** Check for leaking gas while turning on cylinders.

   Rationale: A faulty Bodock seal can lead to gas leaks.

6. **Action:** Open and close the flowmeter valves.

   Rationale: Ensure that the ball or bobbin can move and rotate freely in its cylinder.

7. **Action:** Check the low oxygen alarm by turning the oxygen cylinder off and pressing the oxygen flush valve. Turn the oxygen back on.

   Rationale: The alarm should sound as the oxygen pressure falls to a dangerously low level. The flow of fresh gas through the oxygen flush valve is also confirmed.

8. **Action:** Check that the correct vaporiser is fitted and that it is full.

   Rationale: The control valve should move freely. If more than one vaporiser is fitted, check each one, then ensure that only one of them is left on.

9. **Action:** Connect the correct circuit, having checked it carefully for faults.

   Rationale: Leaks may result from disconnected inner tubes in coaxial circuits or from leaking reservoir bags.

10. **Action:** Connect scavenging. Switch active systems on.

    Rationale: Anaesthetic machines must not be used without some form of scavenging system.

Procedure: Shutting down the anaesthetic machine

1. **Action:** Check contents of gas cylinders and remove any empty ones. Replace them with full cylinders.

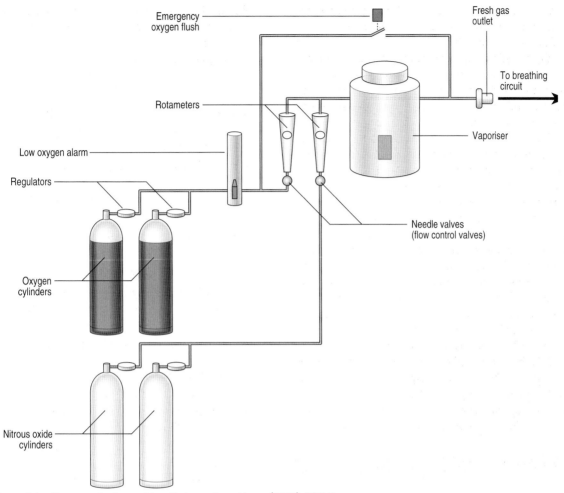

Figure 6.1 The anaesthetic machine. Redrawn from Moore (1999), BSAVA.

Rationale: To ensure that the machine is ready for the next use.

2. **Action:** Open the oxygen flowmeter and allow to flow at 2 litres/min. Close the nitrous oxide cylinder and turn on the nitrous oxide flowmeter until the flow indicator has fallen to 0. Close the flowmeter control.

    Rationale: This will flush all nitrous oxide from the pipes. Any gas in the pipes could register when the flowmeter is switched on, implying that the cylinder is open.

3. **Action:** Turn the oxygen cylinder off and press the oxygen flush valve until no pressure reads on the pressure gauge.

    Rationale: All oxygen must be flushed from the pipes for the same reason as in step 2.

4. **Action:** Wipe the anaesthetic machine with disinfectant.

    Rationale: This minimises the risk of contamination.

PATIENT PREPARATION

Procedure: Pre-anaesthetic instructions

1. **Action:** No food to be given for 12 hours prior to surgery.

    Rationale: Animals that are not fasted may vomit as a result of the anaesthetic drugs. This may lead to fatal aspiration, as the swallowing reflex is reduced or lost during anaesthesia.

Table 6.1   Parts of the anaesthetic machine

Component	Description	Function
Gas supply	Oxygen cylinders are black with a white collar. Nitrous oxide cylinders are blue. Smaller cylinders, such as E and F, can be incorporated into the anaesthetic machine. Larger cylinders, J and G, may be kept separate and gas supplied to the anaesthetic machine through pipes in the wall	Supplies fresh oxygen and nitrous oxide to the patient
Pressure-reducing valve or regulator	Usually incorporated into the yolk and is therefore impossible to identify	Reduces the pressure of the gas leaving the cylinder to ensure a constant flow to the anaesthetic machine regardless of the pressure changes within the cylinder. It provides a safe operating pressure for the machine
Pressure gauge	Usually attached to the anaesthetic machine. As the pressure in the cylinder falls so does the pressure reading, indicating the amount of gas remaining in the tank. When using nitrous oxide, no pressure change will be seen until the cylinder is almost empty because the pressure does not fall until all the liquid has evaporated. This is not a reliable method for measuring the cylinder content of nitrous oxide – the cylinder should be weighed instead	Indicates the pressure of gas being delivered. It will read zero when the tank is empty or when the tank is switched off and the gas in the pipe evacuated
Flowmeters or rotameters	Consist of a tapered glass tube with the flow rate written on it and either a glass ball or bobbin in the tube. Provided that the ball or bobbin can rotate freely within the tube, it will give an accurate reading of the gas flow rate. A bobbin must be read from the top, a ball from the middle. Flowmeters are gas specific and control knobs are usually colour coded: they should never be over-tightened as the valve seat is easily damaged	Control and measure the flow of gas in litres per minute
Vaporisers: uncalibrated	The Boyle's bottle (Fig. 6.2) is an example of an uncalibrated vaporiser: whilst output can be varied, it fluctuates with temperature and gas flow changes	Deliver concentrations of volatile anaesthetic, in a vapour form, to the patient
Vaporisers: calibrated	The Tec and Penlon vaporisers (Fig. 6.3) are calibrated. They remain accurate despite temperature and gas flow changes. They are agent specific	Deliver a known concentration of anaesthetic vapour to the patient
Back bar	Flowmeters and vaporisers can be attached to the backbar in series. This allows more than one volatile agent to be available. The 'Selectatec' manifold allows swift attachment or removal of Tec 3 and 4 vaporisers	Supports the flowmeters and vaporisers
Common gas outlet	Location varies between anaesthetic machines	Connects anaesthetic circuits, ventilators or oxygen supply devices to the machine
Oxygen flush valve	Oxygen reaches this valve swiftly, bypassing the vaporiser. High flow rates are produced. The valve may be locked open in some cases, by rotating it 90°	Provides oxygen in emergency situations and purges anaesthetic from the circuit before disconnection to minimise pollution
Low oxygen alarm	An alarm sounds or, in some cases, a light flashes when oxygen levels become dangerously low	Warns the anaesthetist of low oxygen levels

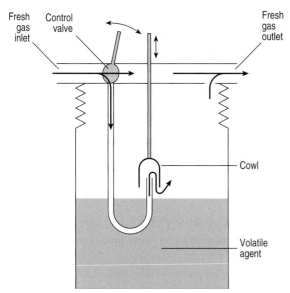

Figure 6.2   Boyle's bottle vaporiser. Redrawn from Moore (1999), BSAVA.

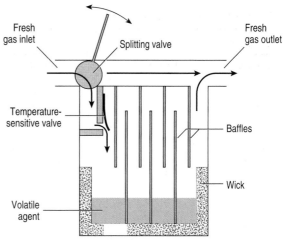

Figure 6.3   Tec and Penlon type vaporisers. Redrawn from Moore (1999), BSAVA.

2. **Action:** Cats should be kept inside overnight with a litter tray until ready to go to the practice the next morning.

   Rationale: This prevents the cat from disappearing before being taken to the practice.

3. **Action:** Dogs should be walked prior to admittance.

   Rationale: This allows the pet to urinate and defecate before going into a kennel.

4. **Action:** Cats must be brought to the surgery in a secure cage or basket. Dogs must wear a secure collar and a lead.

   Rationale: To minimise the risk of escape.

5. **Action:** The client is given a time to arrive at the surgery.

   Rationale: This enables the nursing team to plan the surgery list and allow time for each patient to be admitted.

Procedure: Admitting the patient

1. **Action:** Check that the patient is included on the operating list and confirm the procedure.

   Rationale: A consent form should have been prepared if the patient is booked in for surgery.

2. **Action:** Take the client and pet into a consulting room.

   Rationale: This is more professional than dealing with the client in a busy waiting room.

3. **Action:** Weigh the patient.

   Rationale: The weight is essential for accurate administration of premedicant and induction drugs.

4. **Action:** Obtain a complete history (Table 6.2).

   Rationale: An accurate history is vital in order to evaluate the patient's anaesthetic risk.

5. **Action:** Obtain a signature on the consent form (Fig. 6.4).

   Rationale: The owner or agent of the patient must read, understand and sign the consent form. They must be over the age of 18 years.

6. **Action:** Obtain a contact phone number for the duration of the patient's stay.

   Rationale: It is vital to be able to contact the owner or an agent of the owner in the event of an emergency.

7. **Action:** Identify any lumps to be removed (if relevant).

   Rationale: This will save time searching the patient for them later.

8. **Action:** Transfer the patient to a kennel, making sure the animal cannot escape on the way.

Table 6.2 Questions to ask when obtaining a history

Question	Significance
1. How old is the pet?	This should be on the client records but should be checked: an older pet is a greater anaesthetic risk
2. When did the animal last eat?	If food has been consumed within 12 hours of surgery, there is an increased risk of vomiting during the anaesthetic
3. Has the animal had any previous illnesses and, if so, what treatment was given?	Client records should supplement this information; any condition involving the major body systems may increase the anaesthetic risk
4. Has the animal shown signs of any of the following in the past 24 hours: coughing, sneezing, vomiting, diarrhoea, anorexia; if so, how frequently and has the animal recovered?	The patient may be an increased anaesthetic risk due to dehydration, fever or electrolyte imbalance. They may also introduce pathogens to the environment
5. How well does the patient tolerate exercise?	Poor exercise tolerance may indicate cardiovascular or respiratory problems
6. Is the animal on any medication: if so, has it had any today?	Some drugs may alter the affects of the anaesthetic
7. Is there any history of allergies or drug reactions?	Prolonged recovery from a previous anaesthetic or anaphylactic reactions to any medication should be noted
8. When was the patient last vaccinated?	Up-to-date vaccinations should prevent the spread of contagious diseases
9. Is the patient entire or has it been spayed/castrated; if an entire female, is the animal in season or pregnant?	Particularly significant if the patient is in for ovariohysterectomy as surgery time may be prolonged and there may be an increased risk of haemorrhage
10. Has the owner noticed any of the following: abnormal bleeding, bruising, fainting, seizures, dysuria, tenesmus?	The presence of any of these may indicate a serious illness

Rationale: It is best to ask the owner to leave before their dog is taken through so that the dog accompanies you more willingly.

Procedure: Pre-anaesthetic check – carried out by the veterinary surgeon

1. **Action:** Assess the function of the cardiovascular system using auscultation of the heart and palpation of the pulse. (For normal values see Table 2.1.)

   Rationale: The cardiovascular system is affected by anaesthesia. Note the heart rate and rhythm, abnormal heart or lung sounds, pulse rate and presence of a pulse deficit.

2. **Action:** Assess the function of the respiratory system.

   Rationale: This is also affected by anaesthesia. Note the rate and any signs of dyspnoea.

3. **Action:** Palpate the abdomen.

   Rationale: This may detect the presence of an enlarged liver or abnormally small kidneys, either of which may lead to inefficient excretion of anaesthetic agents.

4. **Action:** Palpate superficial lymph nodes.

   Rationale: Enlarged lymph nodes may indicate the presence of infection, allergy or neoplasia.

5. **Action:** Take the body temperature (see Table 2.1).

   Rationale: Note any temperature outside the normal range.

6. **Action:** Check teeth, claws, ears, skin, coat, anal glands.

Name:

Address:

Contact telephone number today:

Species: Dog/Cat/Rabbit/Rodent/Bird/Reptile/Other

Pet's Name: Breed: Age:

Sex: MALE/FEMALE   Neutered: YES/NO   Weight:

Insured: YES/NO   Company: Microchipped: YES/NO

Vaccinated: YES/NO   Wormed: YES/NO   Treated for fleas: YES/NO

Procedure:

Pre-anaesthetic blood screen: YES/NO

Check teeth: YES/NO

Check claws: YES/NO

Any other comments:

Estimate:

I understand that payment is due at the time the animal is discharged:

Method of payment: Cash/Cheque/Credit/Debit card

I hereby give permission for the administration of an anaesthetic to the above animal and to the surgical procedure on this form, together with any other procedure that might prove necessary.

I understand that anaesthetic techniques and surgical procedures involve some risk to the animal.

I have read and understood the above statement: YES/NO

Signature of owner or authorised agent: Date:

Figure 6.4   An example of a consent form.

Rationale: The owner may wish to have any disorders corrected whilst the patient is anaesthetised.

7. **Action:** Check the sex of patients in for neutering.

   Rationale: It is far better to discover a mistake prior to surgery.

8. **Action:** Identify a cryptorchid patient prior to castration.

   Rationale: The owner can be informed of an increased fee in advance.

9. **Action:** Assess pain, if relevant, prior to the administration of a premedicant.

   Rationale: Most premedicants contain an analgesic, which may mask signs of pain in conditions such as lameness, rendering further physical examination useless.

10. **Action:** Take a blood sample to run a pre-anaesthetic blood screen, if required

    Rationale: Biochemistry blood tests can give a good indication of the function of the patient's liver and kidneys. A packed cell volume (PCV) is also useful.

11. **Action:** Administer a premedicant.

    Rationale: The premedicant may be administered by subcutaneous, intramuscular or intravenous injection, depending on the type of drug, speed of onset required and status of the patient (Table 6.3).

STAGES OF ANAESTHESIA

Anaesthesia – defined as a reversible state of unconsciousness – may be considered to occur in two stages:

1. induction
2. maintenance.

Induction

During the induction period, the patient passes from consciousness into unconsciousness. During this time the risk of cardiac arrest is increased and the whole process may be unpleasant for the patient. The signs displayed during induction or stage I of anaesthesia are described in Table 6.4.

A smooth induction passes swiftly through stages I and II and the signs may be missed. However, when induction is done by a mask or where a premedicant has not been administered, the signs are more obvious.

Induction may be carried out by intravenous or intramuscular injection, using one of the induction agents described in Table 6.5 or by using a mask and inhalation anaesthetic agent. The advantages and disadvantages of each method are discussed in Table 6.6.

Maintenance

During this period, the state of unconsciousness is maintained by the use of drugs, which may be given intravenously, intramuscularly or by the inhalational route. Inhalational agents are delivered to the patient by means of, ideally, an endotracheal tube connected to an anaesthetic circuit and machine. In some cases an anaesthetic mask may be useful. The common inhalation agents are described in Table 6.7.

Procedure: To intubate a patient

After induction, an endotracheal tube (a breathing tube) may be placed in the patient's airway (intubation). This tube conducts anaesthetic gases and oxygen from the anaesthetic machine to the trachea and lungs, bypassing the nasal passages and pharynx. The patient must be sufficiently anaesthetised in order to carry out intubation. This is indicated by the following signs.

- The jaw is relaxed.
- The tongue can be held with no resistance.
- There is no gagging or swallowing reflex on introduction of the tube.

Equipment Required: Selection of suitably sized cuffed tubes, lubricant to facilitate intubation, laryngoscope, local anaesthetic spray to prevent laryngeal spasm in cats, syringe or cuff inflator, stylet to aid difficult intubations, gauze bandage to tie tube in place.

1. **Action:** Select several endotracheal tubes of varying sizes and measure the required length against the patient's head and neck.

Table 6.3   Common premedicant drugs

Premedicant	Family	Use	Warnings
Atropine	Anticholinergic	Traditionally used to counteract the hypersalivation caused when using ether. Used during dentistry to reduce salivation. Used to treat bradycardia during anaesthetic emergencies	
Acepromazine	Sedative/ataractic: phenothiazine	Calms the patient prior to induction Used with opiate analgesics to produce neuroleptanalgesia	May cause seizures: avoid using in patients suffering from epilepsy or undergoing myelography Boxers are very sensitive to the effects of acepromazine – use with caution at very low dose rates
Diazepam	Sedative/ataractic: benzodiazepine	Calms the patient prior to induction Used as a premedicant for sick patients and to treat seizures Can be combined with pethidine or morphine for optimum results	May not always cause sedation in animals: may cause excitement in fit, healthy dogs
Xylazine	Sedative: alpha-2-agonist	May be used on its own as a sedative for minor procedures Can be used as a premedicant Reduces the required dose of intravenous induction agent by 80%	Alpha-2-agonists have a profound effect on the cardiovascular system of dogs and cats They cause extreme bradycardia Use caution when using prior to intravenous induction agents: they increase the delay between injection of an intravenous agent and its effects being seen
Medetomidine	Sedative: alpha-2-agonist	As for xylazine Atipamezole is the licensed reversal agent	As above
Pethidine Morphine Buprenorphine	Analgesic: opioid	Produce pain relief If given prior to surgery, it is more effective and leads to increased post-surgical analgesia	
Butorphanol	Analgesic	As above	
Carprofen	Analgesic	As above	
Ketoprofen	NSAID	As above	Renal and gastric toxicity
Meloxicam	NSAID	As above	Less likely to cause renal and gastric problems
Flunixin	NSAID	As above	Renal and gastric toxicity although an excellent analgesic with anti-endotoxin effect
Phenylbutazone	NSAID	As above	Gastric irritation

NSAID: non-steroidal anti-inflammatory drug.

Table 6.4 Stages of anaesthesia

Stage	Signs	Suitable for
Stage I: Voluntary excitement	Fear, apprehension, resists induction Becomes disorientated Increased pulse rate Increased respiratory rate Breath holding may occur Dilated pupil Possible salivation, vocalisation, defecation, urination All reflexes present, possibly exaggerated	Lasts from induction until the patient is unconscious
Stage II: Involuntary excitement	Hyperactive cranial nerve activity Dilated pupil with eye central, then rotating ventromedially Swift pedal reflex Respiration irregular and gasping, then becoming regular	Begins with unconsciousness and lasts until breathing becomes rhythmic
Stage III: Surgical anaesthesia	*Plane I:* Deep, regular respiration Slight cardiovascular depression Swift pedal reflex Palpebral reflex slows Corneal reflex swift Eye rotated ventromedially Third eyelid moves across the corneal surface	Superficial skin surgery: wound suture, minor lumpectomy
	Plane II: Heart rate and blood pressure slightly reduced Respiratory rate may be increased or decreased Pedal reflex slows then becomes absent Palpebral reflex slows then may become absent Corneal reflex continues Eye remains rotated ventromedially Marked muscle relaxation	Most surgery except laparotomy and thoracotomy
	Plane III: Heart rate and blood pressure reduces Respiratory rate increases, tidal volume decreases Intercostal lag Corneal reflex present Eyeball becomes central, eyelids begin to open Abdominal muscles are relaxed	All procedures
Stage IV: Overdosage	Progressive respiratory failure Weak, thready pulse Eyeball central with dry corneal surface Pupils dilated Cyanosis Prolonged capillary refill time Accessory respiratory muscle activity leads to agonal gasping	To be avoided: may lead to prolonged recovery time Can also cause cardiopulmonary depression which in turn leads to poor organ perfusion. This can cause postoperative organ failure and ultimately result in cardiac arrest

Table 6.5   Common induction agents

Induction agent	Effects and use	Warnings
Pentobarbital (pentobarbitone)	A medium-acting barbiturate Slow onset of action Longer duration of anaesthesia Used to control status epilepticus At higher doses, used for humane euthanasia Produces approximately 30 minutes of anaesthesia	Perivascular injection can cause severe skin reaction Recovery can take up to 18 hours in dogs, 72 hours in cats Excitement is sometimes seen on induction because the drug is slow to cross the blood–brain barrier It should be used with caution in weak or toxaemic patients
Thiopental (thiopentone)	A short-acting barbiturate 2.5% concentration available for small animals in a crystalline form made up with sterile water Recovery is mostly through redistribution of the drug into the patient's fat and not through metabolism Produces approximately 20 minutes of anaesthesia	Perivascular injection can result in severe skin slough Reconstituted solution should be discarded after 24 hours Prolonged recovery in sight-hounds due to their limited fat stores It is cumulative and therefore cannot be used as a maintenance agent It should not be used in animals under 3 months of age
Methohexital (methohexitone)	A short-acting barbiturate Rapidly metabolised, therefore not so cumulative as thiopental: small boluses may be administered as required to maintain anaesthesia Twice as potent as thiopental Produces approximately 10 minutes' anaesthesia	Perivascular injection can cause irritation A brief period of apnoea follows induction Reconstituted solution must be discarded after 24 hours Excitement is seen on recovery in patients that have not been premedicated
Alfaxalone and Alfadolone	These two steroids are combined to form Saffan Can be given by intramuscular injection Licensed for cats, goats and ferrets Suitable for use in many exotic species Produces approximately 10 minutes of anaesthesia	The steroids are contained in the solvent Cremophor EL which causes severe anaphylaxis in dogs Causes histamine release in cats which can lead to swelling of paws and ears Laryngeal oedema may occur in some cats
Ketamine	A dissociative agent Produces mild anaesthesia with profound analgesia Combined with alpha-2-agonists, opioid analgesics and benzodiazepines to produce anaesthesia in cats, dogs, rabbits and small rodents Combined with alpha-2-agonists to induce horses	Unsuitable for patients suffering from renal or hepatic abnormalities
Propofol	A substituted phenol Produces rapid induction when injected intravenously Rapidly metabolised in the liver and therefore not so cumulative as thiopental: further increments may be administered as required to maintain anaesthesia Sight-hounds recover more quickly than when given thiopental Produces approximately 15–20 minutes of anaesthesia	Severe muscle twitches are sometimes seen after prolonged use A brief period of apnoea and a fall in blood pressure may be seen on induction Vials should be discarded once opened

Table 6.6   Methods of induction

Method	Advantages	Disadvantages
Mask induction A tightly fitted black rubber/clear plastic mask is fitted on the animal's face. 100% oxygen is administered for 2–3 minutes to allow the patient to adjust to the mask The anaesthetic concentration is then gradually introduced until it is 3–4%	The patient's airway is not damaged Induction is smooth when patients are depressed or heavily sedated Used for administering oxygen and inhalation agents when endotracheal intubation is not possible Useful for birds and small mammals	May be very distressing for the patient Masks increase the mechanical deadspace Atmospheric pollution is a significant hazard Airway obstruction can occur
Chamber induction The conscious patient is placed inside the chamber, which should be large enough for the animal to lie with its neck extended. Oxygen and the anaesthetic agent at a concentration of 4–5% is then delivered via an air inlet. The patient is removed when it loses its ability to stand	Induction chambers are useful for small mammals Ideal for uncooperative patients	Only suitable for small patients Risk of vomiting Cardiopulmonary function cannot be monitored Risk of atmospheric pollution
Intravenous The induction agent is injected into the cephalic vein over a 10–15 second period, as a 'bolus': half the calculated dose is administered. If the patient is not sufficiently anaesthetised to allow intubation after 15–30 seconds, a second dose is administered (one-fourth of the calculated dose). This is repeated until the required depth is reached	Smooth, rapid induction The induction agent can be given to effect so minimal quantities are used Most induction drugs can only be given intravenously	Patients must be restrained well Risk of perivascular injection, particularly with thiopental sodium
Intramuscular This method can only be used in certain drugs such as ketamine/xylazine mixtures, neuroleptanalgesics and opiates. Recovery is usually prolonged	Technically easier than intravenous injection Useful in fractious patients when intravenous access is not possible	The patient is given the induction agent according to weight Cannot dose to effect so easily Slower onset

Rationale: This will enable the veterinary surgeon to select the one best suited for the patient and avoid excessive mechanical deadspace.

2. **Action:** Inflate the cuff and check for excessive wear and the patency of the tube.

   Rationale: Rubber tubing can perish over time, causing malfunction of the cuff. If the cuff does not inflate, the anaesthetic gases may leak around it during anaesthesia and fluid and debris may be inhaled. Patency is essential for the delivery of oxygen and anaesthetic gases.

3. **Action:** Lubricate the tube with sterile lubricant.

   Rationale: This allows smooth, atraumatic introduction of the tube.

4. **Action:** Restrain the patient in lateral or ventral recumbency.

5. **Action:** Ask an assistant to extend the neck and hold the patient's head so that the nose is pointing upwards (Fig. 6.5).

6. **Action:** Hold the upper jaw stationary whilst the tongue is pulled out and down so that it lies between the lower canines. Pull the lower jaw downwards by pulling the tongue down until the epiglottis can be clearly seen.

Table 6.7   Common inhalation agents

Inhalation agent	Properties	Effects and use	Warnings
Halothane	Relatively low solubility Colourless, volatile liquid Decomposed by light Contains the preservative thymol	Fairly rapid induction and recovery Modest muscle relaxation Poor analgesic	Sensitises the heart to adrenaline and therefore may cause arrhythmias Fall in cardiac output and subsequent hypotension Respiratory depression Lowered body temperature Up to 20% may be metabolised by the liver following retention in fat stores Thymol may cause the vaporiser settings to stick
Isoflurane	Very low solubility Colourless, volatile liquid No preservatives are required	Even more rapid induction and recovery Good muscle relaxation Poor analgesia Inhalation agent of choice for patients with cardiac, liver or kidney disease plus neonatal and geriatric patients	Little effect on cardiac output Respiratory depression Less than 0.2% may be metabolised by the liver due to the low fat solubility of isoflurane
Enflurane	Very similar to isoflurane	Very similar to isoflurane	Marked respiratory depression Induces seizure-like muscle spasms and should be avoided in epileptic patients
Methoxyflurane	High solubility Preservatives required	Slow induction and recovery Good muscle relaxation Considerable analgesia	Decreases cardiac output Marked respiratory depression Over 50% is metabolised by the liver and excreted through the kidneys Must not be used in patients given flunixin – it will lead to severe renal damage

Rationale: In this position the visibility of the anatomy of the pharynx is maximised (Fig. 6.6).

7. **Action:** Using the selected tube, push the soft palate away dorsally if necessary. Push the epiglottis down with the tip of the tube and then insert it between the vocal folds into the trachea (Fig. 6.7).

   Rationale: The soft palate sometimes obscures the view of the epiglottis, which in turn covers the opening into the trachea.

8. **Action:** If intubating a cat, spray a topical local anaesthetic onto the larynx and introduce the tube during inhalation, at which point the vocal folds are open.

Rationale: The larynx of a cat is very sensitive so local anaesthetic is used to desensitise it, preventing laryngospasm.

9. **Action:** In cats and brachycephalic breeds of dog, a laryngoscope is sometimes used to assist intubation.

   Rationale: The smooth blade of the handle enables the operator to move the epiglottis aside and the light source illuminates the pharyngeal area.

10. **Action:** The tube must not be introduced too far or endobronchial intubation may occur (Fig. 6.8).

    Rationale: This results in the ventilation of only one lung.

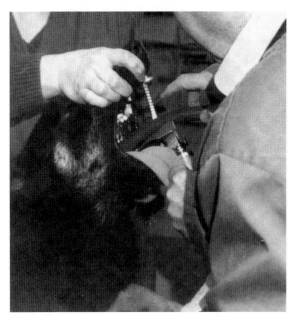

Figure 6.5 Position of an animal for intubation. Reproduced, with permission, from McKelvey and Hollingshead (2000), Mosby.

11. **Action:** Once the tube is inserted, confirm correct placement in the trachea (rather than the oesophagus) by ventilating the patient with 100% oxygen and applying pressure to the reservoir bag. Observe the movements of the chest wall.

    Rationale: Oesophageal intubation results in oxygen and anaesthetic gas being delivered to the stomach rather than the lungs. The stomach will inflate and the patient is unlikely to remain anaesthetised.

12. **Action:** Inflate the cuff of the tube just enough to prevent oxygen escaping around the cuff.

    Rationale: Over-inflation can damage the tracheal mucosa or cause occlusion of the tube. Under-inflation may enable the patient to breathe around the tube and foreign material may pass into the trachea.

13. **Action:** To avoid accidental extubation, secure the tube in place using a piece of gauze bandage. This is tied around the end of the tube over the plastic connector then secured over the mandible or the top of the patient's head with a quick-release bow.

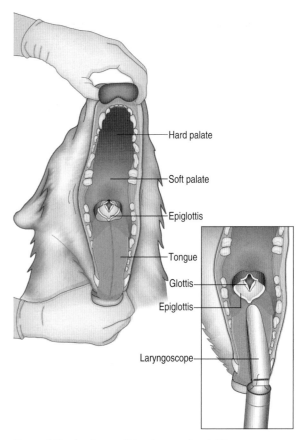

Figure 6.6 Anatomy of the pharynx. Inset: When the epiglottis is depressed, the glottis is exposed. The endotracheal tube is advanced through the glottis. Redrawn from McKelvey and Hollingshead (2000), Mosby.

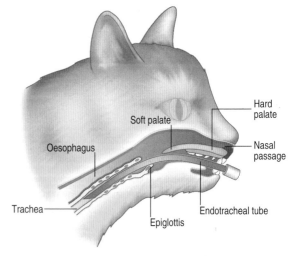

Figure 6.7 Intubation of a cat. The anatomy is illustrated. Redrawn from McKelvey and Hollingshead (2000), Mosby.

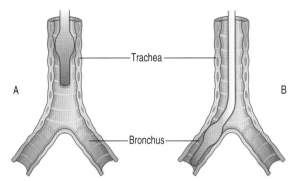

Figure 6.8   Placement of endotracheal tube in the trachea: A, correct placement; B, endobronchial intubation (incorrect). Redrawn from McKelvey and Hollingshead (2000), Mosby.

Rationale: The plastic connector will support the tube, preventing it from collapse when the tie is pulled tight. A quick-release fastening such as a bow is used for easy removal in an emergency.

Procedure: To remove the endotracheal tube – extubation

1. **Action:** Untie the piece of gauze bandage holding the endotracheal tube in place.

   Rationale: This is usually untied before signs of arousal are seen so the tube can be removed quickly when swallowing occurs.

2. **Action:** Deflate the cuff.

   Rationale: Deflation of the cuff is essential as an inflated cuff can easily damage the tracheal mucosa. After oral surgery, the cuff may be left partially inflated to dislodge debris and blood in the proximal trachea as the tube is withdrawn.

3. **Action:** In dogs, the tube is left in place until the swallowing or gag reflex returns.

   Rationale: The swallowing reflex helps protect the animal from aspiration in the event of vomiting.

4. **Action:** Cats should be extubated before the swallowing reflex returns. Signs of impending arousal include tail, limb or head movements or an active palpebral reflex.

   Rationale: Delayed extubation may lead to laryngospasm.

Procedure: Care of endotracheal tubes

Care and maintenance of endotracheal tubes is dependent on the type of material.

1. **Action:** Rinse the tubes in running water.

   Rationale: Any debris and fluid that would otherwise deactivate a detergent will be removed.

2. **Action:** Soak in a detergent solution.

   Rationale: This will soften any residual debris.

3. **Action:** Scrub the tubes inside and out using specialist brushes.

   Rationale: All debris and mucus will be removed.

4. **Action:** Thorough rinsing is essential.

   Rationale: All traces of detergent must be removed to prevent chemical or ischaemic tracheitis.

5. **Action:** Dry thoroughly and check for patency, cuff inflation and general wear. Discard any faulty tubes.

   Rationale: This ensures that no animal is intubated with a faulty tube, which could compromise the anaesthetic or threaten the patient's life.

6. **Action:** The method of sterilisation will depend on the type of material: red tubes should be sterilised using ethylene oxide but must be aired for at least 48 hours before use; polysiloxane tubes can be autoclaved.

   Rationale: Heat will damage red tubes so they should not be autoclaved. Airing after sterilisation with ethylene oxide is essential to avoid chemical tracheitis.

7. **Action:** Store the tubes in a dry, cool environment away from direct sunlight.

   Rationale: Correct care and storage of the endotracheal tubes will prolong their life.

ANAESTHETIC MASKS

There may be some instances where an anaesthetic mask can be used. Masks come in a range of sizes and are made either of clear plastic or malleable black rubber.

They can be used to:

- supply oxygen quickly, in a first aid situation
- provide gases for maintenance in short procedures
- supply gases to induce neonates
- provide oxygen throughout surgery when intravenous drugs have been used for maintaining anaesthesia.

Unfortunately IPPV cannot be carried out using a mask. Gas flow rates also need to be quite high, therefore increasing the risk of atmospheric pollution.

ANAESTHETIC CIRCUITS

The anaesthetic circuit connects the patient to the anaesthetic machine. The most common circuits used today fall into two categories: rebreathing and non-rebreathing. All circuits have advantages and disadvantages depending on the clinical situation so it is recommended that a practice should have a range of circuits available for use.

Anaesthetic circuits have three functions:

- delivering oxygen and anaesthetic gases to the patient
- carrying carbon dioxide away from the patient
- removing potentially harmful gases from the operating theatre via a scavenging system.

Circuit: Jackson Rees modified T-piece (non-rebreathing) (Fig. 6.9)

Equipment: 0.5 litre reservoir bag (open ended if no pop-off valve), expiratory limb (corrugated tubing), fresh gas (narrow gauge plain tubing), pop-off valve (used with a closed bag).

Advantages
- Intermittent positive pressure ventilation (IPPV) can be carried out.
- Bag movement acts as a respiratory monitor.
- Minimal apparatus deadspace and resistance.

Disadvantages
- High gas flow rates required.
- The incorporation of a pop-off valve increases resistance.
- Scavenging is difficult when an open bag is used.

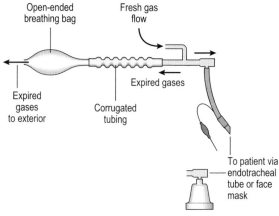

No valves therefore little resistance to breathing. A flow rate of 2.5–3 times the minute volume is required

Open-ended breathing bag — Fresh gas flow — Expired gases — Expired gases to exterior — Corrugated tubing — To patient via endotracheal tube or face mask

Figure 6.9 Jackson Rees modified T-piece anaesthetic breathing system.

Suitable for: Small dogs (under 8 kg), cats, neonates and birds.

Flow rates: 2.5–3 × minute volume.

Circuit: Magill (non-rebreathing) (Fig. 6.10)

Equipment: 2 litre reservoir bag, corrugated tubing, expiratory (Heidbrink) valve, 2 × 'T' connectors.

Advantages
- Efficient, general-purpose circuit.
- Readily maintained and sterilised.

Disadvantages
- The location of the Heidbrink valve is inconvenient for scavenging and surgery around the head area.
- Cannot be used for prolonged IPPV because rebreathing will occur, causing hypercapnia.
- Offers considerable resistance and increased mechanical deadspace.

Suitable for: Patients over 8 kg.

Flow rates: 1–1.5 × minute volume.

Circuit: Lack and parallel Lack (non-rebreathing) (Fig. 6.11)

Equipment: 2 litre reservoir bag, coaxial tubing (outer inspiratory limb) or parallel corrugated tubing, expiratory valve.

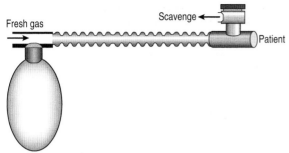

Figure 6.10   The Magill anaesthetic breathing system. Redrawn from Lane and Cooper (2003), Butterworth-Heinemann.

Advantages
- The valve position allows improved access to the head and to scavenging attachments.
- The length of the circuit (1.5 m) allows the anaesthetic machine to be positioned away from the patient.
- Lightweight, exerting less drag than the Magill circuit.

Disadvantages
- Cannot be used for prolonged IPPV.
- The coaxial tubing may become disconnected, causing rebreathing.

Suitable for: Patients weighing between 10 and 60 kg.

Flow rates: 1–1.5 × minute volume.

Circuit: Modified Bain (non-rebreathing) (Fig. 6.12)

Equipment: 2 litre reservoir bag, coaxial tubing (inner respiratory limb), expiratory valve.

Advantages
- Can be used for continuous IPPV.
- The length of the circuit (1.8 m) improves access to the patient.
- The expired air passing through the outer tubing warms the inspired air so conserving the patient temperature.
- Low drag and reduced mechanical deadspace.

Disadvantages
- Inner limb disconnection could cause rebreathing; this can be checked by plugging the end with a syringe while oxygen is flowing – the flowmeter indicator will fall if the tubing is connected.
- High flow rates are required.

Suitable for: Patients weighing 8–30 kg.

Flow rates: 2.5–3 × minute volume.

Circuit: To and fro (rebreathing) (Fig. 6.13)

Equipment: 2 litre rebreathing bag, Waters canister containing soda lime, fresh gas inflow, expiratory valve.

Advantages
- Greater heat conservation (although hyperthermia may occur with prolonged use).
- Bi-directional flow improves the removal of carbon dioxide.
- As there is a low circuit volume, denitrogenation is achieved rapidly and gas concentrations can be altered quickly.
- High gas efficiency.
- IPPV can be carried out.
- Inexpensive (compared with a circle system).

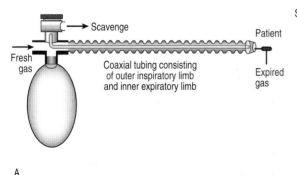

A

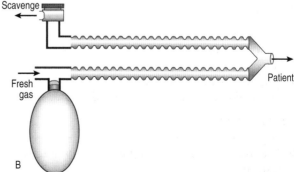

B

Figure 6.11   A, The Lack anaesthetic breathing system; B, The parallel Lack anaesthetic breathing system. Redrawn from Lane and Cooper (2003), Butterworth-Heinemann.

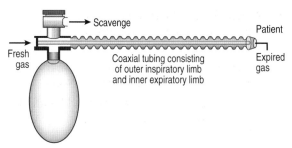

Figure 6.12 The modified Bain anaesthetic breathing system. Redrawn from Lane and Cooper (2003), Butterworth-Heinemann.

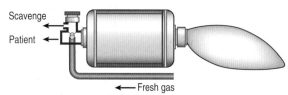

Figure 6.13 Horizontal to and fro anaesthetic breathing system. Redrawn from Lane and Cooper (2003), Butterworth-Heinemann.

Disadvantages
- Channelling may occur if the soda lime does not completely fill the canister.
- Mechanical deadspace increases during surgery as the soda lime is exhausted.
- Bronchiolitis may occur as a result of aspiration of alkaline dust from the soda lime. This can be minimised by placing a gauze filter at the patient end of the canister.
- Sited close to the patient, which may be inconvenient during head surgery.
- Bulky and can cause considerable drag on the tubing.
- Cannot use nitrous oxide in the mixture.

Suitable for: Patients weighing over 15 kg.

Flow rates: There is no circuit factor for the to and fro and minute volume is not required. The flow rate is: 10 ml × bodyweight per minute.

Circuit: Circle system (rebreathing) (Fig. 6.14)

Equipment: Fresh gas inflow inlet, inspiratory and expiratory one-way valves (unidirectional), 'Y' connector to patient, pressure relief valve incorporating scavenging equipment, rebreathing bag, soda lime canister.

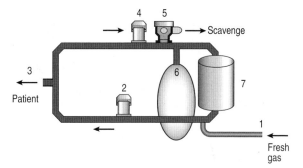

Figure 6.14 Circle anaesthetic breathing system. 1, Fresh gas inflow; 2, Unidirectional valve; 3, Y-connector to patient; 4, Unidirectional valve; 5, Pressure-relief valve; 6, Reservoir bag; 7, Soda lime canister. Redrawn from Lane and Cooper (2003), Butterworth-Heinemann.

Advantages
- Mechanical deadspace remains unchanged during surgery.
- Bronchiolitis is unlikely because the soda lime canister is much further away from the patient.
- High gas efficiency.
- IPPV can be carried out.
- Less circuit inertia than with the to and fro.

Disadvantages
- Expensive.
- High resistance.
- Cannot use nitrous oxide.
- Complex, bulky and difficult to clean.

Suitable for: Patients weighing over 15 kg.

Flow rates: There is no circuit factor for the circle system and minute volume is not required. The flow rate is: 10 ml × bodyweight per minute.

Circuit: Humphrey ADE system (rebreathing and non–rebreathing) (Fig. 6.15)

Equipment: Four-phase ADE exhaust valve, reservoir bag, soda lime canister, fresh gas inlet.

Advantages
- Semi-closed mode selected for small animals under 10 kg.
- Rebreathing mode, therefore economical to use.
- Simplicity: one system for all animals.

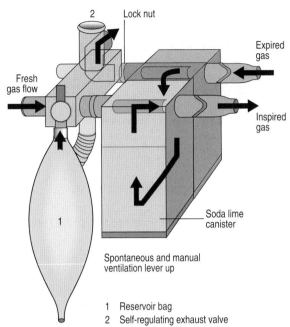

1 Reservoir bag
2 Self-regulating exhaust valve

Figure 6.15 Diagram to show set-up for the Humphrey ADE system. 1, Reservoir bag; 2, Self-regulating exhaust valve.

Disadvantages

- Expensive to buy.
- Cannot use nitrous oxide.
- Difficult to clean.

Procedure: Replacing soda lime

Soda lime is used to absorb the carbon dioxide formed in rebreathing circuits such as the circle system and the to and fro system. It consists of:

- 80% sodium hydroxide ('soda')
- 18% calcium hydroxide ('lime')
- silicates – these help to bind the soda lime and reduce the formation of irritant dust
- pH indicators – these change colour as the soda lime becomes exhausted (either pink to white or white to lilac).

1. **Action:** Put on protective clothing including gloves, apron and goggles. A mask may also be used.

   Rationale: Soda lime is caustic and must be handled with caution. A mask will reduce inhalation of dust.

2. **Action:** Follow the manufacturer's instructions when filling the canister in a circle system.

   Rationale: Circle systems vary – some canisters are designed to be used once only.

3. **Action:** The soda lime canister must be filled completely – do not try to save soda lime by partial filling.

   Rationale: The removal of carbon dioxide depends on the exhaled air being in close contact with the soda lime during the expiratory pause. If there is insufficient soda lime, the exhaled air will pass straight through the canister.

4. **Action:** Compact the soda lime tightly in the 'Waters' canister of the to and fro circuit.

   Rationale: Exhaled gas may pass over the top of the soda lime (channelling) if it does not completely fill the canister. This may result in hypercapnia.

CALCULATING ANAESTHETIC GAS FLOW RATES

An accurate flow rate should be calculated for each anaesthetic procedure to prevent hypoxia and hypercapnia and to ensure that the patient remains anaesthetised. Several factors must be taken into account when calculating flow rates including the patient's tidal volume and respiratory rate and the circuit being used.

- *Respiratory rate* is the number of breaths taken per minute.
- *Tidal volume* is the amount of gas passing into and out of the lungs in each respiratory cycle. It is estimated as follows:

$$\text{Cats/small dogs} = 15\text{ml/kg}$$
$$\text{Medium/large dogs} = 10\text{ml/kg}.$$

- *Minute volume* is the amount of gas passing into and out of the lungs in 1 minute and is calculated from the tidal volume and respiratory rate of the patient:

$$\text{minute volume (ml/kg)} = \text{tidal volume} \times \text{respiratory rate}$$

Table 6.8 Circuit factors

Type of circuit	Circuit factor
Jackson Rees modified T-piece (Ayer's)	2.5–3 × minute volume
Bain	2.5–3 × minute volume
Magill	1–1.5 × minute volume
Lack	1–1.5 × minute volume
To and fro – closed	No circuit factor: calculate flow rates using 10 ml/kg/min
Circle – closed	No circuit factor: calculate flow rates using 10 ml/kg/min
To and fro – partial rebreathing	No circuit factor: calculate flow rates using 25 ml/kg/min
Circle – partial rebreathing	No circuit factor: calculate flow rates using 25 ml/kg/min

(Approximately 200 ml/kg/minute using an average tidal volume of 10 ml/kg and an average respiratory rate of 20 breaths per minute.)

- *Circuit factor* – the factor by which the minute volume must be increased in order to prevent rebreathing (Table 6.8). These values are used to calculate the correct settings for the anaesthetic machine in relation to the particular patient.

1. Calculating the maintenance flow rate of anaesthetic gas to the patient

The formula is:

Bodyweight (kg) × tidal volume (ml) × respiratory rate (no. of breaths/min) × circuit factor = gas flow rate (ml/min)

Example: The gas flow rate for a 30 kg labrador with a respiratory rate of 20 breaths/min on a Magill circuit would be calculated as follows:

30 kg × 10 ml × 20 breaths/min × 1–1.5 = 6000 ml–9000 ml (6–9 litres)/min

2. Combining gases

When nitrous oxide, an effective analgesic, is used in a circuit the amount of oxygen delivered to the patient is limited by the fact that in order to prevent hypoxia oxygen levels must not drop below 33% of the total inspired gas. When calculating flow rates a 2:1 ratio of nitrous oxide:oxygen is required, i.e. nitrous oxide is run at 66%.

Example: A 12 kg spaniel with a respiratory rate of 20 breaths/min is connected to a parallel Lack circuit. Nitrous oxide is to be used. The gas flow rates would be:

Bodyweight (kg) × tidal volume (ml) × respiratory rate (breaths/min) × circuit factor = gas flow rate

12 kg × 10 ml × 20 breaths/min × 1–1.5 = 2400–3600 ml (2.4–3.6 litres)/min

2400–3600 ml ÷ 3 = 800–1200 ml oxygen

800–1200 ml × 2 = 1600–2400 ml nitrous oxide

3. Circle and to and fro circuits

A patient on either of these circuits is rebreathing the same gas continually so very low gas flow rates are required. Neither of these circuits has a circuit factor so the calculation of flow rate using the circuits as closed systems uses 10 ml/kg/min as the minimum oxygen requirement for an animal (Table 6.8). Flow rates of 25 to 50 ml/kg/min are recommended if using the circuits as partial rebreathing systems.

4. Induction

As a general rule, higher flow rates are used during induction. This is particularly important if a mask or induction chamber is being used as a higher flow rate enables the gas and anaesthetic to saturate the anaesthetic circuit and dilute the exhaled gases of the patient.

5. Recovery

Gas flow rates are increased at the end of an anaesthetic, once the vaporiser is turned off, in order to flush exhaled gas from the circuit.

NB. Monitoring anaesthesia: It is vital that the status of the central nervous and cardiopulmonary systems is monitored throughout anaesthesia at 5-minute intervals. All data should be recorded on anaesthetic monitoring records. In order to minimise cardiopulmonary depression the animal should be maintained at a depth of anaesthesia that just prevents a response to surgery. Signs indicat-

Table 6.9   Methods of monitoring the patient during anaesthesia

Method	Used to measure	Description
Palpation of superficial arteries	Heart rate and rhythm Pulse quality	The arteries used in an anaesthetised animal are the femoral, lingual, facial, digital and coccygeal. Use of the peripheral arteries is recommended because they will be the first to indicate developing hypotension
Palpation of the apex beat	Heart rate and rhythm	Used in small mammals or when peripheral pulses are not palpable due to hypotension
Auscultation	Heart rate and rhythm, myocardial contractility and valve action	Oesophageal stethoscopes are recommended because they remain in place throughout anaesthesia – the tip is positioned next to the heart
Electrocardiography (ECG)	Heart rate and rhythm	ECGs demonstrate the electrical activity of the heart and show arrhythmias. They give no indication of cardiac output
Cardiac monitor	Heart rate	A simplified ECG that gives an audible bleep when it registers an 'R' wave
Pulse oximetry	Pulse rate and haemoglobin levels	The device is attached across the tongue and measures arterial oxygen saturation
Blood pressure monitors	Blood pressure	An inflatable cuff is placed on a limb proximal to the site of a distal artery. The cuff abolishes arterial blood flow distal to the cuff. As the cuff is deflated the returning blood flow is detected
Mucous membranes	Hypotension, perfusion, vasoconstriction, cyanosis, hypercapnia	Mucous membrane colour should be salmon pink and can be assessed by looking at the gingiva, conjunctiva, anus, vagina or penis
Capillary refill time (CRT)	Hypovolaemic shock, cardiovascular depression	A mucous membrane is blanched and the time taken to return to normal is the CRT
Respiratory monitors	Respiratory rate	Detect the difference between the inspired (cool) air and expired (warm) air. They do not register respiratory depth
Apnoea alert monitors	Apnoea	An alarm is triggered after a period of apnoea. The trigger period can be set by the operator
Temperature	Hypothermia	Feeling the patient's extremities and taking the rectal temperature will give an indication of peripheral circulation
Pedal reflex	Depth of anaesthesia	This reflex is caused by pinching in between the digits. It is usually lost by stage III, plane II
Palpebral reflex	Depth of anaesthesia	The eyelids will blink when the medial canthus is touched. It is usually lost during stage III, plane II

(Continued)

Table 6.9   Methods of monitoring the patient during anaesthesia—**Cont'd**

Method	Used to measure	Description
Corneal reflex	Anaesthetic overdose	The cornea is very sensitive and should only be tested as a last resort. If absent, anaesthetic overdose has occurred
Blood loss	Hypotension	Calculate the weight of a dry swab. The amount of blood loss can be calculated by weighing the blood-soaked swabs and subtracting their dry weight: 1 g = 1 ml
Saliva and tears	Anaesthetic depth	As anaesthetic depth increases, these secretions slow until they are absent

Table 6.10   Changes in respiratory pattern seen during anaesthesia

Term	Definition	Cause	Action
Bradypnoea	Below normal respiratory rate	Effects of the anaesthetic drugs Anaesthesia too deep	Lighten anaesthesia
Tachypnoea	Above normal respiratory rate	Anaesthetic insufficient Awareness of pain	Deepen anaesthesia Administer analgesics
Dyspnoea	Difficulty breathing	Obstruction in the thorax Obstruction of the anaesthetic circuit	Check that the patient has a patent airway Check circuit is attached: watch the bag for respiratory movements
Apnoea	Absence of respiration	Effects of some induction agents such as propofol, thiopental and methohexital Respiratory arrest	Check that the patient's airway is patent: check tube positioning and for blockage Perform IPPV with 100% oxygen at a rate of 20–30 breaths per minute

Table 6.11   Changes in heart rate seen during anaesthesia

Term	Definition	Cause	Action
Bradycardia	Heart rate lower than normal	Effects of drugs such as medetomidine and acepromazine Increasing depth of anaesthesia Illness	Monitor closely Lighten anaesthesia Administer atipamezole if necessary
Tachycardia	Heart rate higher than normal	Effects of drugs such as atropine and ketamine Insufficient anaesthesia Decreasing depth of anaesthesia	Monitor closely Deepen anaesthesia
No heart rate		Cardiac arrest	Thoracic massage at a rate of 60–80 compressions per minute Apply a compression bandage around the chest to increase venous return to the heart

Table 6.12 Changes in pulse rate seen during anaesthesia

Pulse	Cause	Action
Increased rate	Stress	Premedicate with ataractics such as acepromazine
	Pain	Administer analgesics
	Light anaesthesia	Deepen anaesthesia
	Pyrexia	Administer antipyretics
	Hypoxia	Check oxygen flow rates
	Hypercapnia	Check that no rebreathing is occurring
Decreased rate	Anaesthesia too deep	Lighten anaesthesia
	Systemic illness	Administer atipamezole if necessary
	Effects of anaesthetic drugs such as medetomidine	
Weak, thready	Poor circulation: possible hypovolaemic shock	Administer fluid therapy
	Administration of alpha-2-agonists	
	Peripheral venous constriction	
Strong, jerky	Congenital heart defects: patent ductus arteriosus, pulmonary/aortic stenosis	Monitor closely
	Malfunction of heart valves	

Table 6.13 Changes in the colour of mucous membranes seen during anaesthesia

Colour	Cause	Action
Pale	Hypovolaemic shock	Administer fluid therapy
	Hypotension	
	Anaemia	
	Haemorrhage	
Cyanotic	Respiratory obstruction	Check airway, breathing, circulation
	Cardiac arrest	Remove obstruction
	Administration of nitrous oxide with little	Perform IPPV and thoracic massage as required
	or no oxygen	Administer 100% oxygen
Icteric	Hepatic abnormalities	Monitor closely
Brick red	Carbon monoxide poisoning	Administer 100% oxygen
	Toxaemia	

ing the depth of anaesthesia are described in Table 6.4. These should be used in conjunction with accurate monitoring using methods described in Tables 6.9, 6.10, 6.11, 6.12 and 6.13.

PATIENT RECOVERY

Once surgery has been completed, switch off the vaporiser and nitrous oxide. Run through 100% oxygen to prevent hypoxia if nitrous oxide has been used. The circuit should be flushed with oxygen before final disconnection to avoid atmospheric pollution.

It is essential to monitor the patient closely throughout the recovery period – postoperative mortality occurs when attention relaxes. The patient should be placed in a warm, quiet, accessible kennel with emergency equipment close to hand. The length of time taken to recover depends on various factors including:

- age of the patient
- health of the patient
- anaesthetic agent given
- duration of the anaesthetic
- environmental and body temperatures.

Procedure: Care of the patient during recovery

1. **Action:** Monitor vital signs.

   Rationale: A change can be detected swiftly and acted upon immediately.

2. **Action:** Keep the patient calm.

   Rationale: Excitement on recovery causes increased blood pressure, which may dislodge clots and cause haemorrhage.

3. **Action:** Keep orifices and surgical sites clean and dry.

   Rationale: To minimise the risk of contamination.

4. **Action:** Keep the patient warm.

   Rationale: Hypothermia will delay recovery.

5. **Action:** Administer postoperative medication.

   Rationale: Analgesics should be administered before recovery begins, to maximise their effect.

6. **Action:** Prevent patient interference with wounds.

   Rationale: Apply dressings, bandages or an Elizabethan collar as necessary.

7. **Action:** Assess the patient for postoperative discomfort.

   Rationale: If there are any signs of pain such as vocalisation, panting, abnormal posture, dilated pupils or tachycardia, inform the veterinary surgeon immediately.

8. **Action:** Monitor fluid and nutritional intake.

   Rationale: If the patient is on intravenous fluids, maintain at the given rate. Otherwise allow access to water and give a small amount of a recovery diet.

9. **Action:** Allow the patient opportunity to urinate and defecate.

   Rationale: Urinary catheterisation may be indicated if prolonged recovery is expected.

10. **Action:** Discharge the animal.

    Rationale: This should only occur once the veterinary surgeon is satisfied that the patient has fully recovered.

Procedure: Discharging a patient

1. **Action:** Make sure that all drugs, instructions and invoices are prepared in advance.

   Rationale: The reception staff can take payment and make follow-up appointments, while the owner is waiting for a veterinary nurse or veterinary surgeon to speak to them.

2. **Action:** Take the client into a consulting room.

   Rationale: This ensures privacy and minimal distraction.

3. **Action:** Give directions regarding feeding, exercise, medication, care of dressings, care of wounds, follow-up appointments, stitch removal and possible complications.

   Rationale: Directions should be given verbally and backed up with written instructions to which the owner can refer once they are at home.

4. **Action:** Make any follow-up appointments and take payment (if not already carried out).

   Rationale: The client should take this opportunity to ask any questions.

5. **Action:** Return the pet to its owner, making sure wounds are clean and no catheters are left in place.

   Rationale: This should be the last step because the client will not take in any information once reunited with their pet!

ANAESTHETIC EMERGENCIES

An anaesthetic emergency is anything that poses a threat to the patient's life. Constant monitoring is essential to detect the early warning signs of a potential emergency such as a gradual decrease in respiratory rate prior to respiratory arrest.

Table 6.14 Contents of an anaesthetic emergency kit

Contents	Reason	Indication
Adrenaline (epinephrine) 0.05–0.1 mg/kg	Increases the heart rate and the force of the contraction (therefore increasing cardiac output)	Cardiac arrest Unresponsive hypotension
Atropine 0.02–0.05 mg/kg	Vagolytic	Bradycardia
Doxapram 5–10 mg/kg	Respiratory and central nervous system stimulant	Apnoea Respiratory arrest
Dobutamine 1–5 μg/kg/min	Increases the force of cardiac contractions	Hypotension
Lidocaine (lignocaine) Dogs 1–6 mg/kg Cats 0.25–1.0 mg/kg	Antidysrhythmic	Ventricular premature contractions and ventricular tachycardia
Naloxone 0.01–0.02 mg/kg	Narcotic antagonist	Reverse accidental overdose of Small Animal Immobilon, pethidine, fentanyl, morphine, etorphine
Dexamethasone 1–2 mg/kg	Anti-inflammatory	Treatment of shock
Atipamezole Dogs 0.05–0.2 mg/kg Cats 0.5 mg/kg	Alpha-2-agonist antagonist	Reverse accidental overdose of medetomidine, xylazine and detomidine
Sodium bicarbonate 1.0 mmol/kg	Alkaline	Treatment for metabolic acidosis
Tracheostomy tube	To perform emergency tracheostomy	Laryngeal/oropharyngeal obstruction
Syringes and needles	To administer drugs	
Intravenous catheters, giving set, tape	To administer intravenous fluids	Hypovolaemic shock
Swabs, surgical kit, dressing materials	To perform cardiac massage	Cardiac arrest

The outcome of an emergency depends on:

- correct preparation of an emergency kit
- early observation of warning signs
- correct assessment of the problem
- prompt action.

Table 6.14 describes the contents of an anaesthetic emergency kit, which should be regularly checked for out-of-date drugs and restocked. It should be kept near the theatre and be readily available. Table 6.15 illustrates possible emergencies and the action to be taken.

Intermittent positive pressure ventilation (IPPV)

IPPV is carried out when a patient is not breathing for itself.

1. **Action:** Squeeze the reservoir bag (which is full of fresh gas) on a suitable circuit (circle, Bain or T-piece).

    Rationale: This will oxygenate the patient's lungs and remove carbon dioxide.

2. **Action:** Carry this out at a rate of 10–12 times per minute.

Table 6.15   Anaesthetic emergencies

Emergency	Signs	Action
Apnoea	Absence of breathing Irregular gasping with twitching neck muscles Spasmodic diaphragm contractions Dilated pupils Cyanosis No movement of reservoir bag	Administer 100% oxygen by IPPV Give respiratory stimulants (may have side effects)
Airway obstruction	Non-productive respiratory effort Inspiratory snoring Cyanosis Eventual cardiac arrest	Locate and remove the obstruction If not possible, perform emergency tracheostomy Intubate and administer 100% oxygen by IPPV
Cardiac arrest	Agonal breathing Possibly respiratory arrest No femoral pulse Dilated pupils	Start cardiopulmonary resuscitation (CPR) (refer to Chapter 9)
Bradycardia	Very slow heart rate	Administer 100% oxygen Give vagolytic drugs such as atropine
Haemorrhage	Blood at surgical site Tachycardia Pale mucous membranes Increased CRT Weak, thready pulse	Administer fluid therapy: plasma volume expanders
Hypothermia	Cold extremities Low body temperature Bradycardia Pale mucous membranes Cardiac arrest	Minimise surgical time Keep patient as dry as possible Irrigate exposed viscera with warmed fluids Increase operating room temperature Insulate the patient to prevent further heat loss
Hypotension	Increased CRT Pale mucous membranes Weak pulse	Administer fluid therapy Give adrenaline (epinephrine) or dobutamine

Rationale: This mimics the average respiratory rate of the patient, so enabling adequate oxygenation, removal of carbon dioxide and provision of anaesthetic gas.

3. **Action:** Reduce the concentration of anaesthetic agent slightly.

Rationale: This avoids deeper anaesthesia than is required.

4. **Action:** At the end of anaesthesia, reduce the ventilation rate gradually.

Rationale: Carbon dioxide levels will rise and stimulate the patient's normal respiration.

SPECIALISED TECHNIQUES

Local anaesthesia

In practice, local anaesthetics are most commonly used in large animal work, but they may be used in small animal practice for the following:

- superficial surgery
- to facilitate certain procedures
- during surgery to reduce the depth of general anaesthesia
- as a means of diagnosis.

Table 6.16   Local anaesthetic techniques

Technique	Description	Use
Surface	Gels, ointments, sprays and drops which are applied to the skin or mucous membranes	Drops can be applied to the eye to facilitate ocular examination Gel can be applied to urinary catheters and endotracheal tubes to facilitate placement Ointment can be applied to the skin prior to intravenous catheterisation Spray can be applied to the larynx in cats to prevent laryngeal spasm on endotracheal intubation
Infiltration	Injection of local anaesthetic along the line of surgical incision	Facilitates the suture of small skin wounds
Regional: perineural	Local anaesthetic is injected around the major nerves that provide sensation to the operation site	Diagnosis of lameness by performing a nerve block Cornual nerve block used for disbudding calves
Regional: intravenous	A tourniquet is placed around a limb and local anaesthetic is injected intravenously, distal to the tourniquet. Results in good analgesia of the distal limb. Effective after 5 minutes and lasts until the tourniquet is removed	Surgery on the feet of cattle Occasionally used in limb surgery in dogs
Spinal: epidural	Local anaesthetic is injected into the space between the dura mater and the periosteum lining the spinal cord. It blocks nerves as they leave the spinal canal, resulting in loss of motor and sensory function	Used to provide muscle relaxation and pain relief during pelvic limb orthopaedic procedures and providing analgesia to the anus and perineum

The most widely used local anaesthetic drug is lidocaine (lignocaine). It can be obtained in the form of a topical gel or cream, aerosol and injectable solution with preservative ± adrenaline (epinephrine).

Local anaesthetics work by blocking local nerve transmission to the area, thus reducing sensation. Table 6.16 describes the local anaesthetic techniques in common use.

Muscle relaxation

Many drugs including general anaesthetics produce muscle relaxation to a certain degree. However, at times absolute relaxation is required and specific neuromuscular blocking agents are used. These act directly on the neuromuscular junction and stop the transmission of motor nerve impulses to striated muscle. They have no effect on smooth or cardiac muscle. They do not cross the blood–brain barrier and so do not alter consciousness. Neuromuscular blocking agents will eliminate some of the obvious signs of inadequate anaesthesia such as movement, eye position and cranial nerve reflexes, so care must be taken to ensure that the depth of anaesthesia is appropriate to the procedure being undertaken.

Other signs of inadequate anaesthesia that are not affected by neuromuscular blocking agents include:

- mydriasis
- lacrimation
- salivation
- tachycardia
- hypertension.

Table 6.17   Indications for the use of muscle relaxants

Use	Description
Thoracic surgery	The intercostal muscles are thoroughly relaxed, minimising damage by rib retractors which leads to less post-surgical pain. Access into the surgical site is made easier
Ophthalmic surgery	Muscle relaxants keep the eye in a central position throughout general anaesthesia, making corneal surgery possible There are no eye reflexes to disturb delicate eye surgery being carried out
High risk cases	The amount of general anaesthetic required is reduced when muscle relaxants are used, which in turn reduces the degree of cardiovascular depression
Oesophageal foreign bodies	The striated muscle of the oesophagus of the dog is completely relaxed, which makes the removal of an oesophageal foreign body easier
Orthopaedic surgery	Reduction of dislocations is eased when muscle relaxants have been administered

Table 6.18   Common muscle relaxants

Drug	Effects	Warnings
Depolarising: Suxamethonium	Very short-acting	Evidence of muscle pain on recovery
Non-depolarising: Pancuronium	Long duration of action	Causes modest tachycardia Cumulative so cannot be topped up
Vecuronium	Intermediate duration of action (20–30 minutes) Non-cumulative Has little cardiovascular effect	
Atracurium	Rapid onset Intermediate duration of action (30–40 minutes) Breaks down spontaneously in the body, can therefore be used in animals with poor liver and kidney function	Inactivated by thiopental and other alkaline solutions so thoroughly flush catheters before administration

When a muscle relaxant is used, the respiratory muscles are blocked and the patient is unable to breathe normally. Some means of supporting ventilation such as IPPV must be available and the patient should be intubated and connected to an anaesthetic machine.

The indications for the use of muscle relaxants are listed in Table 6.17 while the common muscle relaxants are described in Table 6.18.

CONTROL OF POLLUTION – SCAVENGING

Anaesthetic gases must be scavenged from the anaesthetic system to avoid atmospheric pollution and potential damage to in-contact theatre personnel. Disorders such as malignancies, abortion and infertility, and liver damage have been linked to exposure to the gases. Under the COSHH Regulations (Control of Substances Hazardous to

Health) employers must assess the risk of exposure and take appropriate action to protect their employees.

Scavenging can be achieved in two ways – active scavenging and passive scavenging. In both cases a scavenge tube is connected to the expiratory valve, pressure-relief valve or expiratory limb of an anaesthetic circuit to conduct waste gases away from the theatre to a safe site.

Active scavenging

Gas is drawn along the scavenge tube by negative pressure generated by an extractor fan. An air brake receiver prevents the fan exerting negative pressure on the anaesthetic circuit and it also allows several systems to be scavenged from one extraction unit.

Passive scavenging

Passive systems either direct the gas into an activated charcoal canister or pass it straight to the air outside the building through ducts in the wall. These systems rely on the combined effects of gas flowing into the anaesthetic circuit, expiratory effort and elastic recoil from the reservoir bag to propel the gas along the tubing. The scavenge tube must not be excessively long or it will offer too much resistance to expiration. Activated charcoal canisters do not absorb nitrous oxide. They must be weighed frequently in order to assess when they are saturated.

REFERENCES AND FURTHER READING

Aspinall V 2006 The Complete Textbook of Veterinary Nursing. Elsevier, Oxford

Lane D R, Cooper B (eds) 2003 Veterinary Nursing, 3rd edn. Butterworth-Heinemann, Oxford

McKelvey D, Hollingshead K W 2000 Small Animal Anaesthesia, 2nd edn. Mosby, London

Moore M (ed) 1999 Manual of Veterinary Nursing. BSAVA, Gloucester

Simpson G (ed) 1991 Practical Veterinary Nursing. BSAVA, Gloucester

Chapter 7

Theatre practice

Pip Millard

CHAPTER CONTENTS

Introduction   135

Sterilisation   136
Use of the ethylene oxide steriliser   137
Monitoring the efficacy of sterilisation   137
Packing materials for sterilisation   138
Packing an item for sterilisation   138
Maintaining the theatre environment   139
Daily cleaning routine   140
Weekly cleaning routine   140
The surgical scrub   141
General handwashing routine   141
Surgical scrub   141
Drying hands after the surgical scrub   142
Theatre attire   143
Folding a surgical gown for sterilisation   144
Putting on a back-tying surgical gown   145
Putting on a side-tying gown   147
Closed gloving   148
Open gloving   148
The plunge method of gloving   148
Preparation of the surgical site   148
Clipping   150
Preparation of the skin   151
Draping the patient   152
Packing drapes for sterilisation   152
Draping with four plain drapes   152
Draping a limb   154
Draping with a fenestrated drape   154

Instrumentation   155
Preparation of the instrument trolley   155
Draping a trolley using Cheatle forceps   155
Laying out an instrument trolley   155
Assisting during surgery   155
Handling and passing instruments   156
Swabbing   156
**Care and maintenance of surgical
    instruments**   157
Cleaning and maintaining instruments   157
Surgical kits   157
Care of specialist equipment   159
Preparation of diathermy equipment   159
Preparation for cryosurgery   159
Cleaning an endoscope   160

INTRODUCTION

The management and maintenance of the theatre environment is of prime importance in a situation where patients, already weakened by their existing condition, are further subjected to procedures that may be painful, bewildering and traumatic.

The main focus in running an efficient operating theatre is on maintaining a good aseptic technique. This must be applied not only to the more obvious care of instruments, preparation of the surgical site and scrubbing-up techniques, but also to the daily routine of maintaining the hygiene of the theatre and associated preparation areas and to the personal hygiene of all who work in the area. It takes very little upset in any of the procedures to compromise asepsis and introduce infection which could in turn lead to wound breakdown, systemic infection, reduced surgical success rate and inevitably an effect on the reputation of the practice.

It is usually the responsibility of the veterinary nurse to organise all matters concerned with the operating theatre and its efficient function and it is to the nurse and her management routines that the veterinary surgeon will turn if things go wrong.

STERILISATION

Sterilisation can be defined as the process by which instruments and drapes are rendered aseptic (or sterile) by the destruction or removal of all microorganisms including spores. This can be achieved by various methods including:

- heat sterilisation:
  hot-air oven
  autoclave
- cold sterilisation:
  ethylene oxide
  radiation.

Boiling cannot be considered to be a method of sterilisation because it does not reach a high enough temperature to destroy bacterial spores.

Chemical solutions based on chlorhexidine or glutaraldehyde will kill bacteria if items are soaked in them. They may be used for surgical equipment, which cannot be sterilised using any other method. However, they should only really be considered to be a method of disinfection.

1. Hot–air oven

Hot-air ovens produce a dry heat. Microorganisms are more resistant to dry heat so high working temperatures are required for a long period of time (Table 7.1). Long cooling periods are also required and the very high temperatures may damage metal items. A safety device should be fitted to the door to prevent accidental opening before the oven is cool. Care should be taken not to overload the oven, as air will be unable to circulate freely.

Use is limited by the long period of time required for sterilisation and cooling. However, hot-air ovens are useful for items damaged by moist heat such as glassware, powders, oils and sharp cutting instruments.

2. Autoclave

This is the most common method of sterilisation used in veterinary practice. In normal circumstances, water cannot reach temperatures greater than 100 °C (boiling point) before producing steam. If water is boiled under pressure, the boiling point is raised so the temperature of the steam is greater. This steam produces heat which penetrates to the innermost layer of the packs. The moisture increases the permeability to the heat. Care should be taken to avoid overloading or blocking the inlet and outlet valves. Items to be autoclaved should be free from grease and protein in order to achieve effective penetration of steam.

The majority of autoclaves designed for modern veterinary practice incorporate a drying cycle. Steam is exhausted and replaced by filtered air which dries the packs (Table 7.2).

Autoclaves are used for sterilising instruments, drapes, gowns, swabs and some rubber or plastic items.

Table 7.1 Hot–air ovens: working temperature and time ratios

Item	Temperature (°C)	Time (minutes)
Glassware and non–cutting instruments	180	60
Powders and oils	160	120
Sharp cutting instruments	150	180

Table 7.2   Autoclaves: working temperature, time and pressure ratios

Pressure (kg/cm²)	Pressure (psi)	Temperature (°C)	Time (minutes)
1.2	15	121	12
1.4	20	126	10
2	30	134	3.5

3. Ethylene oxide

Ethylene oxide gas sterilises by inactivating the DNA in the cells of the pathogen, thus preventing their replication. It is, however, toxic, irritant to tissues and very inflammable. In order to comply with COSHH regulations manufacturer's instructions **must** be followed.

The steriliser, a plastic container fitted with a ventilation system, should be located in a well-ventilated area, such as a fume cupboard away from working areas. Room temperature must be kept at a minimum of 20 °C during the cycle.

Procedure: Use of the ethylene oxide steriliser

1.   **Action:** Place individually packed items into a polythene liner bag.

     Rationale: Liner bags are supplied with the steriliser.

2.   **Action:** Place a scored ampoule containing ethylene oxide liquid inside the liner bag and seal the bag with a metal twist tie.

     Rationale: The bag must be sealed in order to keep the gas circulating around the contents.

3.   **Action:** Put the liner bag into the steriliser unit.

4.   **Action:** Snap the ampoule from outside the bag to release the gas.

     Rationale: To minimise exposure to gas.

5.   **Action:** Close and lock the door to the steriliser unit and turn the ventilator on.

     Rationale: Accidental opening of the unit can be prevented if the unit is locked.

6.   **Action:** After 12 hours turn on the pump.

     Rationale: This aerates the unit before it is safe for the operator to open.

7.   **Action:** Two hours after aerating, remove sterilised items.

     Rationale: This will ensure that any toxic gas has been removed.

8.   **Action:** Store items for a further 24 hours in a well-ventilated room.

     Rationale: This makes sure that all the ethylene oxide has dissipated.

Sterilisation by ethylene oxide is suitable for anaesthetic tubing, endotracheal tubes, fibreoptic equipment, optical instruments, plastic items such as catheters and syringes, high-speed drills and battery-operated drills.

Everyday items such as instruments, gowns and drapes may also be sterilised in this manner but the length of the cycle restricts its use.

4. Radiation

Sterilisation is achieved using gamma irradiation. It can only be carried out under controlled conditions within industry. Many pre-packaged items used in practice such as needles, syringes and catheters are sterilised in this way.

MONITORING THE EFFICACY OF STERILISATION

It is essential that the effectiveness of any sterilisation method be constantly monitored to ensure that all microorganisms including bacterial spores are destroyed. Different sterilisation methods require different working conditions in terms of time and temperature. It is also important to choose the correct method of monitoring efficacy of sterilisation (Table 7.3).

Table 7.3 Methods of monitoring the efficacy of sterilisation

Method	Description	Use
Chemical indicator strips	Paper strips which change colour when the correct temperature and time have been reached. They are placed in the centre of the pack prior to sterilisation	Autoclave – select the correct strip for the cycle Ethylene oxide
Browne's tubes	Small glass tubes filled with an orange liquid which turns green when the correct temperature is reached and maintained for the correct time	Autoclave Hot-air oven
Bowie-Dick indicator tape	A beige tape impregnated with chemical stripes that change to black when the correct temperature has been reached (121°C). It does not indicate that the pack has been exposed for the correct time; therefore it is not a reliable method	Autoclave
Ethylene oxide tape	As above only the tape is green with lines that change to red on exposure to ethylene oxide	Ethylene oxide
Spore strips	Strips of paper impregnated with spores (usually *Bacillus stearothermophilius*) are placed in the load. After sterilisation, they are cultured for 72 hours. Provided that sterilisation has been achieved, no growth will be visible. This is an accurate method although the delay in obtaining the results is a major disadvantage	Autoclave Ethylene oxide Hot-air oven
Thermocouples	Electrical leads with temperature-sensitive tips which are placed in the autoclave with the leads passed out and attached to a recording device. The temperature is checked throughout the cycle and the results are recorded	Autoclave

PACKING MATERIALS FOR STERILISATION

There are a number of different packing materials available for the preparation of items to be sterilised. Selection will depend largely on the method of sterilisation but factors such as cost and personal preference may also be taken into account (Table 7.4).

Procedure: Packing an item for sterilisation

1. **Action:** Select the appropriate packaging material for the method of sterilisation to be used.

   Rationale: A packing material that is non-permeable to steam would not be suitable for an autoclave.

2. **Action:** Select the correct size for the item to be sterilised.

   Rationale: Some methods of packing such as self-seal pouches can be costly to use so do not choose too large a pouch.

3. **Action:** Label the pack with the contents.

   Rationale: This will save opening incorrect packs, which would then require re-sterilisation.

Table 7.4 Packing materials for sterilisation

Packing material	Advantage	Disadvantage	Method of sterilisation
Self-seal pouches	Easy to pack Clear front to view contents Paper back with sterilisation indicator Ideal for individual instruments	Puncture by heavy or sharp instruments (double packing will prevent puncturing but increase the cost)	Autoclave Ethylene oxide
Nylon film	Cheap May be reused Sealed with Bowie-Dick tape	Repeated use leads to brittleness and can cause tiny holes which can go unnoticed	Autoclave
Polythene bags supplied by ethylene oxide manufacturers	Easy to pack Strong	Overpacking can lead to poor gas circulation	Ethylene oxide
Linen drapes	Conforming Used to pack surgical equipment Strong Reusable	Permeable to moisture Require laundering Liable to wear	Autoclave (with a drying cycle) Ethylene oxide (if not too tightly packed)
Paper drapes	Water-repellent Disposable Used to pack surgical equipment	Non-conforming Can tear easily	Autoclave (with a drying cycle) Ethylene oxide (if not too tightly packed)
Metal tins	Long-lasting Useful for gowns, drapes, swabs, instruments Cannot be punctured	Expensive to buy Require a large autoclave Often multi-use, which may lead to contamination of contents	Autoclave (with a drying cycle) Hot-air oven
Cardboard cartons	Reusable Cannot be punctured easily Sturdy Useful for specialised kits	Expensive to buy Bulky to store	Autoclave (with a drying cycle)

4. **Action:** Write the date on the pack.

  Rationale: Sterilised items should be repackaged and sterilised again if not used within 3 months.

5. **Action:** Write name of the person preparing the pack on the pack label.

  Rationale: This allows any problems with the packing to be traced.

MAINTAINING THE THEATRE ENVIRONMENT

It is vital to have a strict cleaning regime in the operating theatre and preparation room to maintain a high standard of asepsis. Both daily and weekly cleaning procedures are essential. In addition to this, there are some general rules for maintaining asepsis in the theatre (Table 7.5).

Table 7.5 Maintaining an aseptic theatre

Action	Rationale
1. The least number of people should be present and movement kept to a minimum.	1. Any movement will increase the risk of wound contamination by airborne particles.
2. Personnel must wear the correct theatre attire at all times.	2. This will avoid contamination from clothing, skin and hair.
3. Clip and disinfect the patient away from the theatre.	3. Hair and debris would contaminate the theatre.
4. Use a new set of instruments for each surgical procedure.	4. Cross-contamination between patients must be avoided.
5. Carry out 'clean' operations before contaminated procedures.	5. Contamination from high-risk procedures should then not occur.
6. Discard any instrument that becomes contaminated.	6. The remaining surgical instruments must remain aseptic.
7. If asepsis is broken by any member of the surgical team it must be rectified.	7. Further contamination can then be avoided.

Procedure: Daily cleaning routine

1. **Action:** Damp dust all surfaces and equipment using dilute disinfectant.

   Rationale: Using a dry cloth would merely move dust around the room.

2. **Action:** Wipe the table and surfaces in between patients, with dilute disinfectant. Clean the floor if it is soiled.

   Rationale: This prevents cross-contamination from one patient to the next.

3. **Action:** Remove used instruments, drapes, etc. after each procedure.

   Rationale: To avoid contaminating the next surgical site.

4. **Action:** At the end of the day, vacuum to remove debris and hair.

   Rationale: Fine particles will be collected more efficiently using a vacuum.

5. **Action:** All waste material and soiled equipment must be removed.

   Rationale: The warm operating theatre is an ideal breeding ground for microorganisms.

6. **Action:** All surfaces, including lights and sinks, must be thoroughly cleaned using dilute disinfectant.

   Rationale: Contaminated dust particles will settle on all surfaces and must be removed.

Procedure: Weekly cleaning routine

1. **Action:** Remove all portable equipment from the operating theatre.

   Rationale: Dirt and debris quickly build up in less accessible areas such as those behind equipment.

2. **Action:** Clean the equipment including the castors.

   Rationale: Castors soon fail to run smoothly if they are not cleaned regularly.

3. **Action:** Scrub the ceiling, walls, floor and all fixtures thoroughly using a disinfectant with detergent properties.

   Rationale: Detergent will remove any organic matter which could otherwise inactivate the disinfectant.

4. **Action:** Use cleaning utensils that are specifically designed for the operating theatre. They should be sterilised or washed in a washing machine after use.

   Rationale: This will minimise cross-contamination from other areas of the veterinary practice.

THE SURGICAL SCRUB

The surgical scrub is performed to reduce the levels of both resident and transient microbes on the hands. The hands come into the closest contact with the surgical site and although sterile gloves may be worn, these cannot be relied on entirely as they may be punctured before surgery is complete.

The correct equipment should be prepared in advance so the complete process from scrubbing to gowning and gloving can be carried out in an aseptic manner. The equipment required is:

- sink with elbow, knee or foot controls
- cleansing agent dispenser
- disposable nail file or orange stick
- sterile scrubbing brush
- sterile towels
- sterile gown
- sterile gloves.

Ideally, a general handwashing procedure is carried out at the beginning of the day. A full surgical scrub is then carried out, lasting up to 10 minutes, prior to the first surgical procedure, then a shorter scrub may be carried out in between subsequent procedures provided there has been no major contamination of the hands.

Before beginning any handwashing procedure, all jewellery and watches must be removed. Nails should be short and free from varnish.

Procedure: General handwashing routine

1. **Action:** Turn on the water and adjust to a warm temperature.

2. **Action:** Allow the water to wash over the hands and drain from the wrists to the fingertips.
   Rationale: This will remove any gross contamination.

3. **Action:** Clean the fingernails with an orange stick or nail file.
   Rationale: Once this has been carried out each day, it may be omitted from further washing procedures.

4. **Action:** Apply plain soap and massage into the hands, from the wrists to the fingertips, in a circular motion including the backs of the hands.

Rationale: It is important to remove all traces of dirt because these may inactivate the antiseptic solution used in the surgical scrub.

5. **Action:** Rinse, allowing the water to drain from the fingertips. Repeat step 4.
   Rationale: Repeating the washing procedure will ensure the removal of any residual organic matter.

6. **Action:** Turn off the water.
   Rationale: The hands must not touch the tap so if the elbow, foot or knee cannot operate it, an assistant may be required. If this is not possible, a paper towel may be used and then discarded.

7. **Action:** Dry hands thoroughly with paper towels.
   Rationale: Air hand-dryers are unsuitable because they spread microorganisms around the environment. Reusable towels are unsuitable because they harbour microorganisms.

Procedure: Surgical scrub (Fig. 7.1)

1. **Action:** Turn on the tap to produce a gentle stream and adjust the temperature.
   Rationale: A gentle stream will minimise splashing.

2. **Action:** Keeping forearms higher than the elbows at all times, wet the arms and hands and apply plain soap.
   Rationale: It is important to keep the hands above the elbows to allow any water to run away from the scrubbed area to avoid recontamination.

3. **Action:** Work the soap into a lather and spread over the hands and arms to 5 cm above the elbow.
   Rationale: Any surface dirt and grease will be removed.

4. **Action:** With the fingers under the stream, clean the nails with a file or orange stick.
   Rationale: Discard the file by dropping it into the sink.

5. **Action:** Repeat step 3 using a surgical scrub solution.

6. **Action:** Take a sterile brush, moisten it under the stream and apply the surgical scrub solution.

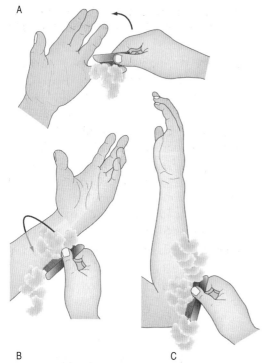

Figure 7.1 The surgical scrub sequence. A, Starting with the little finger and working across to the thumb, scrub each surface of each digit. B, Scrub the forearm, again scrubbing the entire circumference. C, Scrub elbow area to 5 cm (2 inches) above the elbow, including all surfaces.

7. **Action:** Scrub the nails using a straight stroke.

   Rationale: Make sure the bristles of the brush clean under the nails.

8. **Action:** Starting with the little finger, scrub each of the four planes of each finger in straight strokes.

   Rationale: Include the interdigital spaces.

9. **Action:** Clean the palm of the hand and back of the hand using a circular motion.

   Rationale: Care must be taken not to over-scrub the back of the hand because the skin is more delicate and therefore more susceptible to trauma.

10. **Action:** Scrub to 5 cm above the elbow using a circular motion.

    Rationale: Maintain a lather at all times, adding water and scrub solution as necessary.

11. **Action:** If using two brushes, discard the brush into the sink and take the second brush with the scrubbed hand. If not, rinse the brush and add scrub solution before transferring to the other hand.

    Rationale: Once one hand is scrubbed, it must not become recontaminated, otherwise the procedure must be repeated.

12. **Action:** Repeat the process for the remaining hand and forearm.

    Rationale: Use the same method to ensure that no part of the skin is missed.

13. **Action:** Maintaining the hands above the elbows, rinse both hands thoroughly and allow the water to drain into the sink.

    Rationale: Avoid getting water onto clothing because this may lead to strike-through.

14. **Action:** Wash the hands and arms again, using surgical scrub solution, but this time do not include the elbows.

    Rationale: This ensures that the hands do not come into contact with any area that has not been scrubbed.

15. **Action:** Rinse, then dry hands using a sterile towel (see following procedure).

    Rationale: Hold hands above the elbows with palms facing the chest. Do not allow the hands to touch each other.

Procedure: Drying hands after the surgical scrub (Fig. 7.2)

1. **Action:** Stand clear of any surfaces and pick up the corner of the towel with the right hand.

   Rationale: Avoid touching any surface with the sterile towel or scrubbed hands.

2. **Action:** Allow the towel to unfold without shaking it.

   Rationale: Shaking the towel will increase the risk of it touching a surface and will also circulate airborne microbes.

3. **Action:** Let the towel fall over the palm of the right hand and use the first quarter to dry the fingers, palm and back of the left hand. Dry each finger separately and ensure the interdigital areas are included.

   Rationale: The right hand is used to support the towel and dry the left hand, taking care

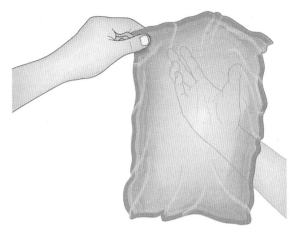

Figure 7.2 Drying hands after the surgical scrub.

not to touch the top side of the towel or come into contact with the left hand itself.

4. **Action:** Using the second quarter of the towel, dry the left forearm and elbow.

   Rationale: By using a separate quarter for each hand and arm, the degree of asepsis achieved is increased.

5. **Action:** With the dry left hand, pick up the towel by the fourth quarter, which is hanging free, and drape it over the palm of the left hand.

Rationale: The procedure followed for drying the left hand is repeated for the right hand.

6. **Action:** Dry the right fingers, palm and back of the hand with the fourth quarter and the arm and elbow with the third quarter.

   Rationale: In some cases, two towels are available. In this case, use one-third of the towel for the fingers, one-third for the palm and back of the hand and the remainder for the arm and elbow. The process is repeated for the other hand with the second towel.

7. **Action:** Discard the towel and proceed to gowning and gloving.

   Rationale: The hands must not be allowed to touch the part of the towel used to dry the arms and elbows.

THEATRE ATTIRE

In order to achieve asepsis, outdoor clothing should be replaced with specific theatre attire by all the surgical team. Whilst nothing except the surgical gown is actually sterile, the clothing acts as a barrier to microorganisms (Table 7.6).

Table 7.6 Theatre attire

Item	Description
Scrub suits	A top and trousers, worn only in the operating room. The top should be tucked into the trousers and the trousers should either have cuffed legs or be tucked into surgical boots. They should be changed daily or more often if soiled. Sterilise periodically.
Footwear	Shoes or boots designed to be non-slip, anti-static, comfortable and easily cleaned. Not to be worn outside of the theatre. Alternatively shoe covers may be used.
Headwear	Hair can be a major source of contamination, so it should be completely covered in the operating room. There are various types of theatre hats available, some paper-based designed as single use and others lint-free machine-washable.
Face masks	Face masks filter air from the nose and mouth but must be close fitting to avoid bacteria entering the surgical environment through the sides of the mask. They should be changed between operations.
Surgical gowns	Surgical gowns are sterile and worn over the scrub suit. Ideally they should be long-sleeved with cuffs. Both reusable and disposable gowns are available. Reusable gowns require the correct folding technique prior to sterilisation in order for the veterinary surgeon to put the gown on in an aseptic manner.
Surgical gloves	Surgical gloves should be worn for all surgical procedures. They come pre-packed in a variety of sizes and are sterile. Gloves without powder are recommended because the powder acts as a foreign body and may cause wound healing problems.

Procedure: Folding a surgical gown for sterilisation (Fig. 7.3)

1. **Action:** Lay the gown flat on a work surface with the inside of the gown face down.

   Rationale: In this position, all creases can be removed, ties identified and sleeves straightened. The outer surface of the gown will be folded in so that when it is put on, ungloved hands will not contaminate it.

2. **Action:** Fold one side of the gown into the centre, tucking the ties in.

   Rationale: Ties must be tucked in to avoid accidental contamination when gowning.

3. **Action:** Fold the other side of the gown right across to the other side, also tucking ties in.

   Rationale: This enables the gown to be folded neatly into a sterile pack but still unfold easily when put on.

4. **Action:** Making sure that the inside collar of the gown is on top, concertina the rest of the gown lengthways until it is the size required to fit into the sterilising pack.

   Rationale: When gowning in an aseptic manner, the gown must be picked up by the inside shoulders and allowed to gently unfold.

Another method of folding a gown ready for sterilisation is shown in Figure 7.4.

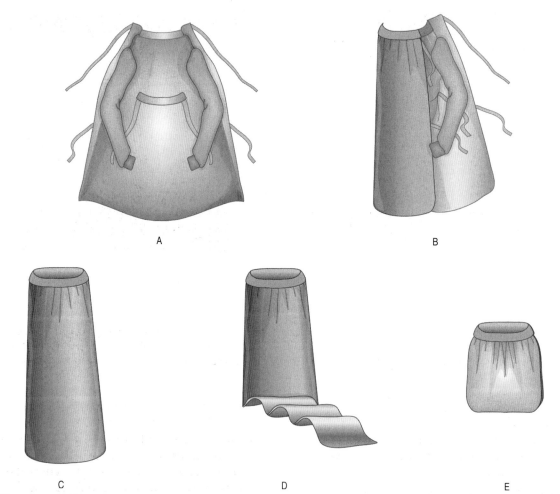

C   D   E

Figure 7.3 Folding a gown. A, Lay flat out. B, Fold side to middle. C, Fold over other side of edge. D, Concertina lengthways. E, Pick up by inside of collar after autoclaving. Redrawn from Lane and Cooper (2003), Butterworth-Heinemann.

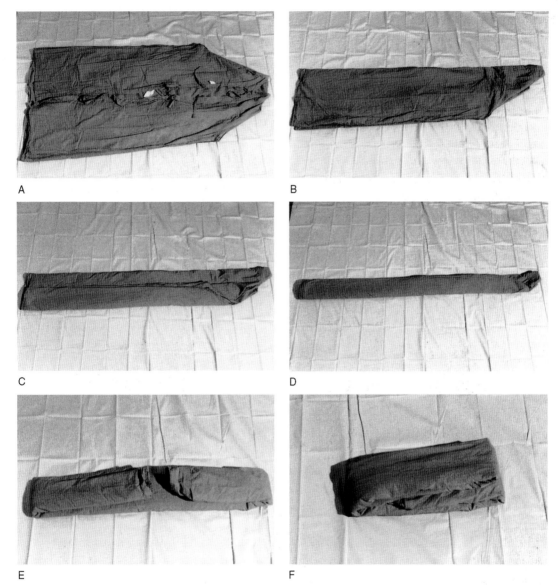

Figure 7.4   Alternative method of folding a gown. The gown in folded inside out (A), folded in half lengthways (B), folded in half lengthways again (C), and again in half lengthways (D); the top and bottom edges are folded to the middle (E), and the gown is then folded in half again (F). Reproduced, with permission, from Lane and Cooper (2003), Butterworth-Heinemann.

Procedure: Putting on a back–tying surgical gown (Fig. 7.5)

1. **Action:** Remove the sterile gown from its pack, hold by the shoulders and allow to gently unfold.

    Rationale: Holding the gown correctly allows the sleeves to be clearly identi-fied. Allowing the gown to gently unfold minimises air movement and the risk of contaminating the gown.

2. **Action:** Slip one hand into each sleeve and push up to but not through the cuff. Arms should be opened wide but no attempt to adjust the gown over the shoulders should be made.

    Rationale: Hands should remain in the sleeves of the gown to avoid contamination. Efforts

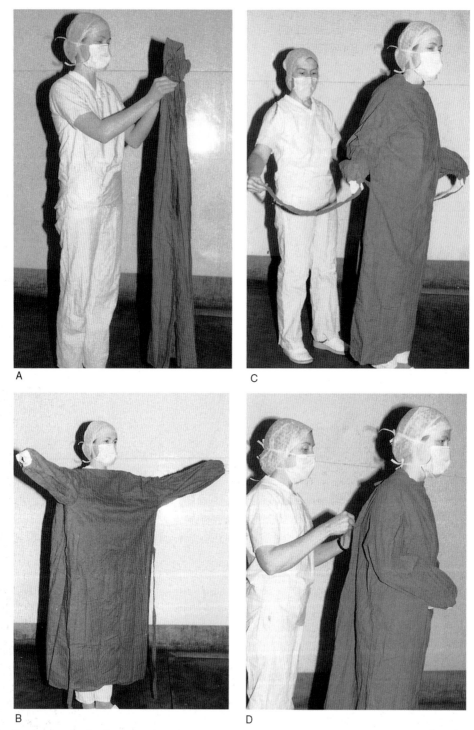

Figure 7.5   Putting on a back-tying surgical gown. Reproduced, with permission, from Lane and Cooper (2003), Butterworth-Heinemann.

to pull the gown over the shoulders create a contamination risk.

3. **Action:** An unscrubbed assistant, touching only the inside of the back of the gown, should pull the gown over the shoulders and secure the ties at the back.

   Rationale: The inside of the gown is no longer considered sterile and can therefore be handled.

4. **Action:** With hands still inside the gown sleeves, pick up the waist ties and hold them out to the sides. The assistant grasps the ends and secures them at the back taking care not to touch any part of the gown.

   Rationale: The back of the gown is now considered non-sterile and should not come into contact with any sterile equipment or drapes.

Procedure: Putting on a side-tying gown (Fig. 7.6)

1. **Action:** Follow points 1–3 above.

2. **Action:** Keeping hands within the sleeves, pass the side tie, which is attached to a paper tape, to the assistant.

   Rationale: There is no risk of contamination if the hands are kept inside the sleeves.

3. **Action:** The assistant passes the tie around the gown. Take the tie back, leaving the assistant holding the paper tape, and tie the gown at the side.

   Rationale: The assistant has not contaminated the gown because he or she has only held the paper tape. The gown is now sterile all the way around, not just at the front as with the previous method.

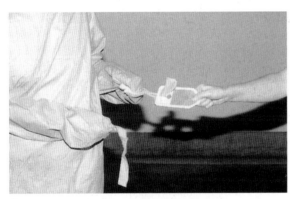

A

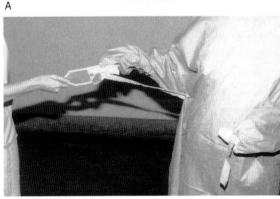

B

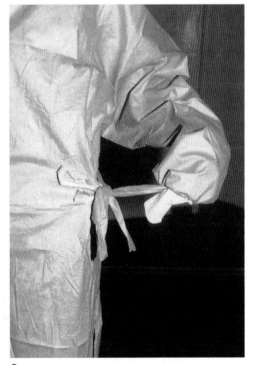

C

Figure 7.6 Putting on a side-tying surgical gown. Reproduced, with permission, from Lane and Cooper (2003), Butterworth-Heinemann.

Procedure: Closed gloving (Fig. 7.7)

1. **Action:** Keeping the hands inside the sleeves of the gown, turn the glove packet so that the fingers face towards the body.

   Rationale: The risk of contamination is minimised because the outsides of the gloves do not have the chance to come in contact with the skin.

2. **Action:** Pick up the right glove (which is on the left) by the rim of the cuff with the right hand.

   Rationale: By turning the glove packet round the right glove is on the left and vice versa.

3. **Action:** Turn the hand over so that the palm is upwards with the fingers of the glove facing towards the body (Fig. 7.7C).

   Rationale: The glove will be in the correct position to be pulled on.

4. **Action:** Using the left hand, grasp the other rim of the glove and pull it over the right hand until it covers the cuffs of the gown.

   Rationale: Both hands still remain within the sleeves of the gown to prevent contamination of the outer surface of the glove.

5. **Action:** The left hand, within the sleeve of the gown, can adjust the fingers of the right glove until comfortable.

   Rationale: The glove must fit snugly but not too tightly.

6. **Action:** Pick up the left glove with the left hand and repeat the same process.

   Rationale: At no time will the skin of the hands have come into contact with the outside of the gloves, thus minimising contamination.

Procedure: Open gloving (Fig. 7.8)

1. **Action:** Push both hands through the cuffs of the gown.

   Rationale: A disadvantage of using the open method of gloving is that the gloves may be contaminated by skin contact.

2. **Action:** With the pack of gloves facing forward, pick up the right glove with the left hand, touching only the inner folded-down surface of the glove.

   Rationale: The inside of the glove may be touched freely because it should never come into contact with other sterile items such as gown and drapes.

3. **Action:** Pull the glove onto the right hand, leaving the cuff folded back, and hook over the thumb.

   Rationale: This will avoid touching the contaminated inner surface by the gloved left hand when unfolding to cover the gown cuff.

4. **Action:** Slide the gloved fingers of the right hand under the left cuff and pull onto the left hand. Hook the thumb under the folded cuff as above.

   Rationale: Only the sterile outer surface of the glove may be touched by the gloved right hand to avoid contamination.

5. **Action:** The gloved fingers of the left hand are then slid under the fold of the right glove. Unhook the thumb and pull the folded part of the glove over the cuff of the gown.

   Rationale: By covering the cuff of the gown, no skin contact is possible thereby minimising any risk of contamination.

6. **Action:** Repeat for the left hand.

Procedure: The plunge method of gloving (Fig. 7.9)

1. **Action:** A scrubbed assistant holds the sterile glove open while the hand is inserted, whilst still in the sleeve of the sterile gown. Repeat for the second hand.

   Rationale: The high risk of contaminating both personnel involved is a disadvantage of this method and it is therefore rarely used in veterinary practice.

PREPARATION OF THE SURGICAL SITE

The skin and coat of the patient are major sources of wound contamination because it is impossible to remove all bacteria. However, careful preparation of the surgical site will minimise the risks.

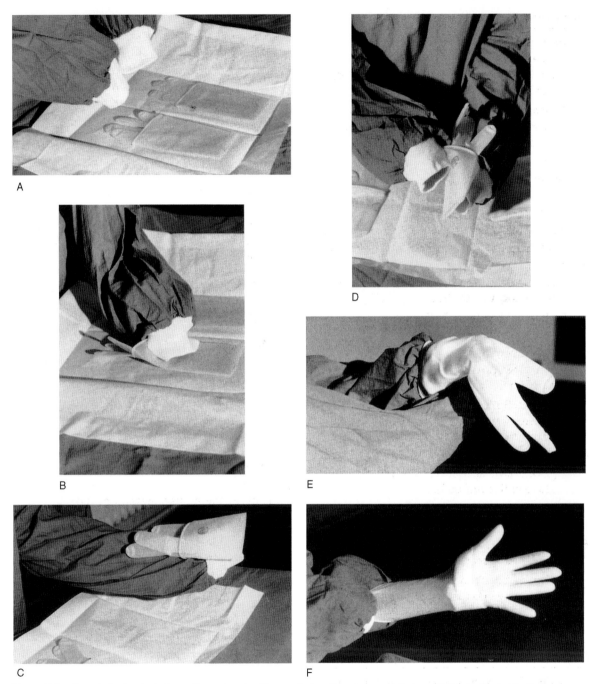

Figure 7.7 Closed gloving technique. Reproduced, with permission, from Lane and Cooper (2003), Butterworth-Heinemann.

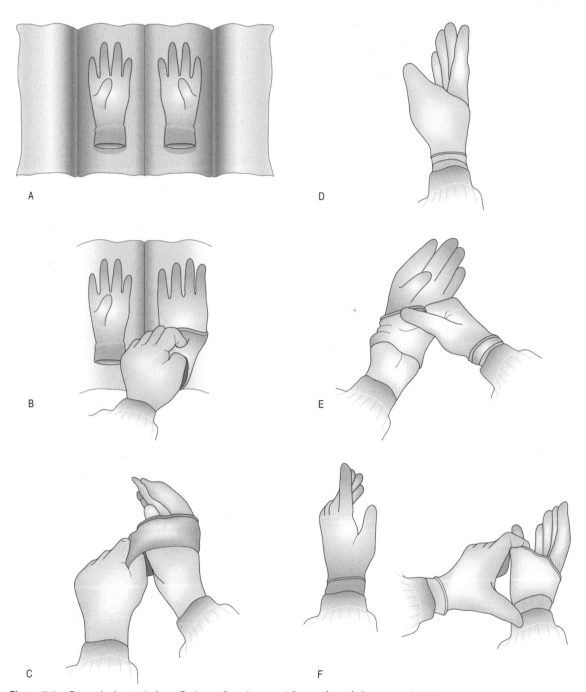

Figure 7.8 Open gloving technique. Redrawn from Lane and Cooper (2003), Butterworth-Heinemann.

Clipping the area surrounding the surgical site is best carried out with the patient anaesthetised. If the patient is considered an anaesthetic risk, clipping the patient prior to induction can reduce anaesthetic time.

Procedure: Clipping

1. **Action:** Ensure the clippers are clean and in good working order.

   Rationale: Poorly maintained clippers are more likely to nick the skin and cause irritation.

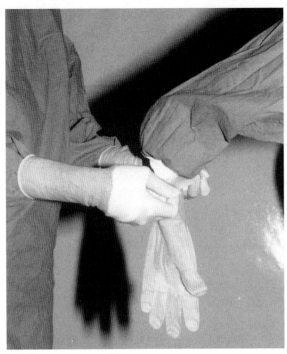

Figure 7.9 Plunge gloving method. Reproduced, with permission, from Lane and Cooper (2003), Butterworth-Heinemann.

2. **Action:** Clip with the grain of the hair first, then clip against the hair.

    Rationale: Removal of long, thick hair is easier with the grain. For a closer clip, cutting against the hair is most effective.

3. **Action:** Clip 5–15 cm beyond the line of the incision.

    Rationale: The surgeon will be able to extend the incision if necessary.

4. **Action:** Make sure all edges are neat.

    Rationale: Clients will not be impressed if the clipping is untidy.

5. **Action:** If clipping around an open wound or near the eyes, apply an appropriate gel or ointment first.

    Rationale: Tiny hairs will act as foreign bodies in an open wound and are very difficult to remove. They cause intense irritation if they get into the eye.

Procedure: Preparation of the skin

1. **Action:** Carry out steps 2–7 in the preparation area.

    Rationale: Contamination of the theatre is avoided.

2. **Action:** Put on surgical gloves – they do not need to be sterile at this stage.

    Rationale: This will protect the patient's skin from contamination by the nurse's hands and protect the hands from the antiseptic solutions.

3. **Action:** Use a chlorhexidine or povidone iodine solution.

    Rationale: They both have antiseptic and detergent properties.

4. **Action:** Use lint-free swabs.

    Rationale: They will not contaminate the site by leaving tiny particles or threads.

5. **Action:** With the 'clean' hand, select a fresh swab and pass it to the 'dirty' hand.

    Rationale: It is good practice to keep one hand 'clean' to prevent contamination of fresh swabs by the other hand, which will scrub the patient, and therefore be 'dirty'.

6. **Action:** Starting at the incision site, scrub the skin working in a circular pattern out towards the edge of the clipped area.

    Rationale: By moving in a circular pattern no area should be missed.

7. **Action:** Once the edge has been reached, discard the swab, select a fresh swab with the 'clean' hand and repeat until there is no discoloration on the swab.

    Rationale: Care must be taken not to return a 'dirty' swab to the centre of the area. The hair at the edge of the area should be included in the scrub to remove debris and flatten hair out of the way but be careful not to make the patient too wet to avoid strike-through or hypothermia.

8. **Action:** Transfer the patient to the theatre and position for surgery.

    Rationale: The site is likely to have become contaminated in the move.

9. **Action:** Wearing sterile gloves and using sterile swabs and water, repeat the scrub procedure described above.

    Rationale: Sterile equipment is used to create an environment that is as aseptic as possible.

10. **Action:** The final skin preparation is carried out by a member of the surgical team, again using sterile swabs, this time held by Rampley sponge-holding forceps. An alcoholic solution of skin disinfectant is applied and left to dry on the skin.

    Rationale: The alcohol solution will remove any remaining detergent and provide residual bactericidal activity. Do not apply to open wounds or mucous membranes. Do not use diathermy if an alcohol solution has been applied.

DRAPING THE PATIENT

The patient is draped to maintain asepsis during surgery. The entire patient must be covered leaving just the surgical area exposed. In order to maintain asepsis, a member of the surgical team who is gowned and gloved carries out the draping (Table 7.7).

PACKING DRAPES FOR STERILISATION

When preparing a drape for sterilisation, the aim is to ensure that all parts are sterilised evenly and when the drape is handled by the surgical team it will unfold easily. This can be achieved by either folding the drape in a concertina fashion or folding it corner to corner. Both methods are illustrated in Figure 7.10.

When folding a fenestrated drape, it is important to use a similar method to that for a plain drape but the fenestration should end up on top of the drape so it can be clearly identified in the sterilisation packaging.

Procedure: Draping with four plain drapes (Fig. 7.11)

1. **Action:** Pick up the first drape and allow it to unfold away from the trolley or table.

    Rationale: The sterile drape must not be allowed to become contaminated by touching a non-sterile area.

2. **Action:** Fold back the edge of the drape underneath itself. This will line the edge of the incision.

Table 7.7 Types of drape

Drape	Advantages	Disadvantages	Comments
Disposable	Water resistant Pre-packed and folded Pre-sterilised Will prevent strike-through Lint free Always in perfect condition	Expensive Less conforming Large stock required Less accurate fenestration size	Can be used under or over a cloth drape Ideal for surgery where fluid is likely to be present Can be secured with sterile spray or may be self-adhesive
Reusable	Cheaper Conforming Required size fenestration using four plain drapes	Porous, which can lead to strike-through Labour intensive: washing and drying Become poor quality with repeated use Require an autoclave with an effective drying cycle	Secured to the skin with towel clips: if the tips puncture the cloth they are no longer sterile and must be replaced

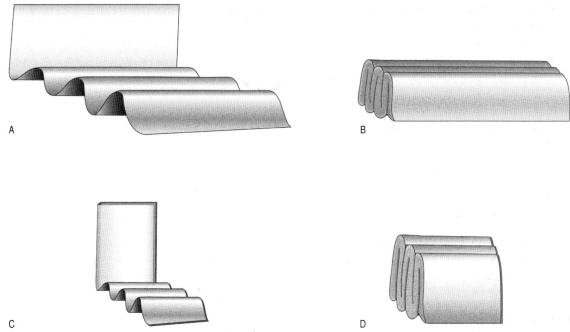

A

B

C

D

Figure 7.10 Folding surgical drapes. A, Concertina cloth widthways (B). C, concertina lengthways. D, Pack cloths in autoclave drum or autoclave bags sealed with indicating tape. Redrawn from Lane and Cooper (2003), Butterworth-Heinemann.

Rationale: This will produce a double layer at the edge of the draped area protecting it from strike-through.

3. **Action:** Hold the drape along the folded edge with the hands inside the drape.

Rationale: This will prevent the hands from touching the patient when the drape is placed.

4. **Action:** Apply the first drape on the surgeon's side.

Rationale: This prevents contamination of the surgeon when leaning over the patient to place the subsequent drapes.

5. **Action:** Place the second drape on the opposite side to the first drape.

Rationale: The surgeon may place this drape by leaning across the patient, or the assistant may place it from their side.

6. **Action:** The third and fourth drapes are placed at either end of the surgical site.

Rationale: They can be placed in any order.

7. **Action:** Apply further drapes to cover any remaining exposed areas of the patient or table.

Rationale: It is very important to cover the patient, the entire table and the area between the surgical site and instrument trolley.

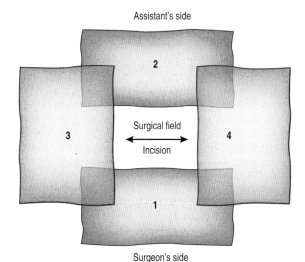

Figure 7.11 Draping with four plain drapes. Redrawn from Moore (1999), BSAVA.

8. **Action:** Place a towel clip diagonally across each corner with one tip on each drape. Secure by picking up a small fold of skin.

   Rationale: Care must be taken not to contaminate the clips by piercing the drape.

9. **Action:** Cover the clips with the corner of each drape.

   Rationale: This will stop the clips getting accidentally caught and pulled.

Procedure: Draping a limb (Fig. 7.12)

1. **Action:** Cover the lower part of the limb with a bandage and hold it upright. It may either be held by an assistant or secured to a drip stand.

   Rationale: The lower part of the limb is a source of contamination. The limb is held

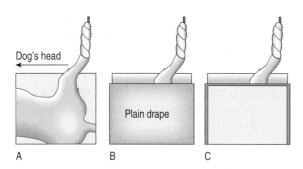

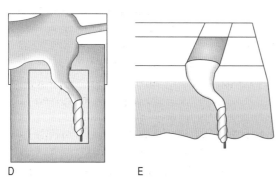

Figure 7.12 Draping a limb for surgery. A, The lower limb is bandaged and attached by tape to a transfusion stand; B, a plain drape is laid over the body and the opposite limb of the patient; C, a smaller plain drape is laid on top of this; D, the tape is then cut and the limb lowered onto the inner drape; E, the drape is carefully wrapped around the limb and secured with a towel clip. Plain drapes or a fenestrated drape is then applied over the surgical site.

upright to allow further drapes to be placed.

2. **Action:** Place a plain drape over the rest of the body and the opposite limb of the patient.

   Rationale: This reduces the risk of contamination from the rest of the body.

3. **Action:** Place a smaller drape on top of the initial drape and lower the limb.

   Rationale: The limb should only be in contact with the second drape.

4. **Action:** Wrap the second drape around the limb and secure with a towel clip.

   Rationale: The limb now has two layers covering it to avoid it contaminating the surgical area.

5. **Action:** Further drapes are placed around the surgical site.

   Rationale: The patient should now be fully draped with only the surgical site visible.

Procedure: Draping with a fenestrated drape

1. **Action:** Pick up the drape and allow it to unfold away from the trolley or table.

   Rationale: Avoid touching anything that will break the sterility of the drape. If asepsis is broken, discard the drape and start again with a new one.

2. **Action:** Hold the drape along the edge with hands inside the drape.

   Rationale: The hands must not touch the patient's skin or coat.

3. **Action:** Looking through the fenestration, place the drape over the surgical site.

   Rationale: If the fenestration is too large, apply further plain drapes over the top to reduce it. If the fenestration is too small, discard the drape and start again with a fresh one.

4. **Action:** Secure the drape with towel clips at each corner.

   Rationale: The clips cannot be concealed under the drape and are therefore more likely to get caught on instruments during surgery.

INSTRUMENTATION

PREPARATION OF THE INSTRUMENT TROLLEY

The instrument trolley can be prepared by the scrub nurse or by the circulating nurse using Cheatle forceps. It should be prepared immediately prior to use and if there is a delay in the start of surgery, the instruments must be covered with a sterile drape to minimise the risk of contamination from the environment.

The top of the instrument trolley will not be sterile. It should be covered with a waterproof sterile drape, to prevent bacterial strike-through in the event that the trolley gets wet, followed by a cloth drape. It is common to pack instruments within a waterproof drape and cloth drape, which can then be unfolded to cover the base of the trolley. Where instruments are taken from multi-use sterilisation drums, two layers of cloth drapes are necessary.

Procedure: Draping a trolley using Cheatle forceps

1. **Action:** Pick up the pairs of Cheatle forceps, one in each hand, using the thumb and ring finger with the tips of the forceps pointing down.

    Rationale: The middle two fingers of each hand can then be used to support the forceps.

2. **Action:** Using one of the forceps to steady the drape, open the other forceps and pick the drape up keeping it folded.

    Rationale: If the drape is allowed to unfold too soon, it is likely to touch a non-sterile surface and become contaminated.

3. **Action:** Move away from any surfaces. With the free forceps, grasp one corner of the drape and with arms held out in front, remove the first forceps and allow the drape to gently unfold.

    Rationale: It is essential to stand clear of anything that may contaminate the drape including yourself. The drape must not be shaken unfolded as this increases the air movement and risk of contamination.

4. **Action:** Select the adjacent corner with the other forceps, straighten the drape and carefully pass it behind the instrument trolley so the trolley is between you and the drape.

    Rationale: Draping the trolley towards you prevents contamination from your clothing because you do not have to lean over the trolley to place the drape.

5. **Action:** Gently bring the drape towards you, covering the trolley. When the trolley is covered, release the drape before your arms drop below waist level.

    Rationale: If you allow the Cheatle forceps to drop below waist level there is an increased risk of touching a non-sterile surface.

6. **Action:** Return the Cheatle forceps to their sterile container.

    Rationale: Whilst the handles of the forceps are non-sterile, the tips must remain sterile or be discarded.

Procedure: Laying out an instrument trolley

1. **Action:** Identify the instruments and equipment required for the surgical procedure to be carried out.

    Rationale: Having all equipment prepared in advance can reduce surgery time and therefore anaesthetic time.

2. **Action:** Place the instruments onto the trolley in order of use from left to right.

    Rationale: This enables the surgeon or scrub nurse to select the required instrument quickly and efficiently.

3. **Action:** Place a sterile drape over the trolley until it is ready to be used.

    Rationale: The risk of environmental contamination is minimised.

ASSISTING DURING SURGERY

Throughout a surgical procedure there should ideally be two nurses assisting – one acting as a circulating nurse, the other as a scrub nurse. The circulating nurse, whilst in a scrub suit, is not gowned and gloved. The scrub nurse is gowned and gloved in order to assist the surgeon during the procedure. Their individual roles are as follows:

The circulating nurse

- Assist in the preparation of the theatre, instruments and equipment
- Adjust and tie the gowns of the surgical team
- Position the patient on the operating table
- Prepare the surgical site
- Connect equipment such as diathermy and suction
- Unwrap suture material and extra equipment required
- Record suture material and swabs used
- Assist the anaesthetist if required
- Prepare and apply postoperative dressings when necessary
- Maintain the cleanliness of the theatre in readiness for the next procedure.

The scrub nurse

- Prepare the instrument trolley
- Pass instruments to the surgeon as required
- Swabbing as required
- Removing soiled instruments or swabs from the surgical area
- Retract tissue and cut sutures when required
- Counting swabs, needles and sutures as they are used and at the end of surgery.

Procedure: Handling and passing instruments

1. **Action:** Identify the procedure being performed.

    Rationale: The surgeon's instrument requirements can then be anticipated.

2. **Action:** Instruments should be pressed firmly into the surgeon's hand so they are ready for use.

    Rationale: The surgeon will not have to look away from the surgical site.

3. **Action:** Pass ringed instruments into the palm with the points outwards and curves upwards.

Rationale: The instrument is then ready for use and sharp points or blades will not damage the surgical gloves.

4. **Action:** Dissecting forceps and the scalpel are passed into a finger grip.

    Rationale: The instruments are ready for use.

5. **Action:** After use, clean with a swab and replace in the same position back onto the trolley.

    Rationale: Instruments not in use should not be left to clutter the surgical site. If they are returned to the correct position on the trolley they can quickly be found next time they are required

Procedure: Swabbing

1. **Action:** Count all swabs before and during surgery.

    Rationale: It is essential to keep a record of all swabs used and a close watch kept on their whereabouts.

2. **Action:** Use the swabs to blot the viscera.

    Rationale: Do not wipe the blood away, otherwise clots which are forming to control the haemorrhage will be removed, and bleeding may begin again.

3. **Action:** Dispose of used swabs into a bowl.

    Rationale: Do not leave them on the trolley or at the surgical site because they may dampen the drapes and allow bacterial strike-through.

4. **Action:** Count all swabs before the incision is closed.

    Rationale: They should equal the total number used during the procedure. This ensures that none is accidentally left in the wound.

CARE AND MAINTENANCE OF SURGICAL INSTRUMENTS

Surgical instruments are commonly made of either chromium-plated carbon steel or stainless steel. Tungsten carbide inserts are often added to the tips of stainless steel instruments because it improves their hardness and resistance to wear. Instruments with tungsten carbide inserts are identified by their gold-coloured handles.

Good quality instruments are costly but will last for many years if they are handled correctly and maintained properly. New instruments require lubricating prior to use.

Procedure: Cleaning and maintaining instruments

1. **Action:** In accordance with the COSHH regulations, protective clothing such as rubber gloves and an apron must be worn.

   Rationale: The risk of contamination by blood or tissue from a patient with a possible zoonotic disease is minimised.

2. **Action:** Remove instruments from the theatre as soon as surgery is complete.

   Rationale: This minimises the risk of contaminating the fresh set of instruments prepared for the next surgical procedure.

3. **Action:** Remove and dispose of any sharp items such as needles, scalpel blades or glass vials.

   Rationale: These should be placed into sharps containers or glass bins as appropriate.

4. **Action:** Remove any packaging, swabs or suture material.

   Rationale: Dispose of these in the clinical waste.

5. **Action:** Separate any delicate equipment.

   Rationale: This should be cleaned separately to avoid damage.

6. **Action:** Rinse the instruments in cold water to remove blood and tissue as soon as possible.

   Rationale: Blood allowed to dry onto the instruments will lead to pitting of the surface. Hot water should not be used because it causes coagulation of proteins.

7. **Action:** Soak the instruments in warm water containing a specified instrument-cleaning agent.

   Rationale: Dismantle instruments and open box joints and ratchets to free all debris.

8. **Action:** Using a small brush, scrub each instrument under running water, paying particular attention to serrations, joints and ratchets.

   Rationale: Debris may become trapped.

9. **Action:** The instruments may be put into an ultrasonic cleaner after manual cleaning, then thoroughly rinsed.

   Rationale: Ultrasonic cleaners are very efficient at removing debris that is inaccessible to manual cleaning.

10. **Action:** Dry the instruments thoroughly.

    Rationale: Water left in joints and ratchets may lead to corrosion.

11. **Action:** Inspect each instrument for damage, non-alignment of the tips or jaws, stiff hinges, bent ratchets, pitting, corrosion and loose screws.

    Rationale: If any faults are identified, the instrument must be removed from the kit and either repaired or replaced.

12. **Action:** Lubricate the instruments with a suitable instrument lubricant.

    Rationale: The life of the instruments will be prolonged, especially those with joints and ratchets.

13. **Action:** Package ready for sterilisation.

    Rationale: Cover sharp points, identify the instrument and date the pack.

SURGICAL KITS

It is common practice to have a number of surgical kits made up ready for use. Each kit should be clearly identified as to its contents so the correct instruments can be prepared for surgery. Colour-coded autoclavable plastic tape is often used to identify all the instruments belonging to the same kit. Figure 7.13 illustrates some instruments commonly found in general kits.

Although surgical kits will vary according to surgeon preference, some guidelines for general kits are set out below.

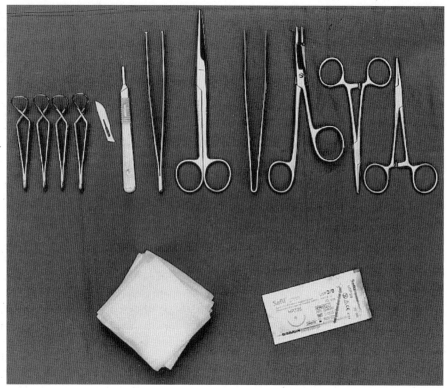

Figure 7.13   Commonly used instruments: a basic suturing kit. Top (left to right): towel clips, scalpel blade and handle, rat-tooth forceps, Mayo scissors, dressing forceps, Gillies needle holders, Spencer Wells forceps. Bottom (left to right): swabs, suture materials. Reproduced, with permission, from Bowden and Masters (2001), Butterworth-Heinemann.

General surgical kit

- Scalpel handle
- Rat-tooth forceps
- Dressing forceps
- Mayo scissors
- Metzenbaum scissors
- 4 × large Spencer Wells artery forceps
- 4 × small Spencer Wells artery forceps
- 2 × Allis tissue forceps
- Gelpi self-retaining retractors
- Langenbeck hand-held retractors
- 4 × Backhaus towel clips
- Needle holders.

This kit would be suitable for laparotomy, gastrotomy, tumour removal, ovariohysterectomy, pyometra, orchidectomy, Caesarean section, hernia or rupture repair.

General eye kit

- Small scalpel handle
- Eyelid retractors
- Micro-corneal forceps
- Micro-dissecting forceps
- Ophthalmic scissors
- Capsular forceps
- Irrigating cannula
- Iris repositor
- Castroviejo needle holders.

This kit would be suitable for enucleation, entropion or ectropion, removal of eyelid tumours, conjunctival flap, distichiasis.

Orthopaedic pinning kit

- Scalpel handle
- Rat-tooth forceps
- Dressing forceps

- Mayo scissors
- 4 × Spencer Wells artery forceps
- 4 × Mosquito artery forceps
- 2 × Allis tissue forceps
- 2 × Hohmann hand-held retractors
- Gelpi self-retaining retractors
- Selection of Steinmann pins
- Jacobs chuck and key
- Orthopaedic ruler
- Hacksaw and blade
- Pin cutters
- Needle holders.

CARE OF SPECIALIST EQUIPMENT

1. Diathermy

Diathermy is used to either cut or coagulate tissues. Unlike electrocautery, which uses an electric current to create a red-hot probe that is applied to the tissue, diathermy relies on alternating high-frequency currents to produce local heat within the tissue at the site of application. It is applied to control haemorrhage and decrease surgical time.

Monopolar or bipolar electrodes can be used to apply diathermy. Monopolar diathermy is used for cutting and coagulation and requires the patient to be 'earthed'. Bipolar diathermy allows more control over the depth and location of coagulation. It does not require the patient to be earthed and it cannot be used for cutting.

Procedure: Preparation of diathermy equipment

1. **Action:** Prepare the diathermy machine by placing a contact plate in a suitable position on the operating table. The plate should be connected to the diathermy machine by a wire.

   Rationale: This is done to 'earth' the patient. Contact gel can be applied to the plate before the patient is placed onto it. Alternatively a rectal probe can be used. The current is transferred via the plate or probe to the ground. Electrical burns to the patient will then be avoided.

2. **Action:** Select the required electrodes.

   Rationale: The cutting electrode can be a flat blade, scalpel blade or wire. A flat blade,

ball electrode or dissecting forceps can be used to achieve coagulation diathermy. Dissecting forceps grasp the tissue and the current is applied by touching the forceps with the electrode.

3. **Action:** Do not prepare the surgical site with alcohol-based surgical solution.

   Rationale: Do not use any inflammable material such as alcohol in conjunction with diathermy as there is a risk of fire.

4. **Action:** Follow the manufacturer's instructions regarding sterilisation, maintenance and operation of the unit.

   Rationale: Some parts such as the handles and attachments can usually be sterilised.

2. Cryosurgery

Cryosurgery is used to kill cells within a specific area with minimal damage to surrounding healthy tissue. This is achieved by the application of controlled extreme cold, which eventually destroys the cells. The cells are damaged by the effects of freezing and later die.

Procedure: Preparation for cryosurgery

1. **Action:** Wear protective clothing: apron, goggles and thick gloves. Avoid splashing yourself.

   Rationale: Liquid nitrogen can cause severe cold burns.

2. **Action:** Do not touch any metal surfaces that have been cooled by liquid nitrogen.

   Rationale: Again, severe cold burns may occur.

3. **Action:** Select a suitable refrigerant – generally liquid nitrogen

   Rationale: A suitable container must be used to store the liquid nitrogen.

4. **Action:** Prepare the surgical site by clipping and cleaning the area.

   Rationale: Surface lesions do not require asepsis. Normal aseptic procedures should, however, be carried out for deeper lesions.

5. **Action:** Protect the surrounding healthy tissue.

Rationale: Apply petroleum jelly or polystyrene to protect healthy tissue from the effects of the freezing.

6. **Action:** Select the correct size probe for the procedure to be carried out.

    Rationale: The most efficient method of applying cryosurgery is under pressure by a spray using a hollow probe.

7. **Action:** Apply the probe to the area and then remove it before applying it again. This cycle must be repeated for optimum effect.

    Rationale: Temperatures below $-20\,°C$ rapidly freeze the tissues. Slow thawing occurs when the probe is removed. The patient may be required to have cryosurgery a number of times before the targeted cells are killed.

8. **Action:** Discuss postoperative care with the client: daily cleaning of the area is necessary, there may be skin sloughing, and a slight discharge, erythema and oedema often occur in the first 24 hours; hair-covered areas may heal with unpigmented hair.

    Rationale: These points should be discussed with the owner prior to surgery commencing. If the patient is a show animal, the change in hair-colour at the affected site could be a problem.

9. **Action:** Wash the probe in mild detergent, gently rubbing discoloured areas.

    Rationale: A build-up of debris, particularly on the tip of the probe, can lead to corrosive deposits building up which damage the probe.

10. **Action:** Do not use corrosive or abrasive solutions.

    Rationale: These cause thinning of the metal components.

11. **Action:** Follow manufacturer's instructions. Some probes may be sterilised.

    Rationale: Not all cryosurgery units can be sterilised.

3. Endoscopes

Endoscopy is the non-invasive visual examination of the interior of a body cavity. A light source is combined with a series of optical lenses and mirrors to create a delicate, expensive instrument.

Two types of endoscope are used in veterinary practice – rigid and flexible. The flexible endoscopes may be fibreoptic or video endoscopes. Fibreoptic endoscopes contain glass-fibre bundles and, although flexible, they are brittle and care must be taken not to break the individual strands.

Procedure: Cleaning an endoscope

1. **Action:** Clean the endoscope immediately after use.

    Rationale: If left covered in dirt, the endoscope will be more difficult to clean and will deteriorate due to the presence of dried blood and mucus.

2. **Action:** Never immerse an endoscope in liquid unless the manufacturer's instructions specifically state that you can. Do not autoclave or place in a hot-air oven.

    Rationale: Considerable damage will occur to the delicate control section or light connector if liquid enters them.

3. **Action:** With the light source still attached, connect the water bottle and suction pump.

    Rationale: Follow manufacturer's instructions.

4. **Action:** Prepare the recommended disinfectant.

    Rationale: Approximately 1 litre is required.

5. **Action:** With the tip of the endoscope in the solution, aspirate by depressing the suction button.

    Rationale: This ensures that patency is maintained.

6. **Action:** Clean the biopsy valve with a cotton bud and the biopsy channel with a specific cleaning brush, then clear rinse using suction.

    Rationale: This area must be cleaned thoroughly to remove any traces of tissue.

7. **Action:** Disconnect the water bottle, block the water inlet and blow all the water out of the channel by depressing the water/air button.

Rationale: Water must not be left in here as it leads to deterioration of the working parts.

8. **Action:** Wipe the insertion tube with lint-free swabs dampened with disinfectant. Rinse with clear water.

   Rationale: Swabs must be lint-free to avoid leaving tiny threads.

9. **Action:** Wipe the light guide tube with dampened swabs.

   Rationale: Remove any residual disinfectant.

10. **Action:** Apply an alcohol solution to the ocular lens and clean carefully.

    Rationale: The alcohol will evaporate quickly without leaving smears.

11. **Action:** Dry the endoscope thoroughly by hanging it up on a secure hook.

    Rationale: Any residual liquid will run downwards away from the controls.

12. **Action:** Store in a carrying case or cabinet.

    Rationale: This will protect the endoscope from damage.

REFERENCES AND FURTHER READING

Aspinall V 2006 The Complete Textbook of Veterinary Nursing. Elsevier, Oxford

Bowden C, Masters J 2001 Quick Reference Guide to Veterinary Surgical Kits. Butterworth-Heinemann, Oxford

Lane D R, Cooper B (eds) 2003 Veterinary Nursing. Butterworth-Heinemann, Oxford

Moore M (ed) 1999 Manual of Veterinary Nursing. BSAVA, Gloucester

Simpson G (ed) 1991 Practical Veterinary Nursing. BSAVA, Gloucester.

Chapter 8

Surgical nursing procedures

Trish Scorer

CHAPTER CONTENTS

Introduction 163

Wound management 164
Bandaging techniques – general points 167
Individual bandaging techniques 168
Robert Jones bandage 168
Velpeau sling 168
Ehmer sling 169
Ear bandage 172
Chest bandage 172
Limb bandage 173
Tail bandage 174
Splinting a limb 176
Casting using plaster of Paris 176
Drainage systems 177
Use of the Penrose drain 177
Fracture management 178
First aid procedure in a case of a suspected
   fracture 178
Suturing techniques 180
Simple interrupted skin suture 180
Biopsy techniques 181
Fine needle aspiration 181
Punch biopsy 183
Dentistry 183
Scaling and polishing the teeth 183

INTRODUCTION

After the diagnosis and treatment of a patient's condition has been completed by the veterinary surgeon it is often the task of the veterinary nurse to dress and bandage the affected area. Depending on the site and type of wound, the aim of bandaging is to cover and protect the area from contamination and the risk of infection and to prevent the patient from interfering with the wound, both of which will delay the rate of healing. Bandaging is also used to immobilise fractured or dislocated bones to reduce discomfort and accelerate healing.

Many wounds will not require bandaging and in some cases a bandage may draw the patient's attention to the area, leading to self-mutilation. This must be considered when deciding whether or not to apply a bandage. In all cases the wound must be cleaned and dressed and the patient placed under observation. At first this may be done by the nurse, and later, when the patient goes home, the owner must be instructed as to how to deal with the wound and the warning signs to watch out for.

This chapter describes the steps involved in wound care and in the various types of bandage. It also covers biopsy techniques and the correct method of scaling and polishing an animal's teeth – a procedure that is often performed by the veterinary nurse.

Procedure: Wound management

1. **Action:** Place the animal in a comfortable position on a table.

    Rationale: If the animal feels uncomfortable it will try to escape.

2. **Action:** Ask an assistant to restrain the animal so that it is relaxed but secure and the wound is accessible for treatment.

    Rationale: The assistant will be able to react quickly should the animal try to escape. The animal may resent the wound being touched.

3. **Action:** Wash your hands with a surgical scrub.

    Rationale: It is important not to introduce infection into the wound.

4. **Action:** Control any haemorrhage. (Refer to Control of haemorrhage procedure in Chapter 9).

    Rationale: Any bleeding should be controlled as a large loss of blood may cause shock.

5. **Action:** Check for signs of shock and treat. (Refer to Treatment of shock procedure in Chapter 9).

    Rationale: If left untreated the animal's condition will deteriorate.

6. **Action:** Assess the type of wound and treat accordingly (Table 8.1).

    Rationale: Different types of wound need different treatment, dressings and aftercare. A general anaesthetic/sedative may be needed.

7. **Action:** For open wounds, fill wound with a sterile lubricant and clip hair away from around the wound.

    Rationale: The lubricant prevents hair from contaminating the wound. The hair is clipped to allow the area to be cleaned aseptically.

8. **Action:** Clean the area surrounding the wound with a surgical scrub and warm water. Clean the wound by lavage with warm, sterile saline in a 20 ml syringe with a 20G needle. Continue until all debris has been flushed away.

    Rationale: Cleaning the wound in this way will provide enough pressure to remove contamination, without damaging the cells.

9. **Action:** Assess the blood supply to the wound. If necessary, debride the wound by using a scalpel blade to remove necrotic tissue and restore blood supply.

    Rationale: Necrotic tissue must be removed. The area must have a good blood supply to start the healing process.

10. **Action:** Close the wound if necessary (Table 8.1). Suturing techniques are covered later in this chapter.

    Rationale: First intention wound healing occurs when the edges of the wound are held together. Second intention or granulation is the healing of an open wound.

11. **Action:** Apply a light dry dressing to first intention wounds. A secondary and tertiary layer may be applied for protection (Tables 8.2. and 8.3).

    Rationale: This will absorb any blood or exudate produced by the wound and protect the wound from infection, trauma and patient interference.

12. **Action:** For second intention wounds, use a moist dressing that will not dry out the wound. The use of a hydrogel applied to the wound before the primary layer is applied is recommended. Apply a secondary and tertiary layer.

    Rationale: A moist dressing will provide the correct environment to promote a healthy bed for granulation and re-epithelialisation. The secondary layer absorbs any exudate and provides support. The tertiary layer acts as a protective outer layer, holding the others in place.

13. **Action:** Ensure that the dressing is comfortable and that the patient will not interfere with it.

    Rationale: Reasons for interference include the bandage being too tight resulting in poor circulation, pain, sutures being too tight, and boredom. An Elizabethan collar, topical sprays or supervised muzzling may be used.

Table 8.1   Wound classification

Type	Comments	Treatment
Open wounds:	There is a break in the covering of the body surface	
Incised	Skin edges are clean and clearly defined. The cut edges may bleed freely. The wound will heal quickly, by first intention. Caused by sharp, cutting materials, e.g. scalpel or glass	Ensure that deeper structures are not damaged before closing the wound. Hold edges together with sutures
Laceration	The wound is irregular in shape, with possible tissue loss. There may be little blood loss. Risk of infection is high. The wound will heal by second intention, with possible scarring	Assess the wound, i.e. is any skin available for closure/partial closure by suturing? Dress the wound
Puncture	Surface wound is small with a deep track running down from it. The surface wound will heal quickly, trapping bacteria and causing an abscess to form. Common causes are bites, air gun pellets and thorns	Remove the cause of the injury. The wound must be kept open to allow infection to escape and granulation tissue to develop at the bottom of the tract. Application of a warm compress or poultice will encourage this
Abrasion	The epidermis has been rubbed off, exposing the dermis. Can be painful as nerve endings are exposed. Although not serious, there is a risk of contamination	Clean and dress the wound with a moist dressing
Abscess	A collection of pus enclosed in an area of inflamed tissue. Commonly results from a puncture wound	The abscess must be lanced (unless already burst), but only when it is 'pointing'. This is the thinning of the skin over the abscess, indicating a point which can be lanced. Placing a warm compress on the area will encourage this. Using a scalpel blade at 90°, incise the wound. Express the pus. Flush the wound with sterile saline until clear. Keep the wound open and continue to flush daily. The wound will heal by second intention
Avulsion	Forceful separation of the tissue from its attachment. Commonly seen in wounds associated with road traffic accidents and dog fights	Assess the wound – is there any free and healthy skin available for closure or partial closure by suturing? Assess whether the patient has suffered any internal damage. Infection may be present and the wound may need to be drained during the healing process. Dress the wound according the degree of damage
Degloving and shearing	Similar to an avulsed wound but with loss of blood to an area resulting in sloughing of the tissue. There may be damage to underlying organs or bones	Assess the wound – is there any free and healthy skin available for closure or partial closure by suturing? A skin graft may be an option. Assess whether the patient has suffered any internal damage. Infection may be present and the wound may need to be drained during the healing process. Dress the wound according the degree of damage

(Continued)

Table 8.1 Wound classification—Cont'd

Type	Comments	Treatment
Closed wounds:	The injury does not penetrate the thickness of the skin	
Contusion	A bruise. Occurs when blood vessels are ruptured due to a blow to the skin surface. May be seen in an open wound	Arrest the internal haemorrhage by applying a cold compress
Haematoma	A collection of blood under the skin causing swelling. The wound is soft and often painless. If left the blood will clot, contract and become 'knobbly'	Arrest the internal haemorrhage by applying a cold compress, and if possible, apply a firm dressing. Surgical intervention may be necessary to drain the haematoma
Other types:		
Skin graft	A portion of skin is taken from one area of the body to fill a deficit in another part. There are two types: a *pedicle graft* involves moving the entire skin thickness to another area. This heals by first intention; a *free skin* graft moves the epidermis and part or all of the dermis. This heals by second intention	Dress according to type
Ulcer	A local excavation of the surface of an organ or tissue. An ulcer contains inflammatory exudate within a crater. This heals by second intention	Remove the cause of the injury, dress with a moist dressing if anatomically possible. Treat bacterial infections
Tumour	Any abnormal swelling in or on part of the body that has no physiological use. May be benign or malignant	Before treatment the type of tumour must be identified. Surgical intervention is often necessary
Fistula	A tract that passes from one skin surface to another and is lined with epithelial cells. Common sites are anal sacs as a result of infection, retrovaginal as a congenital abnormality, and oronasally as a result of extraction of the upper canines	Treatment depends on the site. Surgical intervention may be required
Sinus	A blind ending tract that runs from the skin surface to deep within a tissue. Often results from infection. Commonly caused by penetrating foreign bodies and anal furunculosis	Remove foreign bodies surgically. Anal furunculosis may be treated by surgery, cryosurgery or by the use of immunosuppressant drugs
Hernia	A hole within a muscular wall which allows the passage of organs through it. May result in strangulation of the blood flow to the organs, which can become ischaemic and/or necrotic. Common sites are umbilical, inguinal and perineal	Surgical treatment to replace the organs and remove damaged tissue
Rupture	A tear within a muscular wall. Most commonly seen within the diaphragm following a road traffic accident	Treat for shock and relieve pressure on the chest cavity by lifting the chest higher than the abdomen. Close the diaphragmatic tear surgically when the patient is stable

Table 8.2 Wound dressings

Type	Comments
The primary layer of a bandage is usually a wound dressing which gives the wound the optimum conditions for healing. Materials which can be used for this layer are:	
Lint and gauze	A dry, non-sterile dressing. Can be autoclaved. Soft and absorbent but 'old fashioned'. Can be soaked in Hartmann's solution and used to debride wounds
Gamgee	A cotton wool sheet covered on each side by gauze. Dry and non-sterile
Petroleum gauze	A moist dressing. Gauze impregnated with petroleum jelly. Inhibits epithelial growth
Perforated film dressing, e.g. Melolin	A dry, sterile dressing. Commonly used for surgical wounds (first intention healing). Can be used to debride a larger wound by allowing the necrotic tissue to stick to it and removing it at dressing change. A painful way of debridement
Foam dressing, e.g. Allevyn	A dry, sterile dressing. Good absorbency
Hydrogels, e.g. Intrasite, Biodres	A moist gel applied into and onto the wound. Designed to promote debridement and granulation and reduces bacterial contamination
Hydrocolloids, e.g. Granuflex, Tegasorb	A moist, sterile dressing that rehydrates the wound and promotes debridement and granulation
Alginates, e.g. Kaltostat	A moist, sterile dressing derived from seaweed. A gel is formed over the wound which promotes wound healing
Semi-permeable film dressing, e.g. opsite, Bioclusive, Tegaderm	A sterile film dressing which retains moisture within the wound. No absorbency but can be left in place for longer periods
Poultice	A dry dressing which is soaked in hot water and applied to a wound to draw out infection from the wound

14. **Action:** Explain the aftercare of the wound and dressing to the owner.

    Rationale: Protect from wet and dirt by covering with a bag. Observe for patient interference, odour, sores, discharge and slipping. Change the dressing when advised.

Procedure: Bandaging techniques – general points

1. **Action:** Prepare all equipment necessary for the type of bandage.

    Rationale: This will save time and allow you to complete the bandage without leaving the animal.

2. **Action:** Place the animal in a comfortable position on a table.

    Rationale: If the animal feels uncomfortable it will try to escape.

3. **Action:** Ask an assistant to restrain the animal so that it is relaxed but secure, and the area for bandaging is accessible.

    Rationale: The assistant will be able to react quickly should the animal try to escape. The animal may resent the wound being touched.

4. **Action:** Apply a primary dressing to any wounds (Table 8.2).

    Rationale: This layer is applied directly to the skin surface. It is necessary to ensure the correct environment to protect the wound and encourage healing. Dressings can be moist or dry.

5. **Action:** Apply the bandage. Wherever possible, apply the bandage in a 'reverse wind' method.

    Rationale: This will create a more even tension.

6. **Action:** Ensure that the bandage is comfortable and that the patient cannot interfere with it.

Rationale: Reasons for interference include the bandage being too tight resulting in poor circulation, pain, sutures being too tight, and boredom. An Elizabethan collar, topical sprays or supervised muzzling may be used.

7. **Action:** Explain the aftercare of the wound and dressing to the owner.

   Rationale: Protect from wet and dirt by covering with a bag. Observe for patient interference, odour, sores, discharge and slipping. Change the dressing when advised.

INDIVIDUAL BANDAGING TECHNIQUES (TABLE 8.3)

Procedure: Robert Jones bandage

1. **Action:** Apply two strips of 2.5 cm wide zinc oxide tape to the cranial and caudal aspect of the lower third of the limb. Allow another 10 cm of tape to overhang the toes, and gently stick together.

   Rationale: These strips will later be included in the bandage, and form the 'stirrups' (Fig. 8.1A).

2. **Action:** Apply cotton wool around the entire length of the limb. Pay particular attention to any bony prominences. Use at least three layers, depending on the size of the animal. Ensure that it is of an even thickness throughout.

   Rationale: This layer provides the support. The greater the amount of cotton wool, the more immobilised the limb becomes. Larger animals will require more layers.

3. **Action:** Compress the cotton wool by bandaging it with a conforming bandage, appropriate to the size of the animal. Leave two toenails showing at the bottom.

   Rationale: This must be applied firmly and evenly to gain maximum support. The two toenails can be used as a guide to circulation, and will also encourage the animal to use the limb to some degree.

4. **Action:** Continue applying conforming bandage until sufficient tension has been created.

Rationale: The bandage should be approximately three times the width of the animal's leg. When it is 'flicked' with your finger, it should sound like a ripe melon.

5. **Action:** Separate the zinc oxide tapes from each other. Twist the tape 180° and stick to the conforming layer (Fig. 8.1B).

   Rationale: This will prevent the bandage from slipping down the limb.

6. **Action:** Apply a layer of cohesive bandage over the conforming bandage (see also Figs 8.1C–H).

   Rationale: This will protect the other layers.

Procedure: Velpeau sling

1. **Action:** Apply cotton wool padding to the carpal and metacarpal area of the affected limb.

   Rationale: This area will be held in flexion, and needs to be padded for the comfort of the animal.

2. **Action:** Apply conforming bandage, appropriate to the animal's size, above the carpus for several turns (Fig. 8.2A).

   Rationale: This secures the bandage.

3. **Action:** Flex the elbow and shoulder, and at the same time, take the bandage over the shoulder, under the chest, medial to the other front leg, and back to the carpus.

   Rationale: This will hold the shoulder and elbow in flexion against the body.

4. **Action:** Flex the carpus, and include this in the bandage (Fig. 8.2B). Continue up over the shoulder and under the chest as before.

   Rationale: The carpus, elbow and shoulder should now be held in flexion against the chest.

5. **Action:** Continue in this manner, until the whole limb is held securely.

   Rationale: The animal should not be able to move the limb, but make sure that the sling does not impede respiration.

6. **Action:** Apply a layer of cohesive bandage over the conforming bandage (Fig. 8.2C).

   Rationale: This will protect the other layers.

Table 8.3   Bandaging techniques

Type	Indications	Comments
Robert Jones	Support and immobilisation of fore- and hindlimbs, commonly used in fractures. Reduction of pain, oedema and haemorrhage (Fig. 8.1)	A light, but firm cylindrical bandage
Velpeau sling	Support and immobilisation of the elbow joint following luxation or surgery (Fig. 8.2)	
Ehmer sling	Support and immobilisation of the hip, following reduction of a luxation (Fig. 8.3)	
Ear	Support and protection of the ear following trauma, or postoperatively following resection or haematoma (Fig. 8.4)	One or both ears can be included. Ensure that the ear position is marked with a pen
Chest	Support and protection of wounds and dressings. Useful for holding chest drains in place (Fig. 8.5)	
Limb	Support and protection of wounds, reduction of pain, swelling and movement (Fig. 8.6)	Ensure toes and dewclaws are padded. Work from distal to proximal. Include the whole foot and joint above the injury
Tail	Protection of wounds from environmental trauma and/or self mutilation (Fig. 8.7)	Elastoplast may be applied directly to the hair to prevent this bandage from slipping
Ring	Indicated where there is a foreign body protruding from a wound. A ring bandage protects the wound while preventing further penetration by the object. Usually used in a 'first aid' situation	Ready-made rings can be obtained. To make a ring – wind conforming bandage around your hand five times (size of ring depends on area of wound to be covered). Remove carefully, maintaining the ring shape and with the same bandage wind it around the ring creating a bound circle like a doughnut. Continue until you have the desired size and shape (see Fig. 8.8A–E)
Splint	Immobilisation of an injury below the elbow or stifle	Limited to lower limbs. Immobilisation cannot be achieved above the elbow and stifle due to the large mass of muscle that surrounds the bones. Application is often painful for the patient and therefore limited to a first aid procedure. Common splints used in practice: Gutter splints – made of hard plastic, lined with foam, and snap off to the correct length; Zimmer splints – made of pliable aluminium backed in a foam composite
Cast	Immobilisation of a limb	Common cast material: Plaster of Paris – bandage covered in gypsum (calcium sulphate) that sets hard when water is added. Polyurethane-based and thermoplastic materials – lightweight, waterproof, short drying time and more radiolucent than plaster of Paris

Procedure: Ehmer sling

1. **Action:** Apply cotton wool padding to the metatarsal area of the affected limb.

    Rationale: This is the starting point of the sling, and should be padded to provide comfort for the animal.

2. **Action:** Apply conforming bandage, appropriate to the animal's size, around the padding for several turns (Fig. 8.3A). Ensure that the last bandage turn finishes on the lateral side of the metatarsals.

    Rationale: This secures the bandage.

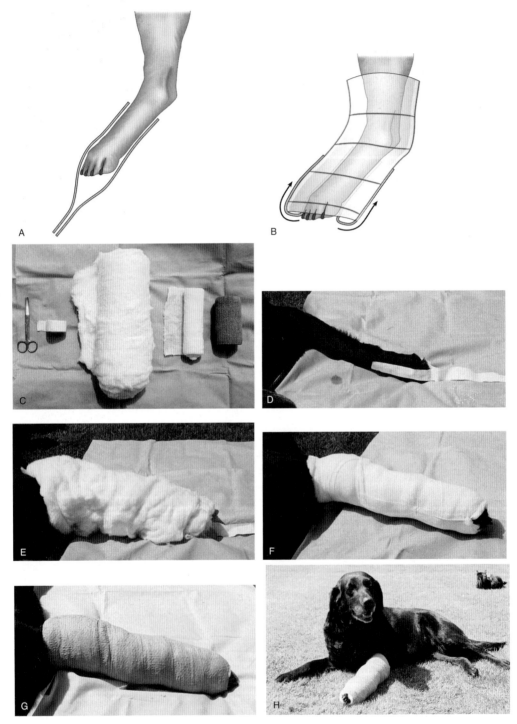

Figure 8.1 The Robert Jones bandage. A, Stick the stirrups gently together. B, Stick the stirrups to the conforming bandage. C, Materials required for Robert Jones bandage. D, Zinc oxide tapes are applied to the limb to act as 'stirrups'. E, Cotton wool is wrapped around the entire length of the limb. F, Conforming bandage is wrapped over the cotton wool and the stirrups are twisted and stuck to the outside. G, Cohesive bandage is applied as a protective layer. H, Patient with a correctly applied Robert Jones bandage.

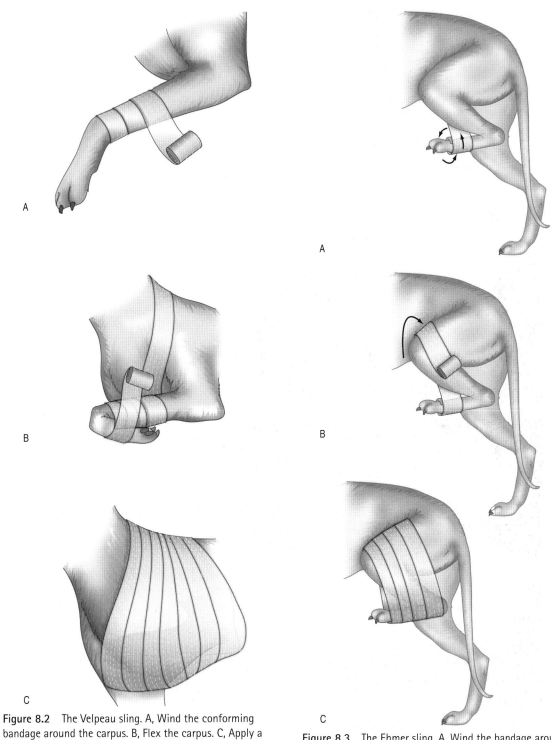

Figure 8.2   The Velpeau sling. A, Wind the conforming bandage around the carpus. B, Flex the carpus. C, Apply a layer of cohesive bandage over the top.

Figure 8.3   The Ehmer sling. A, Wind the bandage around the metatarsals. B, Bring the bandage over the lateral thigh. C, Apply a layer of conforming bandage.

3. **Action:** From this point, take the bandage up the medial aspect of the stifle, pad the top of the femur, and bring the bandage over to the lateral aspect of the thigh (Fig. 8.3B). The limb should be held in flexion.

   Rationale: This is halfway to the complete figure-of-eight that is the aim of the bandage.

4. **Action:** Take the bandage down to the medial aspect of the metatarsals, and around to the lateral aspect. You are back at the starting point.

   Rationale: This figure-of-eight bandage ensures that the foot is rotated inwards, the hock outwards, which in turn pushes the femoral head into the acetabulum.

5. **Action:** Continue in this manner, until the whole limb is securely held.

   Rationale: The animal should not be able to move the limb.

6. **Action:** Apply a layer of cohesive bandage over the conforming bandage (Fig 8.3C).

   Rationale: This will protect the other layers.

Procedure: Ear bandage

1. **Action:** Apply cotton wool padding to the top of the head, above the ear flap. Fold the affected ear(s) up onto the padding.

   Rationale: This will provide comfort and absorb any discharge. One or both ears can be folded on top of the head.

2. **Action:** Cover the ear(s) with cotton wool padding. Ensure that the padding is the same size as the ear flap.

   Rationale: This helps to keep the bandage neat, with no pieces hanging over the face of the animal, but large enough to be effective.

3. **Action:** Apply a layer of synthetic padding. Start at the top of the skull, run cranially around the ear that is down (if any), under the jaw, and back up to the start point.

   Rationale: The idea is to keep the healthy ear exposed. This is achieved by using a fig-ure-of-eight design, winding the bandage cranially then caudally around the healthy ear (Fig. 8.4A).

4. **Action:** Continue as above, but apply the padding caudally around the healthy ear. Ensure that the bandage is not too tight around the larynx and trachea. Continue until the ear(s) and padding are covered.

   Rationale: Check that the bandage does not impede the animal's respiration.

5. **Action:** Apply a cohesive bandage appropriate to the animal's size in the same manner. Continue until the padding layer is covered.

   Rationale: This will secure and protect the other layers.

6. **Action:** Mark the direction of the bandaged ear with an arrow (Fig. 8.4B).

   Rationale: This will help when the bandage is removed. The operator will know where the earflap is and can avoid injuring it.

Procedure: Chest bandage

1. **Action:** Start the bandage between the shoulder blades. Apply a layer of synthetic padding material cranially over the right lateral scapula. Bring the bandage through the front legs, caudal to the left scapula. Bring the bandage up to the start point.

   Rationale: This is halfway to achieving the desired figure-of-eight bandage.

2. **Action:** From the start point, take the bandage caudal to the right scapula, through the front legs, cranial to the left scapula. Bring the bandage over the left lateral scapula back to the start point.

   Rationale: The figure-of-eight is complete.

3. **Action:** Continue in this manner several times, moving the end point caudally, half the width of the bandage.

   Rationale: This style ensures that the bandage does not slip backwards.

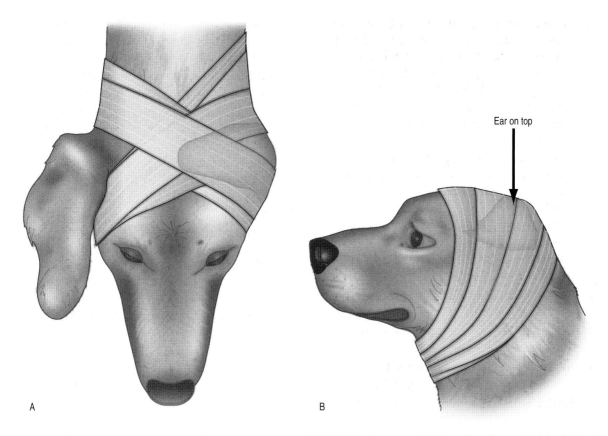

A   B

Figure 8.4   The figure-of-eight design for an ear bandage. A, Wind the bandage around the head in a figure-of-eight. B, Mark the position of the ear with an arrow.

4.   **Action:** Wind the bandage around the chest, working caudally, until the desired size is achieved (Fig. 8.5).

   Rationale: Check at regular intervals that the bandage does not impede the animal's breathing.

5.   **Action:** Apply a cohesive layer appropriate to the animal's size in the same manner. Continue until the padding layer is covered.

   Rationale: This will secure and protect the other layers.

Procedure: Limb bandage

1.   **Action:** Apply cotton wool padding between the digits and pads of the affected limb (Fig. 8.6A).

   Rationale: This will absorb sweat, and prevent the digits from rubbing together.

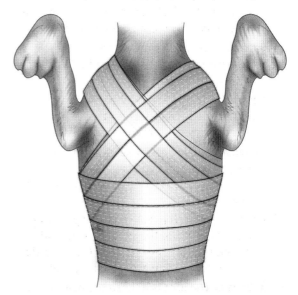

Figure 8.5   Chest bandage.

A

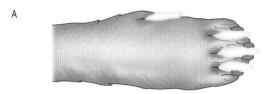

B

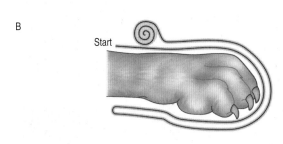

C

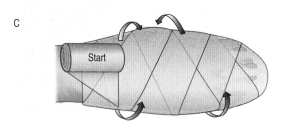

D

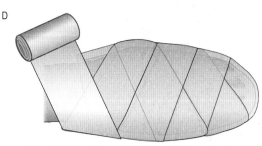

Figure 8.6 Limb bandage. A, Pad the digits and pads with cotton wool. B, Bandage over the toes. C, Twist the bandage through 90°. D, Continue winding the bandage up the limb.

2. **Action:** Apply a secondary layer of synthetic padding. Start on the cranial aspect of the limb, over the toes to the caudal aspect, and return to the start (Fig. 8.6B). Turn the bandage by 90° (Fig. 8.6C) and cover the toes in a figure-of-eight. Work from distal to proximal. Overlap the bandage by half its width.

    Rationale: This layer is used for padding and support. It will also absorb any exudate from the wound.

3. **Action:** Continue up the limb until over the joint above the injury (Fig. 8.6D).

    Rationale: This will provide more support for the limb and in turn hold the bandage in place.

4. **Action:** Apply a tertiary layer, again working from distal to proximal.

    Rationale: This layer is used to hold the other layers in place, and create an outer layer that will withstand daily wear and tear. A layer of conforming bandage, followed by a cohesive layer, is often used. However, the cohesive layer alone is often enough.

Procedure: Tail bandage

1. **Action:** Following the dressing, cover any wounds by placing an empty syringe case over the end of the tail. Ensure the end of the case is pierced with a hole for ventilation (Fig. 8.7).

    Rationale: This will prevent further trauma to the wound should the animal want to wag its tail!

2. **Action:** Apply a layer of cohesive bandage from caudal to cranial over the syringe case.

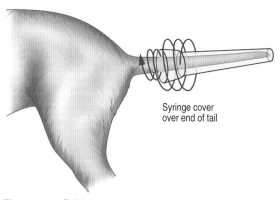

Syringe cover
over end of tail

Figure 8.7 Tail bandage.

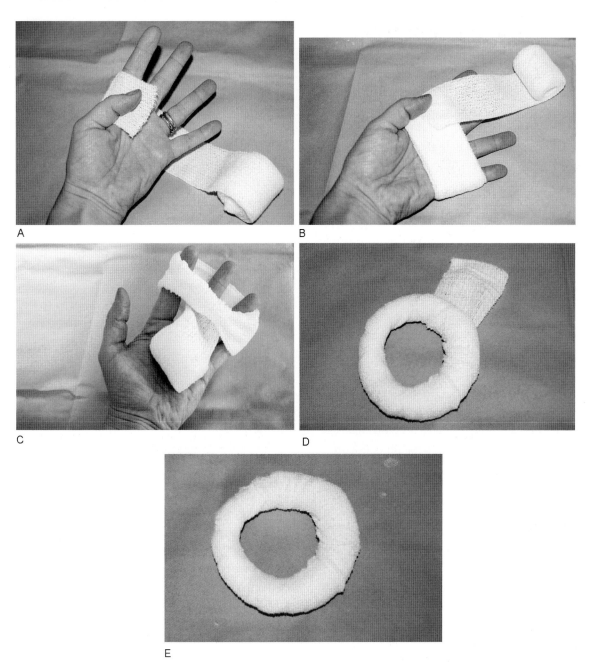

Figure 8.8 Making a ring pad. A, Conforming bandage is placed across the hand. B, Conforming bandage is wound around the hand several times. C, Ring of bandage is carefully removed from hand and remaining bandage is wound around the ring. D, Continue to wind bandage around the ring until desired shape and size is created. E, Finished ring pad which can now be placed over the penetrating foreign body to protect the wound.

Rationale: Cohesive bandage has more grip on the hair than conforming bandage, making it less likely to come off. However, in shorthaired dogs, Elastoplast may have to be used to hold the bandage in place.

3. **Action:** Continue applying the bandage, working the animal's hair into each wind.

   Rationale: This will help the bandage to stay in place.

4. **Action:** Elastoplast may be applied to the top of the tail bandage.

   Rationale: This may be needed for extra grip.

Procedure: Splinting a limb

1. **Action:** Apply two layers of synthetic padding to the affected limb. Cover both the joint above and the one below the injury. Pay particular attention to bony prominences.

   Rationale: To stabilise the injury both joints must be included. The padding provides comfort; however, the splint must be in close contact to provide immobility. Some splints have padding attached but when used less additional synthetic padding is needed.

2. **Action:** Apply the splint to the limb. Ensure that it is long enough to immobilise the joints above and below the injury.

   Rationale: There are many different types of splints available.

3. **Action:** Hold the splint in place with micropore tape in two or three places.

   Rationale: This holds the splint in place.

4. **Action:** Apply a layer of cohesive bandage over the top.

   Rationale: This protects the splint.

Procedure: Casting using plaster of Paris

1. **Action:** Before applying the cast, ensure that the fracture has been reduced.

   Rationale: Reduction is necessary for optimum healing of the site.

2. **Action:** Cover the limb with tubular gauze, appropriate to the animal's size. Ensure that the joints above and below the injury are covered. Allow 2 cm of extra gauze at either end.

   Rationale: This will be folded back later to create a smooth end.

3. **Action:** Apply a layer of synthetic padding, again leaving 2 cm at either end.

   Rationale: This is for the animal's comfort. Apply more padding to joints and bony prominences.

4. **Action:** Unroll the plaster of Paris bandage by 10 cm and immerse in hand-hot water for a few seconds.

   Rationale: The drying time is shortened if warm water is used.

5. **Action:** Squeeze out excess water from the bandage. Apply to the limb, working from distal to proximal. Overlap the bandage by half its width.

   Rationale: Leave the middle two toes protruding from the end of the cast; these can be used as a guide to circulation.

6. **Action:** Ensure even coverage over the joints.

   Rationale: The cast can become weak over these points.

7. **Action:** Turn over the tubular gauze and padding at the ends. Smooth into the plaster of Paris.

   Rationale: This creates a neat and tidy cast.

8. **Action:** Smooth and mould the cast into the correct shape.

   Rationale: Any changes must be made before the bandage dries.

9. **Action:** The bandage must be completely dry before allowing the animal to bear weight on the limb.

   Rationale: Drying times vary; refer to manufacturer's instructions.

10. **Action:** Ensure that the circulation is checked regularly by using the protruding toes as a guide.

    Rationale: The toes should be warm to touch. Cold toes may indicate that the cast is too tight.

DRAINAGE SYSTEMS (TABLE 8.4)

Procedure: Use of the Penrose drain

1. **Action:** Clean and debride the wound. (Refer to Wound management procedure, p. 164.)

    Rationale: This will reduce the risk of infection and increase the blood supply to the wound, increasing the rate of wound healing.

2. **Action:** Using a scalpel blade, make an incision at the top of the wound (Fig. 8.9A), working from the inside to the outside of the wound. The incision should be no wider than the width of the drain. Leave the tip of the blade protruding.

3. **Action:** Using a pair of sterile artery forceps, grasp the tip of the blade. Retract the scalpel blade until the tips of the artery forceps are showing on the inside of the wound (Fig. 8.9B).

    Rationale: This technique maintains the incision.

4. **Action:** Release the blade and dispose of it safely.

    Rationale: This leaves the artery forceps through the incision.

5. **Action:** Attach the end of the Penrose drain to the artery forceps and pull through (Fig. 8.9C). Release when 4–5 cm is showing.

Rationale: This technique inserts the drain without the need to release and return to the incision, thus reducing soft tissue damage and time taken.

6. **Action:** Repeat this procedure at the base of the wound.

7. **Action:** Suture the wound. (Refer to Suturing techniques section, p. 180.)

    Rationale: The wound is separate from the drain.

8. **Action:** Suture the Penrose drain at either end to the skin at the point of the incisions made earlier. Use two single interrupted sutures, preferably in a nylon of a different colour to the wound sutures.

    Rationale: The sutures hold the drain in place. The different colours allow easy identification of the sutures when it comes to removing them.

9. **Action:** Cut the ends of the drain so that 2–3 cm protrude.

    Rationale: A longer length than this increases the risk of contamination.

10. **Action:** The wound can be dressed to absorb any exudate draining from the tubing. Ensure that the site is bathed and the dressing changed daily.

    Rationale: This reduces the risk of contamination and keeps the drain open.

Table 8.4   Drainage systems

Type	Comments
Closed drains	No exposure to the environment. Can be active (suction) or passive (reliant on gravity)
Thoracic – water trap	Fluid or air is drawn out from the thorax by gravity. It is prevented from returning by a water trap placed at least 80 cm away from the animal. Use in non-ambulatory patients only
Thoracic – Heimlich valve	Inlet is attached securely into the animal, whilst the outlet is attached to a giving set and bag
Urinary catheter	Drainage of the bladder. Can be indwelling and attached to a giving set and bag
Needle and syringe	Used in many situations as a low pressure active drain
Open drains	Exposure to the environment. All types are passive
Penrose	Broad, hollow latex tubing. Fluid passes over the surface by capillary action
Seton	Usually a sterile gauze bandage packed into an area. A 'tail' is left protruding
Sump	Similar to a Penrose drain. Air passes inside to the wound whilst fluid passes over the outside. Used in deep abscesses

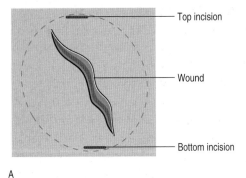

A

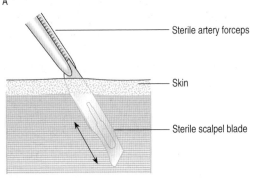

B

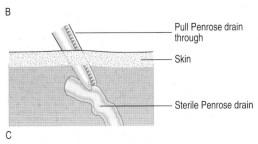

C

Figure 8.9 The Penrose drain. A, Make an incision at the top of the wound. B, incise from inside to outside. C, Pull the drain through.

11. **Action:** If the drain is left uncovered, advise the owner to bathe the site twice daily with salt water.

    Rationale: This removes the exudate, keeps the drain open, and reduces the risk of contamination.

12. **Action:** Advise the owner of the signs that may indicate infection and fluid build-up.

    Rationale: Examine for signs of oedema, redness, pain, irritation and systemic illness.

13. **Action:** Prevent the animal from removing the drain.

Rationale: Use an Elizabethan collar appropriate to the animal's size.

14. **Action:** When removing the drain, prepare the area aseptically.

    Rationale: There is a risk of contamination.

15. **Action:** Remove the sutures on the top site and pull the drain upwards until clean drain is showing.

    Rationale: About 5 mm of clean drain is necessary. This maintains asepsis.

16. **Action:** Cut the drain horizontally at this point.

    Rationale: This ensures that only 'clean' drain enters the wound.

17. **Action:** Remove the sutures at the bottom site and pull the drain through from this point.

    Rationale: The holes left will heal by granulation.

FRACTURE MANAGEMENT

Procedure: First aid procedure in a case of a suspected fracture

1. **Action:** Check the animal's airway, breathing and circulation. (Refer to Treatment of asphyxia procedure in Chapter 9).

   Rationale: This must be done before checking for other injuries. The animal will die within a few minutes without oxygen.

2. **Action:** Restrain the animal in a comfortable position. Gently examine for injuries.

   Rationale: An injured animal is more likely to try to escape and/or bite.

3. **Action:** Control haemorrhage. (Refer to Control of haemorrhage procedure in Chapter 9).

   Rationale: Loss of blood will cause the animal to go into shock. (Refer to Treatment of shock procedure in Chapter 9).

4. **Action:** Examine the patient for fractures. This must be done gently to prevent further injury.

5. **Action:** If possible, clean any wounds and apply a sterile dressing.

   Rationale: This may not be possible if first aid treatment is not in the practice.

6. **Action:** Gently apply a splint or Robert Jones bandage to the affected limb. (Refer to Individual bandaging techniques section, pp. 168 and 176.)

   Rationale: This will immobilise the limb, reducing pain and further damage.

7. **Action:** If necessary, transport the animal to the surgery, constantly monitoring the patient's condition. Ensure that the animal is adequately restrained.

   Rationale: It is often easier to move the animal with two people. A stretcher may be necessary for large animals. If a spinal injury is suspected then always use a rigid stretcher. (see Chapter 1).

8. **Action:** Treat the animal for shock.

   Rationale: Refer to Treatment of shock procedure in Chapter 9.

9. **Action:** Administer analgesia as directed by the veterinary surgeon.

   Rationale: The animal will be in pain.

10. **Action:** When stable the patient may be X-rayed to diagnose the extent of the injuries.

    Rationale: An animal suffering from shock is not a good candidate for sedation/anaesthesia. Treatment for shock is of primary importance to stabilise the patient before administering an anaesthetic.

11. **Action:** Any fractures may then be reduced and a method of fixation performed (Table 8.5).

Table 8.5 Methods of fracture fixation

Type	Comments
External techniques	
Splints	See Individual bandaging techniques and Table 8.3
Casts	See Individual bandaging techniques and Table 8.3
Robert Jones bandage	See Individual bandaging techniques and Table 8.3
Internal fixation	
Intramedullary pins include:	Inserted into the medullary cavity
Steinmann pin	Straight sharpened pins. Choose the correct size, as the pin must be a snug fit
Kirschner wire/nail	As above
Rush pin	Curved pins, used in pairs
Cerclage wire	Made from stainless steel. Can be used as single sutures, in conjunction with pins or plates, or as a tension band for avulsed fractures
Bone plates and screws include:	
Venables plate	Self-tapping screws are inserted into holes in the bone
Sherman plate	Similar to the Venables plate but not as strong
Dynamic compression bone plate and ASIF/AO (Association for the Study of Internal Fixation) and cortical and cancellous screws	A tap is used to cut a thread in the bone for the screws. This gives a stronger hold. The holes in the plate are angled so that when the screws are tightened the fracture site is compressed
Lag screws	Half or fully threaded screws that draw fragments back into position
External/Internal fixation	
External fixator, e.g. Kirschner–Ehmer device and Ilizarov fixator	A series of pins screwed into the bone through the skin, held in place by scaffolding on the outside
Cage rest	Limited movement of the animal. Common treatment for a fractured pelvis

Rationale: There are several methods of treatment. Choice is dependent on location of fracture.

SUTURING TECHNIQUES (FIG. 8.10)

Procedure: Simple interrupted skin suture

1. **Action:** Ensure that the wound to be closed is clean and has a good blood supply. (Refer to Wound management section, p. 164.)

    Rationale: This reduces the risk of infection and increases the rate of wound healing.

2. **Action:** Select an appropriate suture material for the wound (Table 8.6).

    Rationale: This will depend on the type of tissue being sutured.

3. **Action:** Select an appropriate type of needle holders and grasp them using the thumb and ring finger.

    Rationale: This grip aids precision in placing and using the needle.

4. **Action:** Position the threaded needle at a right angle in the needle holder. Grasp the needle along two-thirds of its length.

    Rationale: This will prevent the needle from bending.

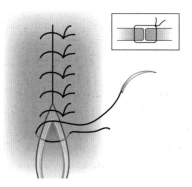

Simple interrupted

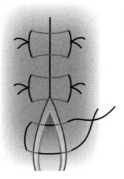

Horizontal mattress

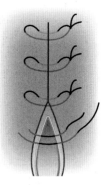

Vertical mattress

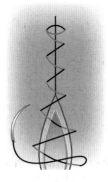

Simple continuous

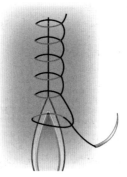

Ford interlocking suture

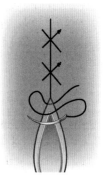

Cruciate mattress

Figure 8.10 Common suture patterns used in the skin. Redrawn from Lane and Cooper (2003), Butterworth-Heinemann.

5. **Action:** Pick up a pair of rat-toothed forceps with the other hand. These should be held like a pencil.

    Rationale: The forceps are used to hold the skin stable.

6. **Action:** Stabilise the skin on the far side of the wound with the forceps. Push the tip of the needle through the skin towards you.

    Rationale: The 'bite', i.e. the distance from the skin edge to the point at which the tip of the needle enters the skin, should be equal to the skin thickness.

7. **Action:** Release the needle and skin. Regrasp the tip of the needle and pull through.

    Rationale: The needle is through the far side of the wound.

8. **Action:** Stabilise the near side of the wound with the forceps. Push the needle through the underside of the skin.

    Rationale: This 'bite' should be the same size as the first.

9. **Action:** Release the needle and skin. Regrasp the tip of the needle and pull through.

    Rationale: The needle has now passed through both sides of the wound.

10. **Action:** Tie the knot. Use a surgeon's knot on the first throw by looping the ends around each other twice. Follow with two single knots. These should be in a reef knot, not a granny knot.

    Rationale: The knot can be tied by hand or by instrument. The latter is less time-consuming with practice. The skin edges should be brought together so that they are just touching. The first throw should never be pulled tight as that is done with the later throws.

11. **Action:** Cut the ends of the suture as short as possible without risk of the knot undoing.

    Rationale: This will help prevent the animal biting the sutures, leading to removal.

12. **Action:** Repeat the suture along the length of the wound.

    Rationale: In a simple wound work the stitches from left to right or right to left. If the wound is irregular then place a few sutures along the wound and fill in the spaces. This will create an even closure.

BIOPSY TECHNIQUES (TABLE 8.7)

Procedure: Fine needle aspiration

1. **Action:** Place the animal in a comfortable position on a table.

    Rationale: If the animal feels uncomfortable it will try to escape.

2. **Action:** Ask an assistant to restrain the animal so that it is relaxed and secure, and the site is accessible.

    Rationale: The assistant will be able to react quickly should the animal try to escape. The animal may resent the site being touched.

3. **Action:** Clean the area selected for the biopsy with surgical scrub and warm water until aseptic.

    Rationale: This reduces the risk of infection.

4. **Action:** Attach a 10 ml syringe to a 23G needle.

    Rationale: These sizes will provide the correct amount of negative pressure to gather the sample.

5. **Action:** Insert the needle into the site and pull back on the plunger. Repeat this five times. Do not withdraw the needle from the site.

    Rationale: This process draws cells from the biopsy site into the needle.

6. **Action:** Maintain slight pressure in the syringe by holding the plunger slightly back. Remove the needle from the site.

    Rationale: This pressure will prevent cells from being pulled out of the needle when removed from the site.

7. **Action:** Remove the needle from the syringe. Pull back on the plunger and replace the needle. Position over a microscope slide.

Table 8.6 Suture materials

Type	Characteristics	Indications
Absorbable		
Chromic catgut	Derived from the intestines of cattle and sheep. A synthetic catgut is available. A monofilament that knots well. Occasional tissue reaction. Strength lasts for 14 days	Subcutaneous, subcuticular and muscle sutures
Polyglactin 910 (Vicryl)	A braided synthetic suture. High tensile strength lasting for 21 days. Totally absorbed in 70–90 days	Subcuticular, subcutaneous, muscle and mucous membrane
Polyglycolic acid (Dexon)	As polyglactin but absorption is longer. Knots can slip undone	Subcuticular, subcutaneous, muscle and mucous membrane
Polydioxanone (PDS*11)	A synthetic monofilament. High tensile strength lasting for 42 days. Causes little tissue reaction	Subcutaneous, subcuticular and muscle sutures
Non-absorbable		
Monofilament nylon (Ethilon)	Minimal tissue reaction, high tensile strength. Knots must have at least three throws for stability	Skin
Braided silk (Mersilk)	A natural suture material. Adequate tensile strength. Can attract infection. Occasional tissue reaction	Skin
Braided nylon (Nurolon)	Produced to mimic silk. Less tissue reaction, high tensile strength	Skin

Table 8.7 Biopsy techniques

Type	Comments	Indications
Fine needle aspirate (FNA)	Simple and quick to perform. Examination will provide information on cell type only. Can be performed on a conscious patient	Swellings, bone marrow and soft tissue
Needle core biopsy (True-cut)	Quick to perform. Requires special needle. More information provided than FNA. Patient may need a general anaesthetic (GA) or sedation.	Swellings and organs
Punch biopsy	Quick to perform. Requires special punch. More information provided than FNA. Patient may need a GA or sedation	Skin, soft tissue and organs
Incisional (wedge)	No special equipment. A portion of the mass is surgically removed. Provides much information on type of mass. Patient will require a GA	Skin, soft tissue and organs
Trephine	Special instrument required. Removes a circular area of tissue. Patient will require a GA	Bone lesions
Excisional biopsy	Removal of entire mass or organ. Provides full information on type. Patient will require a GA	Mass or organ that can be excised completely

Rationale: Pulling back on the plunger draws all the cells in the needle into the syringe. The needle can now be removed without wasting any cells.

8. **Action:** Push down on the plunger. Ensure that all the cells are expressed onto the microscope slide.

   Rationale: The sample is now ready to be made into a smear and examined.

Procedure: Punch biopsy

1. **Action:** Place the animal in a comfortable position on a table.

   Rationale: If the animal feels uncomfortable it will try to escape.

2. **Action:** Ask an assistant to restrain the animal so that it is relaxed and secure, and the site is accessible.

   Rationale: The assistant will be able to react quickly should the animal try to escape. The animal may resent the site being touched.

3. **Action:** Clip the site to be selected for biopsy.

   Rationale: This will make the site more accessible.

4. **Action:** Clean the area with surgical scrub and warm water until aseptic.

   Rationale: This reduces the risk of infection.

5. **Action:** With a 25G needle inject local anaesthetic around the site. Allow sufficient time for the local anaesthetic to work.

   Rationale: This will reduce the pain sensation for the animal.

6. **Action:** Use a sterile punch biopsy to excise the sample. Ensure the full thickness of the skin has been included (Table 8.7).

   Rationale: 4mm and 6mm biopsy punches are available. Choice depends on thickness of skin to be sampled.

7. **Action:** Place the sample in a pot containing 10% formal saline.

   Rationale: This 'fixes' the sample, preventing cell necrosis and aiding cell examination.

8. **Action:** Close the wound left by the biopsy punch with a simple interrupted suture. (Refer to Suturing techniques section, p. 180.)

   Rationale: As the wound has been incised, it will heal quickly by first intention healing.

DENTISTRY

Procedure: Scaling and polishing the teeth

1. **Action:** Make sure that the patient is stable under a general anaesthetic and at the correct depth.

   Rationale: Refer to Chapter 6, Anaesthetic procedures.

2. **Action:** Introduce an endotracheal tube of the correct size into the trachea. Tie the tube to the upper jaw using a length of bandage.

   Rationale: It is essential that the animal is intubated to ensure that no fluid from the procedure enters the lungs. The tube must be secure.

3. **Action:** Apply an eye lubricant to both eyes.

   Rationale: Tear production is reduced when under an anaesthetic and this will help lubrication and decrease the risk of infection from the dental procedure.

4. **Action:** Position the patient in lateral recumbency, the head slightly lower than the body. This can be achieved by tilting the table or raising the shoulders.

   Rationale: This will encourage fluid from the procedure to run out of the mouth.

5. **Action:** Make sure that any fluid is able to drain away from the animal. A tub table is ideal.

   Rationale: This prevents the animal becoming wet and possibly hypothermic.

6. **Action:** Put on a face mask, gloves and goggles (Fig. 8.11).

   Rationale: This prevents bacteria in the mouth, disturbed by the procedure, from entering the operator.

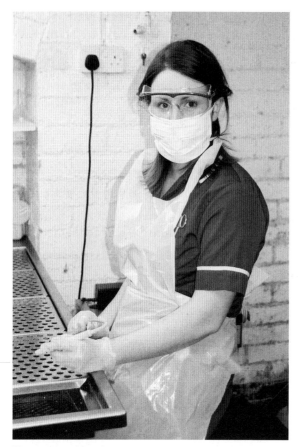

Figure 8.11 Veterinary nurse dressed in apron, mask, goggles and gloves ready to begin a dental scaling.

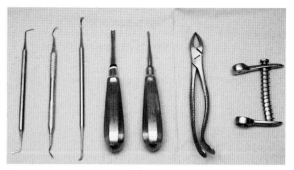

Figure 8.12 Dental instruments from left to right: periodontal probe, dental probe, hand scaler and curette, a pair of luxators, extraction forceps, mouth gag.

7. **Action:** Select a mouth gag appropriate to the animal's size (Fig. 8.12). Insert the top and bottom of the gag into the upper and lower canines respectively.

   Rationale: To keep the mouth open, enabling the operator to work.

8. **Action:** Pack the pharynx with a sterile throat pack appropriate to the animal's size.

   Rationale: To prevent fluid entering the lungs.

9. **Action:** Examine the teeth for signs of periodontal disease (Table 8.8).

   Rationale: Any problems must be referred to the veterinary surgeon.

10. **Action:** Using an ultrasonic scaler, scale the visible teeth on that side (Fig. 8.13). Refer to manufacturer's instructions. Spend no longer than 10 seconds on one tooth.

    Rationale: The vibrating action of the ultrasonic scaler may damage the tooth if used for longer than 10 seconds. You may return to the tooth later if it is still not clean.

11. **Action:** With the aid of appropriate dental instruments (Table 8.9 and Fig. 8.12) check that all calculus (tartar) is removed.

    Rationale: Calculus is the hard brown deposit on the teeth that forms from plaque as a result of bacterial action.

12. **Action:** Mop up any debris and excess fluid with damp cotton wool swabs.

    Rationale: It is important to clean as you work; this prevents the fluid soaking the animal.

13. **Action:** Turn the animal over. Ensure that the anaesthetic circuit does not twist and that the endotracheal tube is not pulled out.

    Rationale: Dislodging or twisting the anaesthetic tubing are common problems when moving the animal. It may be necessary to disconnect the circuit briefly.

14. **Action:** Repeat the scaling process on the other side.

    Rationale: It is possible to reach the inside of the far teeth.

15. **Action:** Polish the teeth with a polishing hand piece (refer to manufacturer's instructions) using prophylactic paste.

    Rationale: Polishing the teeth will leave them smooth, which in turn reduces the ability of bacteria to stick to the surface.

Table 8.8   Periodontal disease

Condition	Description	Treatment
Plaque	A soft layer composed of bacteria in an organic matrix that forms on the surface of a tooth	Brushing pet's teeth at home. Change diet if necessary
Calculus	A calcified deposit that forms on the surface of the teeth as a result of bacterial action on plaque	Scaling and polishing
Gingivitis	Inflammation of the gums, which become swollen and bleed easily. Caused by plaque at the base of the teeth	Removal of plaque and calculus by scaling and polishing. Short-term antibiotics to erase the infection
Periodontitis	Resulting from untreated gingivitis, the gum line recedes away from the base of the tooth	Extraction of the tooth. Treatment for gingivitis
Caries	Decay and crumbling of the tooth due to acid produced by bacteria	Extraction or filling
Fracture of the crown	Caused by trauma to the tooth	Extraction or filling
Retained deciduous teeth	Teeth are not shed before permanent ones erupt. May cause misplacement of new teeth	Extraction

Table 8.9   Dental instruments (Fig. 8.12)

Name	Description	Use
Periodontal probe	A long thin instrument with a 90° bend in the head. It has graduations on the probe. It is blunt ended	Used to examine and measure the subgingival margin, tooth mobility, inflammation and lesions
Dental probe	A long thin instrument with a rounded head. It has a sharp end	Used to examine caries, fractures and lesions
Dental mirror	A long handle with a small, round mirror at the end	Used to visualise the inner and back surfaces of the teeth
Scaler	A long handle with a thin, bent head. It has a sharp, pointed tip	Used to remove supragingival calculus. If used subgingivally it will damage the tissue with its sharp tip
Curette	A long handle with a thin, bent head. It has a rounded tip	Used to remove supragingival and subgingival calculus
Luxator/Elevator	A thick handle with a rounded and/or curved tip. Various sizes available depending on the requirements of the patient	Used to break down the periodontal ligament which holds the tooth in place
Periosteal elevator	A long, thin handle with rounded or straight, and/or curved tips. Various sizes are available depending on the requirements of the patient	Used when a periosteal flap is opened to facilitate the removal of a tooth
Extraction forceps	Various sizes available depending on the shape and size of the tooth	Used to lift a tooth out after being loosened by elevation. Do not use to remove 'set in' teeth as the tooth can snap off leaving the root in place

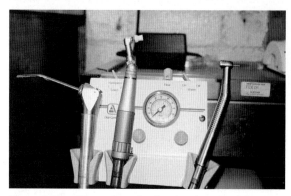

Figure 8.13 Ultrasonic scaler showing the water/air source, the polisher and the drill.

16. **Action:** When both sides have been completed, clean up any excess paste, check that all teeth have been cleaned and remove the throat pack.

    Rationale: It is very important to always check that no teeth have been overlooked.

17. **Action:** Ensure the animal is clean and dry before finishing.

    Rationale: A dental scale and polish is a very wet procedure. If necessary use a hair dryer to dry the animal's fur.

REFERENCES AND FURTHER READING

Aspinall V 2006 The Complete Textbook of Veterinary Nursing. Elsevier, Oxford

Conner J, McKerrel J 1995 A Guide to Animal Bandaging. Millpledge, Retford

Hotson-Moore A (ed.) 1999 Manual of Advanced Veterinary Nursing. BSAVA, Gloucester

Lane DR, Cooper B (eds) 2003 Veterinary Nursing, 3rd edn. Butterworth-Heinemann, Oxford

Tracy DL (ed) 1994 Small Animal Surgical Nursing, 2nd edn. Mosby, London

Chapter 9

First aid procedures

Trish Scorer

CHAPTER CONTENTS

Introduction 187

Evaluation of the emergency patient 187
Control of haemorrhage 188
Treating burns and scalds 191
Treating frostbite 191
Treatment of asphyxia 192
Tracheotomy 193
Artificial respiration in the intubated
    patient 194
Artificial respiration with no endotracheal
    tube in place – assume no damage to
    chest wall 194
Mouth to nose resuscitation – assume chest wall
    is damaged 194
Cardiac massage 195
Treatment of poisoning 196
Treatment of bites and stings 202
Treatment of electrocution 203
Treatment of shock 203
Dystocia–difficult birth 209
Diagnosis of dystocia 209

INTRODUCTION

Under the Veterinary Surgeons Act 1966 anyone may perform first aid on an animal to save life, prevent suffering or prevent the condition from deteriorating but only until such time as a veterinary surgeon is able to attend to the animal. Although, by law, lay people and veterinary nurses are able to perform the same procedures, the veterinary nurse will have the greater knowledge and training to be able to assess the situation and deal with the frightened animal and the clinical experience to apply the relevant techniques.

Procedure: Evaluation of the emergency patient

1. **Action:** Call a veterinary surgeon as soon as possible.

   Rationale: This must be done at the first available opportunity. While you are waiting you can assess for 'airway, breathing and circulation'.

2. **Action:** Ensure that the environment is safe to treat the animal.

   Rationale: Do not attempt to treat the animal if there is any risk to you, e.g. fire, electrocution, traffic, radiation or falling masonry.

3. **Action:** Stand back from the animal and evaluate the situation. What are you presented with?

Rationale: You must remain calm and in control. The owners are likely to be panicking. Avoid rushing in to help before you have assessed the situation.

4. **Action:** Make sure that the patient is restrained appropriately. If the animal is breathing normally, it may be necessary to apply a tape muzzle (see Chapter 1).

    Rationale: This is made easier if you have an assistant. The animal is likely to be frightened and in pain and its immediate reaction is to escape and/or bite.

5. **Action:** Check that the animal has a patent airway. (Refer to Treatment of asphyxia procedure.)

    Rationale: The animal may be trying to breathe but if the airway is blocked, respiration will be difficult.

6. **Action:** Check the animal is breathing. If not, check that the heart is beating, and begin artificial respiration. (Refer to Treatment of asphyxia procedure.)

    Rationale: Lack of oxygen to the body will kill the animal within a few minutes.

7. **Action:** Check that the animal has a heartbeat. If not start cardiac massage and artificial respiration. (Refer to Treatment of asphyxia procedure.)

    Rationale: If the heart is not beating, blood will not circulate around the body to supply the vital organs.

8. **Action:** Once the patient is stable, check for haemorrhage and control it. (See Control of haemorrhage procedure, below.)

    Rationale: Loss of blood may cause the animal to go into shock.

9. **Action:** Examine the patient for fractures and immobilise. (See Fracture management in Chapter 8).

    Rationale: This must be done before attempting to move the patient to reduce pain and prevent the injury deteriorating.

10. **Action:** Check the patient's capillary refill time, mucous membrane colour, pulse and temperature. Record all the information (see Chapter 2).

Rationale: These all indicate the condition of the animal.

11. **Action:** Examine the patient for other wounds.

    Rationale: These can be cleaned and dressed as appropriate.

12. **Action:** Treat for shock.

    Rationale: Refer to Treatment of shock.

Examples of conditions requiring emergency treatment are shown in Table 9.1.

Procedure: Control of haemorrhage

1. **Action:** Place the animal in a comfortable position on a table or at a comfortable height for you.

    Rationale: If the animal feels uncomfortable it will try to escape.

2. **Action:** Ask an assistant to restrain the animal so that it is relaxed and secure and the wound is accessible for treatment.

    Rationale: The assistant will be able to react quickly if the animal tries to escape. The animal may resent the wound being touched.

3. **Action:** Clean your hands with a surgical scrub.

    Rationale: It is important not to introduce infection into the wound.

4. **Action:** Assess what type of haemorrhage you are presented with (Table 9.2).

    Rationale: The extent of the haemorrhage depends on the type of blood vessels that have been damaged, e.g. an arterial bleed is much more serious than a capillary bleed.

5. **Action:** Control the haemorrhage using one of the methods described in Table 9.3.

    Rationale: The method used will depend on materials to hand, e.g. you may be in the surgery or at the roadside.

6. **Action:** Once haemorrhage has been controlled, check for signs of shock and treat if necessary (see Treatment of shock procedure, p. 203).

    Rationale: Blood loss will reduce the circulating blood volume – hypovolaemic shock. This must be treated or the animal may die.

Table 9.1   Conditions requiring emergency first aid

Condition	Definition	Symptoms
Death	Absence of a heartbeat for more than 3 minutes. Until death is confirmed, emergency treatment must continue. (See Cardiac massage procedure)	No heartbeat No respiration (Cheyne–Stokes respiration may be present) Pupil is fixed and dilated No corneal reflex Cornea is dry and glazed Mucous membranes are cyanotic and dry Body temperature cools Rigor mortis sets in after a few hours
Unconsciousness	Occurs when the animal's brain is unable to respond to sound and touch. Usually the patient is flaccid and still but occasionally the brain becomes overactive, e.g. epilepsy, and the patient's muscles convulse. There are two types of unconsciousness: 1. Stupor – animal is aware of surroundings 2. Coma – patient cannot be roused Treatment starts by evaluating the patient's airway, breathing and circulation (ABC). See Evaluation of the emergency patient, p. 187	Heartbeat present but may be slow Respiration present Pupil may be reactive to light but slow (compare both pupils' reactions as a difference may indicate brain damage) Nystagmus (side-to-side or up-and-down movement) or strabismus (squint) may be present Cornea is moist The eyeball position, as in anaesthesia, can indicate the depth of unconsciousness Muscles are flaccid
Epilepsy	A type of unconsciousness. Occurs when there is abnormal electrical activity in the brain. Various causes include brain damage, poisoning, infection and metabolic disease, e.g. liver or kidney failure Treatment of epilepsy is covered in Chapter 3	There are three phases: 1. Pre-ictal phase – patient may be anxious or excitable 2. Ictal phase – patient collapses and has convulsions. Body is tense with limbs extended and often paddles its limbs. Head and neck are extended. The jaws champ and saliva becomes foamy. Eyes are fixed and stare ahead. Respiratory rate is increased. The patient may urinate and defecate 3. Post-ictal phase – the patient calms down but is dazed and exhausted
Collapse	A collapsed patient is unable and/or unwilling to stand up. Ensure constant monitoring as this can progress into unconsciousness Evaluate the patient's airway, breathing and circulation. See Evaluation of the emergency patient (p. 187)	Vital signs may be normal. It will respond to sound, light and touch
Asphyxia/ respiratory failure	Occurs when the lungs are unable to oxygenate the blood. Causes may include trauma, airway obstruction, neoplasia, anaesthetic overdose and poisoning Evaluate the patient's airway, breathing and circulation. See Evaluation of the emergency patient (p. 187) and Treatment of asphyxia (p. 192)	Cyanosis Dyspnoea Tachypnoea Orthopnoea Tachycardia Collapse leading to unconsciousness

Table 9.2   Types of haemorrhage

Type	Identification	Treatment
Arterial	Bright red and pumps out in spurts. Bleeding point is easy to identify	Very serious. Haemorrhage must be arrested immediately. Use directed digital pressure on the ends of the vessels until a more long-term method can be instigated
Venous	Darker red and flows in a steady stream. Bleeding point is easy to identify	Slightly less serious than an arterial bleed. However, haemorrhage must be arrested quickly. Use direct digital pressure or a pressure bandage
Capillary	Multiple, pinpoint haemorrhages. The wound will ooze with little force. Commonly seen in incisional wounds	Less serious than arterial and venous haemorrhage. However, capillary bleeding over a long period of time can be serious. Use of a pressure bandage is recommended
Mixed	Commonly seen. This is a combination of the above	Treatment depends on the extent of the haemorrhage
External	Haemorrhage on the outside of the body. Easy to identify	Treatment depends on the extent of the haemorrhage
Internal	Haemorrhage inside the body. Difficult to identify and therefore treat	Treatment depends on the area affected. Possible treatments are a pressure bandage, ice pack, immobilisation of the area and/or treatment for hypovolaemic shock

Table 9.3   First aid treatment of haemorrhage

Type	Method	Comments
Direct digital pressure	With a clean finger and thumb apply pressure to the wound on either side. Care must be taken not to push a foreign body or bone fragments deeper	Quick and easy; however, this is a temporary measure and a pressure bandage must be applied as soon as possible
Pressure bandage	Apply direct pressure by using a sterile dressing and firmly applied bandage. Ensure breathing is not impeded	Deep wounds may need packing with sterile gauze before bandaging. If foreign bodies or bone fragments are suspected, use a ring pad to remove the pressure from the site
Pressure points	An artery is pushed against a bone in order to reduce the flow of blood in that vessel. Can be used in the brachial, femoral and coccygeal artery	The artery is not always easy to find. Venous bleeding will still continue. This is a temporary measure and a pressure bandage must be applied as soon as possible
Tourniquet	A ready-made or improvised strap is applied above the haemorrhage on a limb. Pressure should be such that it just stops the haemorrhage	This is used as a last resort. The tourniquet should be applied for no longer than 15 minutes, before resting for 1 minute, and then reapplying closer to the wound

7. **Action:** Monitor the animal closely. If blood soaks through the dressing you have applied, place further dressing material on top of the ones applied previously.

   Rationale: Removing the previous dressing will pull off any clot formed and restart the haemorrhage.

Procedure: Treating burns and scalds

1. **Action:** Ensure the environment is safe to treat the animal.

   Rationale: Do not attempt to treat the animal if there is any risk to you, e.g. fire, electrocution, radiation or falling masonry.

2. **Action:** Place the animal in a comfortable position.

   Rationale: The animal may be in extreme pain and may try to escape and/or bite.

3. **Action:** Ask an assistant to restrain the animal so that it is relaxed and secure, and the burn is accessible for treatment.

   Rationale: The assistant will be able to react quickly should the animal try to escape. The animal may resent the wound being touched.

4. **Action:** Clean your hands with a surgical scrub.

   Rationale: It is important not to introduce infection into the wound.

5. **Action:** Cool the area with cold water. A shower hose is ideal as it covers a large area with little pressure. Continue for at least 10 minutes.

   Rationale: This will cool the area, limiting the number of cells destroyed. The use of an ice pack is not recommended as it puts pressure on the burnt area.

6. **Action:** Keep the patient warm by wrapping it in dry blankets. Care must be taken, as the animal will be in severe pain.

   Rationale: Although the burns must be cooled, the patient must be warmed to reduce shock. Avoid the use of direct heat, i.e. lamps and pads.

7. **Action:** Clean the area gently with sterile saline.

   Rationale: The area is extremely painful and proper cleaning may only be achieved under a general anaesthetic. General anaesthesia is only recommended if the patient is stable.

8. **Action:** Dress the wound with wound gel and/or paraffin tulle.

   Rationale: The wound must be kept moist at all times.

9. **Action:** Apply a light, non-adhesive dressing on top.

   Rationale: Heat must be able to escape, and moisture loss must be avoided so the dressing must be minimal.

10. **Action:** Apply a polythene bag or cling film over the dressing.

    Rationale: This will prevent moisture evaporating from the area.

11. **Action:** Gently place a cold wet towel on top. Replace regularly.

    Rationale: This will keep the area cool.

12. **Action:** Observe and treat for shock.

    Rationale: Fluid therapy is essential to replace the fluid lost from the wound.

13. **Action:** Consult the veterinary surgeon on the administration of antibiotics and analgesia.

    Rationale: A burn is extremely susceptible to infection so antibiotic cover is essential.

Procedure: Treating frostbite

1. **Action:** Ensure the environment is safe to treat the animal.

   Rationale: Do not attempt to treat the animal if there is any risk to you.

2. **Action:** Place the animal in a comfortable position.

   Rationale: The animal will be in pain and will try to escape and/or bite.

3. **Action:** Ask an assistant to restrain the animal so that it is relaxed and secure, and the frost burns are accessible for treatment.

   Rationale: Common places for frostbite are anywhere that the blood supply is reduced, e.g. on the ear tip, nose, paws, pads and scrotum.

4. **Action:** Clean your hands with a surgical scrub.

    Rationale: It is important not to introduce infection into the wound.

5. **Action:** Apply warm water (body temperature) to the areas. Continue until all areas are warmed to body temperature.

    Rationale: This will gradually warm the area, reducing the number of cells destroyed.

6. **Action: Do not rub the area.**

    Rationale: This will shatter frozen cells.

7. **Action:** Observe and treat for shock.

    Rationale: Refer to Treatment of shock procedure.

8. **Action:** Consult the veterinary surgeon on the administration of antibiotics and analgesia.

    Rationale: Frostbite wounds are susceptible to infection so antibiotic cover is essential.

Procedure: Treatment of asphyxia

1. **Action:** Clear any blockages from the mouth and pharynx by opening the mouth and removing any obstruction.

    Rationale: The animal may be unconscious but trying to breathe. Examples of obstructions are vomit, balls, toys, blood, water and leaves (if fallen into water).

2. **Action:** Loosen and/or remove collar.

    Rationale: Be aware that the animal may recover quickly and try to escape. A dog running around without its collar is a stray.

3. **Action:** If the animal has water or a foreign body blocking the trachea then the Heimlich manoeuvre can be used.

    Rationale: This technique is designed to force foreign matter from the trachea.

4. **Action:** Hold the animal up by its hind legs, or for larger animals, hang it upside down over a table or door frame.

    Rationale: The obstructing material may move downwards by gravity.

5. **Action:** Administer a sharp punch to the abdominal wall, above the xiphisternum, angled down towards the diaphragm (Fig. 9.1).

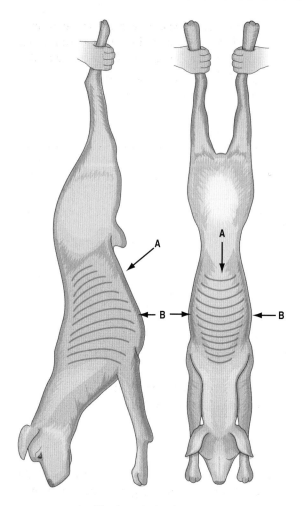

→ Direction and point of impact of blow

Figure 9.1 The Heimlich manoeuvre: A, standard; B, modified version. Redrawn from Lane and Cooper (2003), Butterworth-Heinemann.

    Rationale: This will force air down the respiratory tract, from the lungs to the trachea, and dislodge the blockage.

6. **Action:** Repeat up to four times.

    Rationale: Repeating the procedure too often can inflict damage.

7. **Action:** If attempts to remove the blockage are unsuccessful, provide an emergency airway by pushing a wide gauge needle through the ventral midline of the neck into the trachea.

    Rationale: This will act as an air inlet/outlet until a proper tracheotomy can be performed.

8. **Action:** Prepare the animal for a tracheotomy by clipping and scrubbing the ventral throat area. (See Tracheotomy procedure, below.)

   Rationale: This is a surgical procedure carried out by the veterinary surgeon.

Procedure: Tracheotomy

This procedure creates a temporary opening in the trachea which allows the animal to breathe when there is upper airway obstruction. It is usually done as an emergency procedure under local anaesthetic or sedation. The patient may present with increased inspiratory effort, dyspnoea, cyanosis, open-mouth breathing and orthopnoea (extension of the neck and abduction of the elbows). If the patient has an acute upper airway obstruction and there is no time to prepare for a tracheotomy, i.e. patient is close to death, then a wide gauge hypodermic needle can be pushed through the ventral midline of the trachea as a temporary measure.

1. **Action:** Restrain the patient in sternal recumbency on the table.

   Rationale: This is the optimal position for the procedure. The trachea can be palpated and the skin overlying it is taut.

2. **Action:** Clip and clean the area selected for the tracheotomy, with surgical scrub and warm water, until aseptic.

   Rationale: This is a surgical site and should be aseptic. There may not be time for scrubbing up if the patient's life is at risk.

3. **Action:** A small incision is made in the skin, between the fifth and sixth tracheal rings, in the ventral midline of the neck. This is usually done with a size 15 scalpel blade.

   Rationale: This is the optimal site for the tube. It is away from the larynx and the tube will not be disturbed as the patient moves its neck.

4. **Action:** Separate the pair of longitudinal neck muscles which overlie the trachea.

   Rationale: This exposes the cartilaginous tracheal rings.

5. **Action:** Incise between the tracheal rings and insert the tracheotomy tube.

   Rationale: The incision should be one-third of the circumference of the tracheal rings.

6. **Action:** Secure the tube in place with sutures placed cranially and caudally.

   Rationale: Sutures in this position will ensure equal tension on the tube and prevent it pulling out.

7. **Action:** If the tube is left in place for some time the area must be cared for correctly (Table 9.4).

   Rationale: The wound is liable to infection which may compromise the patient's recovery.

Table 9.4 Care of the tracheotomy tube

1. Patients with a tracheotomy tube require critical care – monitor the patient 24 hours a day
2. Avoid fluffy bedding and cat litter as this can be sucked up into the tube
3. Do not feed sloppy, dry or flaky food
4. Never put a lead or collar on the patient
5. Ensure that the patient does not occlude the tube when sleeping
6. Before beginning any procedure with the tube, administer 100% oxygen to the patient for five minutes
7. Clean the tube regularly, ideally every 2–3 hours
8. Wear disposable gloves when cleaning the tube
9. Clean around the tube entry site with surgical scrub and then dry
10. Unlock and remove the inner tube. Clean thoroughly and rinse through with hot water and shake it dry
11. Replace the inner tube
12. Administer 100% oxygen to the patient for 5 minutes

Procedure: Artificial respiration in the intubated patient

1. **Action:** Place an endotracheal tube of an appropriate size in the larynx and trachea of the unconscious animal.

    Rationale: An endotracheal tube must not be used in a conscious animal as the cough reflex will initiate 'gagging'.

2. **Action:** Check that the endotracheal tube is free from blockages.

    Rationale: The airway must be clear to allow air to pass through.

3. **Action:** Place the animal in the recovery position (Fig. 9.2). Connect the endotracheal tube to an oxygen supply via a closed anaesthetic circuit.

    Rationale: This is the most efficient and hygienic way for the veterinary nurse to perform artificial respiration.

4. **Action:** Squeeze enough oxygen out of the rebreathing bag to raise the chest slightly. Use gentle pressure at approximately two breaths per second.

    Rationale: This rate mimics the patient's own panting.

5. **Action:** Rest every 15 seconds for 5 seconds.

    Rationale: This time allows you to monitor for the recommencement of the animal's own breathing.

6. **Action:** If there is no oxygen supply to hand, then blow down the tube at 1 second intervals.

    Rationale: The carbon dioxide in your own respiration will act as a respiratory stimulant.

7. **Action:** Continue until the animal begins to breathe on its own.

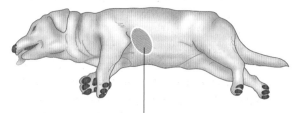

Area to which pressure is applied in artificial respiration

Figure 9.2 The recovery position. Redrawn from Lane and Cooper (2003), Butterworth-Heinemann.

Rationale: This process may be continued for about 30 minutes. If breathing has not restarted by this time the animal may be pronounced dead.

Procedure: Artificial respiration with no endotracheal tube in place – assume no damage to chest wall

1. **Rationale:** Lay the animal on its right side. Extend the head and neck and pull the tongue forwards. Pull the front legs forward so that the upper leg does not lie on the chest.

    Rationale: This is the optimum position for maximum air intake.

2. **Action:** Place the palm of your hand in the middle of the chest wall (Fig. 9.2).

    Rationale: This hand is used to push the chest wall onto the lungs, forcing air in and out.

3. **Action:** Apply firm steady pressure downwards and then release.

    Rationale: The elastic rib cage springs back, drawing air into the lungs.

4. **Action:** Apply the pressure at 1/2 to 1 second intervals, depending on the size of the animal.

    Rationale: The smaller the patient, the faster the respiration rate should be.

5. **Action:** Continue until the animal begins to breathe on its own.

    Rationale: This process may be continued for about 30 minutes. If breathing has not restarted by this time, the animal may be pronounced dead.

Procedure: Mouth to nose resuscitation – assume chest wall is damaged

1. **Rationale:** Lay the animal on its right side. Extend the head and neck and pull the tongue forwards.

    Rationale: This is the optimum position for maximum air intake.

2. **Action:** Grasp the nose firmly in the left hand so that the thumb and fingers curl around

the nose and mouth and hold the mouth closed.

Rationale: This creates an air-tight seal.

3. **Action:** Place the right hand under the lower jaw (Fig. 9.3).

   Rationale: The weight of the head is now supported.

4. **Action:** If possible wear a facemask or use a cloth or handkerchief to blow through.

   Rationale: This method is more hygienic for the veterinary nurse.

5. **Action:** Blow down the nose at 1 second intervals. Turn your head away after each blow to avoid inhaling the expired air and saliva.

   Rationale: This procedure provides the animal with your expired breath. This is rich in carbon dioxide, which acts as a respiratory stimulant.

6. **Action:** Do not over-inflate the lungs. Use just enough air to raise the chest slightly.

   Rationale: Some animals, especially the small and/or young, have very delicate lung tissue that can easily be damaged.

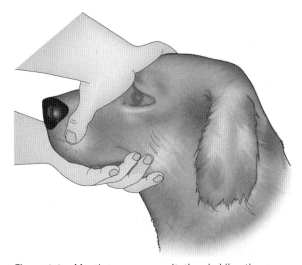

Figure 9.3 Mouth to nose resuscitation: holding the nose. Redrawn from Lane and Cooper (2003), Butterworth–Heinemann.

Procedure: Cardiac massage

1. **Action:** This procedure should be started as soon as possible after lack of a pulse or heartbeat has been detected.

   Rationale: Lack of blood to the cells, pumped around by the heart, very quickly results in cell death and eventually death of the patient.

2. **Action:** Lie the patient in right lateral recumbency.

   Rationale: In this position the heart is situated slightly uppermost and so is easier to palpate.

3. **Action:** Locate the position of the heart.

   Rationale: This is within the rib cage, between ribs 3 and 6.

4. **Action:** Place the fingertips of both hands on either side of the chest, over ribs 3–6. Use rhythmical but gentle compression to push the rib cage down. Use a method appropriate to the animal's size.

   Rationale: For cats and small dogs use pressure with the fingertips of both hands on either side of the thorax. For medium-sized dogs use the lower palm of the hand, and large dogs will require the operator to punch with a closed fist.

5. **Action:** Apply compression at 1/2 to 1 second intervals, depending on the animal's size.

   Rationale: Small dogs and cats have a faster heart rate than larger dogs, so need a faster compression rate.

6. **Action:** Carry out artificial respiration at the same time as cardiac massage.

   Rationale: This is easier with two people.

7. **Action:** If only one person is available, apply cardiac massage for five compressions and inflate the chest three times. Repeat the procedure continuously.

   Rationale: This method requires one operator to do both cardiac massage and artificial respiration, which can be exhausting after a time.

8. **Action:** If the heart does not restart within 3 minutes then the animal may be declared dead.

Rationale: Beyond this time there will be extensive brain damage due to lack of oxygen.

Procedure: Treatment of poisoning

1. **Action:** Take a comprehensive history from the owner of the animal (Table 9.5).

    Rationale: The history may be taken over the telephone or when the animal is brought into the surgery. It will provide information to help identify the poison and the time at which it was taken.

2. **Action:** Inform the veterinary surgeon.

    Rationale: This must be done at the first available opportunity.

3. **Action:** If the animal is still in contact with the poison, then remove it from the source. In the first instance, this is likely to be done by the owner – explain clearly what you expect them to do – they may be panicking.

    Rationale: For example, if the animal has the poison on its coat or is close to the source,

e.g. gas. If the coat is contaminated, wipe the poison away with paper towelling until professional advice can be sought. The use of an Elizabethan collar or towel wrapped around the patient will prevent further ingestion.

4. **Action:** Identify the poison (Table 9.6). Ask the owner to bring in the packet or label if applicable.

    Rationale: The type of poison will determine your actions. The information may be obtained from your questions to the owner.

5. **Action:** Prevent further absorption of the poison. The use of an emetic (Table 9.7) and/or a demulcent (Table 9.8) may be used. **Never** induce vomiting if the poison is corrosive or the patient is unconscious or fitting.

    Rationale: If the identity of the poison is known and it is non-corrosive, then advise the owners to induce emesis at home. Emesis is ineffective if the substance has been ingested for over 4 hours.

Table 9.5   Questions to ask the owner

Question	Rationale
Do you know the cause of the poisoning?	Time is saved if the owner can give you the details of the poison or bring the packet or container to the surgery
Do you know at what time the patient ate, or came into contact with, the poison?	This will determine whether inducing emesis will be effective
Did the patient eat anything unusual prior to the onset of symptoms?	If a sample is available then advise the owner to bring it to the surgery
Was the patient missing prior to the onset of symptoms? If so, then where?	If the owner knows that the patient has been in a certain place, e.g. shut in a garden shed or garage, then this should be searched for a possible source
Is there any substance on the patient's coat, or around or in its mouth?	Advice can be given to obtain a sample and prevent further absorption
Is there any medication, human or animal, which is damaged or missing?	This may help identify the poison. If a sample is available then advise the owner to bring it to the surgery
Did the owner use any product in the house or garden prior to the onset of symptoms?	This may help identify the poison. If a sample is available then advise the owner to bring it to the surgery

If the poison is known, the Veterinary Poisons Information Service can be contacted with the consent of the veterinary surgeon. The telephone number is 020 7635 9195 or 0113 245 0530. A charge will be made for the use of this service; however, many veterinary practices subscribe yearly.

Table 9.6 Toxic agents

Type	Causes	Effects	Treatment
Medicines			
ACP misuse	Accidental overdosing with tablets in the house Idiosyncratic reaction to the drug	Depression or collapse. (Cats may become hyperaesthetic) Vasodilatation leads to decreased blood pressure and increased susceptibility to heatstroke on warm days Brachiocephalic dogs are especially likely to suffer Increased likelihood of fits in epileptic animals	Induce vomiting if many tablets have been eaten (unlikely, since few surgeries prescribe more than a few tablets for specific occasions) Treat symptoms of collapse/ shock, heatstroke and epilepsy
Abnormal response (anaphylactic reaction)	Allergic-type response to medication, e.g. vaccination, antibiotics	Depression, occasionally vomiting and diarrhoea, swelling of injection sites Severe reactions result in collapse, with signs of shock	Swellings may have cold compresses applied Treat for shock if collapsed and maintain if unconscious Prepare corticosteroid injection
Non-steroidal anti-inflammatory drugs (NSAIDs)	Owners using human preparations on their animals (dosing their pets with so-called pain killers). Dogs 'stealing' owners' medications *Aspirin* – particularly toxic in cats *Ibuprofen, flurbiprofen* and *naproxen* – may be rapidly fatal in some dogs *Phenylbutazone* – more toxic to cats than dogs	*Aspirin* – Depression. Gastric irritation, leading to vomiting and anorexia. Cats may show some incoordination. *Ibuprofen* and *flurbiprofen* – Gastric ulceration and perforation in dogs leads to vomiting and haematemesis, followed by diarrhoea with melaena. Kidney damage may cause acute and fatal renal failure. Dehydration due to fluid losses *Naproxen* – Gastric inflammation and ulceration leading to vomiting and melaena Anaemia due to low-grade blood loss Dehydration	Stop medication with the drugs. *Before symptoms show*, induce vomiting as soon as possible. *If showing symptoms*, give absorptive preparations and/or demulcents. Dosing with activated charcoal is vital in cases of aspirin poisoning and should be given immediately after vomiting ceases Prepare intravenous fluids Prepare **cimetidine** for intravenous injection in cases of naproxen poisoning
Paracetamol	Owner-administered dose or tablet packet chewed	Dogs tolerate paracetamol well but cats are easily poisoned by as little as half a 500 mg tablet. Poisoning with paracetamol results in haemoglobin being changed to methaemoglobin, which is incapable of transporting oxygen *Signs* Cyanosis Depression or excitement Incoordination due to hypoxia Facial swelling	Induce vomiting if no symptoms shown Give absorptive material by mouth but NOT before consulting veterinary surgeon – if *N-acetyl cysteine* is to be used, the absorptive material may also prevent the absorption of this antidote

(Continued)

Table 9.6   Toxic agents—Cont'd

Type	Causes	Effects	Treatment
			Provide oxygen if any sign of cyanosis; ensure that the animal rests as much as possible. Prepare **methionine** or *N*-acetyl cysteine (human preparation Parvolex) for oral administration
Salbutamol	Human preparations that are used to treat asthma and for premature labour	Stimulation of the sympathetic nervous system, causing peripheral vasodilatation and rapid heart rate (tachycardia) Panting respiration Muscle weakness	General first aid treatment but beta-blockers may be needed if the heart rate becomes excessively high
Calcipotriol	Vitamin D derivative contained in psoriasis creams and ointments, chewed by pups	Similar to vitamin D overdose. Poisoning leads to hypercalcaemia and hyperphosphataemia, causing acute nephritis and damage to gastrointestinal tract *Signs* Haemorrhagic diarrhoea Polyuria and polydipsia Collapse with or without convulsions Death may occur within 24 hours	Induce vomiting if ingested within 2–4 hours Prepare activated charcoal solution Prepare Hartmann's solution for intravenous administration – it is important to flush the calcium and phosphates through the kidneys to minimise renal damage Prepare furosemide (frusemide) diuretic injection
Herbicides			
Chlorates	Ingestion of weedkillers or drinking from contaminated puddles – this substance does not degrade readily after use	Vomiting and diarrhoea with abdominal pain Cyanosis of mucosae, turning to a muddy brown colour (blood becomes chocolate in colour because poison causes the formation of methaemoglobin – see Paracetamol)	General first aid treatment Prepare **methylene blue** injection
Dinitro compounds	Ingestion of 2,4-dinitrophenol (2,4-D) or dinitro-orthocresol (2,4,5-T)	Depression, listlessness, muscle weakness. Rapid respiration and dyspnoea Hyperthermia with sweating Urine is almost fluorescent yellow/green	General first aid treatment Monitor rectal temperature to detect hyperthermia

Paraquat	Ingesting weedkiller (although this product is rapidly absorbed onto the soil after application, which renders it harmless). Paraquat has been used in malicious poisonings, but most cases are due to accidents	Inflammation of the mouth and tongue Vomiting and diarrhoea, with abdominal pain Depression and progressive respiratory distress and cyanosis over a period of days, resulting in death	**Induce vomiting** as soon as ingestion of this chemical is suspected. Even though this is an irritant poison, the effects of the absorbed poison are so severe that treatment is usually hopeless and the only hope is to remove the poison from the alimentary tract as soon as possible. Administering fuller's earth is also helpful because the poison will bind to the fuller's earth and be rendered inactive
Insecticides			
Borax	Ant killers (e.g. Nippon) which are based on honey and therefore very attractive to dogs	Vomiting and diarrhoea Collapse, convulsions and possible paralysis Poisoning may be fatal	General first aid treatment
Organophosphates	Overdosing with insecticidal sprays, chewing insecticidal collars, etc.	Vomiting and diarrhoea Salivation Constricted pupils Muscular twitching, excitement, followed by weakness, incoordination Depression or convulsions	General first aid treatment Prepare **atropine sulphate** for injection
Organochlorines	Woodworm treatments and other insecticides (aldrin, dieldrin, gamma BHC, etc.) Many products are now withdrawn from sale but old stocks still exist	Involuntary twitching of muscles, especially facial, fore- and hindlimbs and convulsions Behavioural changes, e.g. aggression, pacing, apprehension, frenzy	Wash off contamination Administer absorptive material and/or liquid paraffin to decrease absorption. **Fatty foods and drinks** (including milk) **must not be given** as they may increase absorption of the poison Prepare **barbiturate** injection to control convulsions
Molluscicides			
Carbamate Metaldehyde	See Organophosphates Ingestion of slug bait, which some dogs and cats seem to find very palatable	Incoordination leading to hyperaesthesia and convulsions Rapid pulse and respiration and possibly cyanosis	General first aid treatment Dosing with liquid paraffin may delay absorption of poison as long as it is given before the patient

(Continued)

Table 9.6   Toxic agents—Cont'd

Type	Causes	Effects	Treatment
			shows any symptoms (do not dose the unconscious patient) Prepare **barbiturate** injection to control convulsions
Rodenticides			
Alphachloralose	Rat baits and preparations to control pigeon and seabird populations	Poison acts by lowering the body temperature Progressive depression, incoordination and coma with hypothermia	General first aid treatment but warmth is essential
Calciferol	Ingestion of rat bait	See Calcipotriol (Medicines)	
Anticoagulant preparations	Rat baits. Several different compounds come under this heading: warfarin, coumatetralyl, chlorophacinone, difenacoum, brodifacoum, bromadiolone	Interference with clotting mechanism results in haemorrhages in the mucosae, bruising and haematomas, swollen joints, etc.	General first aid treatment Prepare injections of vitamin K. Large and repeated dosing may be necessary
Household chemicals			
Alcohol	Ingestion of alcoholic drink or fermenting grain (especially likely with pups)	Hyperaesthesia, incoordination, collapse and even death	Induce vomiting and provide general first aid treatment
Chocolate	Ingestion of large amounts of high cocoa content chocolate or cocoa powder. (Not a common poisoning, but causes much public concern)	Nervous excitement progressing to fits and coma Tachycardia Panting	Induce vomiting (may not be effective if chocolate ingested because of its sticky consistency). Gastric lavage may be required Prepare activated charcoal solution Prepare diazepam/ phenobarbital to control fits
Disinfectants Household disinfectants, when diluted to correct strength, do not cause a problem but are often used undiluted or incorrectly diluted by overzealous owners	Phenols – **Cats are particularly susceptible to poisoning by phenols.** Licking paws after walking on wet surfaces recently cleaned with undiluted or incorrectly diluted solutions of disinfectant	These are corrosive poisons with a strong, distinctive odour, e.g. pine disinfectants Convulsions, coma and death in acute poisoning cases Less acute cases may have inflamed mouths (stomatitis) and occasionally ulcers in the mouth	**Do not induce vomiting** General first aid treatment, including thorough washing of contaminated fur As for phenols

	Grooming coat after accidental spraying or splashing with strong disinfectant solutions Quarternary ammonium compounds – as for phenols	Animals may also vomit and have diarrhoea and abdominal pain These are also corrosive poisons but are odourless. Depression and anorexia. Occasionally vomiting Salivation, stomatitis and mouth ulcers, especially on the tongue tip Skin ulcerations if compound not washed off quickly	
Ethylene glycol (antifreeze)	Ingestion of water drained from car radiators (dogs seem particularly prone to drink this)	Incoordination, depression and rapid breathing. Later animal may become uraemic	General first aid treatment **Ethanol** is the specific antidote and intravenous injections may be prepared if available at the surgery
Petroleum products	Usually a problem in cats which have fallen into containers of sump oil, drained from cars Accidental spillages of petrol, paraffin, etc. Caking of tar in the paws	These are very corrosive poisons with a distinctive odour Depression, vomiting, collapse and death if enough ingested If submersed in the liquid, may also suffer an aspiration pneumonia, which is very severe because of the extremely irritant nature of the inhaled liquid Inflammation of the in-contact skin and mouth, especially the tongue if the animal has been allowed to groom	**Do not induce vomiting** General first aid treatment, including giving olive oil by mouth to decrease the absorption of the toxins

ACP, acepromazine. Reproduced with permission from Cooper and Lane (1999), Butterworth–Heinemann

Table 9.7 Emetic agents

Agent	Method
Washing soda crystals	Two crystals on the back of the tongue
Apomorphine	Only given under the direction of the veterinary surgeon; 0.1 mg/kg subcutaneously
Xylazine	Only given under the direction of the veterinary surgeon; 3.0 mg/kg intramuscularly
Mustard	Not as effective as above; 2 teaspoonfuls in a cup of warm water

Table 9.8 Demulcent agents – used to bind poison in gut

Agent	Method
BCK granules	1–3 heaped teaspoons orally. May need to mix with food or water and syringe in
Charcoal	1 g/kg orally. May need to mix with food or water and syringe in
Kaolin	1–2 ml/kg orally

6. **Action:** Collect a clearly labelled sample of any poison, vomit and/or urine/faeces. This may be used for analysis at a later date.

   Rationale: Analysis may aid identification of the substance.

7. **Action:** Treat the symptoms shown by the patient. Administer drugs as directed by the veterinary surgeon.

   Rationale: If the patient is collapsed or unconscious, administer oxygen. If advised, administer demulcents (Table 9.8) to bind the poison.

8. **Action:** Administer an antidote if it is available.

   Rationale: Very few poisons have an antidote. If there is one, it is given under the direction of a veterinary surgeon.

9. **Action:** Administer fluids orally if the animal is conscious, or set up an intravenous drip.

   Rationale: Oral fluids will dilute any poison that has been absorbed. In some cases the administration of fluids will reduce the damage to the tissues as they will flush out the poison in the urine.

10. **Action:** Make the patient warm and comfortable. Monitor the patient's rectal temperature. Ensure that the body temperature is maintained.

    Rationale: Some poisons will depress or raise the body temperature.

11. **Action:** Monitor the patient continually.

    Rationale: Any changes in the patient's condition must be acted upon quickly.

12. **Action:** If the owner implies that this poisoning is malicious, maintain a diplomatic silence and do not express opinions which could be used in a subsequent legal case.

    Rationale: The case history and the laboratory results may be used as evidence in a legal case, should the poisoning be malicious. Make sure that all records are accurate and kept safely.

Procedure: Treatment of bites and stings

1. **Action:** Place the animal in a comfortable position on a table.

   Rationale: If the animal feels uncomfortable it will try to escape.

2. **Action:** Ask an assistant to restrain the animal so that it is relaxed and secure, and the area is accessible for treatment.

   Rationale: The assistant will be able to react quickly should the animal try to escape. The animal may resent the area being touched.

3. **Action:** Clean your hands with a surgical scrub.

   Rationale: It is important not to introduce infection into the wound.

4. **Action:** Assess the type of wound (Table 9.9).

   Rationale: Treatment depends on the cause of the injury. There may be multiple bites or stings.

5. **Action:** Treat the area with the appropriate action.

   Rationale: Refer to Table 9.9.

6. **Action:** Monitor the patient continually.

   Rationale: Any changes in the patient's condition can be acted upon quickly.

Table 9.9 Treatment of bites and stings

Type	Symptoms	Complications	Treatment
Wasp sting	Commonly seen in dogs. Stings are usually around the mouth and nose, and also the feet. The result is a painful swelling and, if in the mouth area, excessive salivation. Stings to the pharynx can inhibit respiration. The sting is **not** left in the animal	Some animals may be allergic to the sting and may show an excessive reaction, anaphylaxis Collapse, dyspnoea and symptoms of shock may be seen	Wash the area with warm water and apply a dilute solution of water and acetic acid (vinegar). If the patient is collapsed then treat as for shock. If the patient is dyspnoeic then treat for asphyxia (see Treatment of asphyxia procedure)
Bee sting	Commonly seen in dogs. Stings are usually around the mouth and nose, and also the feet. The result is a painful swelling and, if in the mouth area, excessive salivation. Stings to the pharynx can inhibit respiration. The sting **is** left in the animal	Some animals may be allergic to the sting and may show an excessive reaction, anaphylaxis. Collapse, dyspnoea and symptoms of shock may be seen	The sting has a pumping sac attached This must be removed carefully to avoid further liquid entering the site. Hold the sting at the point of entry with a pair of tweezers and remove. Wash the area with warm water and apply a solution of water and bicarbonate of soda (1 teaspoon in 1 pint of water)
Snake bite	Commonly seen in dogs. Bites are usually around the head and neck. The area is painful and oedematous. Two fang marks may be visible. The patient may be dull and depressed; may lead to collapse	The severity of the reaction depends on the type of snake, the amount of venom injected and the patient's reaction to the venom	Call a vet. Keep the patient as still as possible. Thoroughly wash with warm water, but **do not** rub. This will push the venom deeper into the tissue. Apply a cold compress to reduce tissue perforation. Administer anti-venom and medication under the directions of the veterinary surgeon
Toad skin venom	Commonly seen in dogs that have picked up the toad in their mouths. Excessive salivation may be seen	Occasionally the animal may swallow the toad	Constant observation of the patient. Occasionally nervous symptoms may develop. Administer medication as directed by the veterinary surgeon

Procedure: Treatment of electrocution

1. **Action:** Assess the environment that you are in – is there any risk to you or to others?

   Rationale: Never touch an electrocuted animal until the power supply is disconnected as you may get an electric shock via the animal.

2. **Action:** If the power cannot be disconnected then push the animal from the source with a **dry, wooden** pole.

   Rationale: Such a pole will not conduct the electricity.

3. **Action:** Check the patient's airway, breathing and circulation. (Refer to Treatment of asphyxia procedure.) Resuscitate as appropriate.

   Rationale: The animal may be found collapsed or even dead. Electric shocks may induce cardiac arrest.

4. **Action:** When stable, examine the patient for burns and other injuries. Treat as appropriate.

   Rationale: Burns may appear on the entry and exit points of the electric current. Pieces of skin that touch other skin, e.g. toes or scrotum, may also be affected.

Procedure: Treatment of shock

1. **Action:** Assess the animal for clinical signs of shock (Tables 9.10 and 9.11).

   Rationale: From this examination you can assess the severity of the problem.

Table 9.10   Clinical signs of shock

Symptom	Reason
Rapid, weak pulse	The heart is working harder because of low blood volume/pressure
Quiet heart sounds	Poor cardiac filling
Pale mucous membranes	Vasoconstriction due to the blood going to the vital organs, e.g. heart, brain and lungs
Increased capillary refill time	Vasoconstriction due to the blood going to the vital organs, e.g. heart, brain and lungs
Cold extremities	Due to vasoconstriction and low metabolic rate
Depressed level of consciousness	Reduced blood flow to the brain
Reduced urine output	Reduced blood flow to the kidneys

Table 9.11   Types of shock

Type	Cause
Cardiogenic	Cardiac output is reduced, e.g. reduced cardiac filling, pericarditis, or reduced cardiac emptying, cardiomyopathy
Hypovolaemic	Low circulating blood volume, e.g. haemorrhage, excessive vomiting or diarrhoea
Vasculogenic	The capacity of the blood vessels increases due to vasodilation
a. Neurogenic – trauma to the central nervous system b. Anaphylactic – an abnormal reaction to an antigen Causes widespread histamine release, which in turn causes vasodilation c. Endotoxic – endotoxins from bacteria release chemicals which cause vasodilation	

2. **Action:** Restore the circulating blood volume to its original level by using intravenous fluid therapy.

   Rationale: This will increase blood pressure and therefore improve the circulation to the body tissues.

3. **Action:** The fluid used should resemble that which is lost. In cases of severe shock the use of a plasma expander is recommended.

   Rationale: Replace blood with blood or a plasma expander, and replace electrolytes with a crystalloid solution such as Hartmann's solution. Plasma expanders increase the osmotic pressure of blood, which draws fluid into the blood vessels, increasing circulating blood volume.

4. **Action:** Provide oxygen to the patient via a closed anaesthetic circuit.

   Rationale: This will correct hypoxia caused by low haemoglobin levels due to blood loss.

5. **Action:** Provide warmth. This should be by indirect heat, i.e. a warm environment and/or conserving body heat with bubble wrap and blankets.

   Rationale: Direct heat will increase surface dilation of the capillaries and take blood away from the vital organs to the skin surface.

6. **Action:** Monitor the patient closely.

   Rationale: Any changes in the patient's condition can be noted and treated.

7. **Action:** Administer medication under the direction of a veterinary surgeon.

   Rationale: Drugs used may include sodium bicarbonate to correct metabolic acidosis, corticosteroids, anticoagulants, adrenaline (epinephrine) and antibiotics.

For treatment of injuries to the different body systems refer to Table 9.12.

Table 9.12   Injuries to the body systems

Area	Possible causes	Symptoms	Treatment
Respiratory system			
Nose	Trauma	Head shaking, epistaxis, mouth breathing crepitus, deformity and/or dyspnoea	Cold compress to control swelling/haemorrhage Oxygenation if dyspnoeic. Rest to lower blood pressure. Constant monitoring in case of concussion
	Foreign body, e.g. grass/grass seed	Sneezing, head shaking, epistaxis, discharge and/or mouth breathing	Remove if visible. Prepare for general anaesthetic (GA)/sedation
	Tumour	Head shaking, epistaxis, mouth breathing crepitus, deformity and/or dyspnoea	Cold compress to control haemorrhage Oxygenation if dyspnoeic. Rest to lower blood pressure
Pharynx and oesophagus	Foreign body, e.g. grass, fish hook, string, balls and sticks	Gagging, retching, salivation, dysphagia, dyspnoea and/or asphyxia	Remove if visible. Prepare for GA/sedation. Fish hooks must be cut out (not pulled). Treat asphyxia (refer to Treatment of asphyxia procedure). The Heimlich manoeuvre may be required
Larynx and trachea	Foreign body, e.g. grass, balls and sticks	Gagging, retching, salivation, dyspnoea and/or asphyxia	Remove if visible. Treat asphyxia (refer to Treatment of asphyxia procedure). The Heimlich manoeuvre may be required
	Trauma, e.g. dog bites, strangulation from a caught collar	Open and closed wounds, pain, swelling, emphysema (air in tissues) dyspnoea, air hissing and/or asphyxia	Clean and dress wounds. Ensure that no fluid enters the trachea. Cover holes into the trachea with clean cling film before dressing. Treat dyspnoea with oxygen. Treat asphyxia (refer to Treatment of asphyxia procedure). Treat for shock
Lungs and chest wall	Trauma, e.g. bites, gun shot wounds	Open and closed wounds, pain, swelling, emphysema (air in tissues) dyspnoea, air hissing and/or asphyxia	Clean and dress wounds. Ensure that no fluid enters the trachea. Cover holes into the trachea with clean cling film before dressing. Treat dyspnoea with oxygen. Treat asphyxia (refer to Treatment of asphyxia procedure). Treat for shock

(Continued)

Table 9.12 Injuries to the body systems—Cont'd

Area	Possible causes	Symptoms	Treatment
	Fluid in the alveolar spaces	Dyspnoea and asphyxia	Treat dyspnoea with oxygen. Treat asphyxia (refer to Treatment of asphyxia procedure). Treat for shock
	Paraquat poisoning	Dyspnoea and cyanosis	Refer to Treatment of poisoning, p. 196
	Trauma resulting in a pneumothorax and/or haemothorax	Open and closed wounds, pain, swelling, emphysema (air in tissues) dyspnoea, air hissing and/or asphyxia	Clean and dress wounds. Ensure that no fluid enters the thorax. **Do not** remove any penetrating foreign bodies. The use of a ring pad will prevent displacement of the foreign body and/or fractures. Cover holes with clean cling film before dressing. Treat dyspnoea with oxygen. Treat asphyxia (refer to Treatment of asphyxia procedure). Treat for shock
Diaphragm	Trauma, e.g. road traffic accident	Commonly seen in cats. Dyspnoea, abdominal respiration and lung collapse	Treat dyspnoea with oxygen. Encourage abdominal organs back into place by lifting the patient up under the shoulders. Rest with the head and shoulders higher than the body
Digestive system			
Mouth	Stings	Swelling and salivation	Refer to Treatment of bites and stings, p. 202
	Foreign body, e.g. bones, sticks, string and fish hooks	Gagging, retching, salivation, dysphagia, dyspnoea and/or asphyxia	Remove if visible. Prepare for GA/sedation. Fish hooks must be cut out (not pulled). Treat asphyxia (Refer to Treatment of asphyxia procedure). The Heimlich manoeuvre may be required.
	Trauma	Fractures, crepitus and/or wounds	Compress wounds if possible. Fractures will need immobilising under GA.
Stomach and intestines	Infection	Vomiting and/or diarrhoea. Pain and dehydration	Supportive therapy such as intravenous fluids. Nil by mouth. Treat shock
	Gastric dilatation and volvulus. The stomach distends with gas and then twists (volvulus) at the cardia and pylorus	Restlessness, vomiting and belching. Swelling of the abdomen, laboured breathing, progressing to collapse and death	Call a vet as soon as possible. Relieve pressure in the stomach by passing a stomach tube. Use a roll of bandage as a mouth guard to prevent chewing. If that is unsuccessful then insert a wide bore needle into the left abdominal wall at the point of maximum distension
	Intussusception or foreign body, e.g. toys, bones and balls	Vomiting, pain and dehydration	Supportive therapy such as intravenous fluids. Nil by mouth. Treat shock. Prepare for X-rays and surgery
Rectum	Prolapse caused by tenesmus or diarrhoea	Protrusion of the rectum through the anal sphincter. Common in hamsters. Can be partial or total. Swelling can occur if left for too long	Moisten the area with warm saline and lubricate with liquid paraffin. Attempt to replace by turning the prolapse back on itself. Ensure that hands are scrubbed. Prevent further straining with an analgesic suppository or local anaesthetic. Prevent self-trauma with the use of an Elizabethan collar

Anus	Impacted faeces or foreign body, e.g. bones	Tenesmus, discomfort, haemorrhage and licking the area	Lubricate the area with liquid paraffin. Remove with fingers or forceps. Wear gloves
Perineum	Fly strike	Smelly, inflamed and burnt area. Eggs and maggots visible	Remove ALL maggots. Clip and clean the area. An application of an insecticide can be used. Treat for shock if extensive
Urogenital system			
Prolapsed uterus and polyps	Sometimes seen at time of oestrus	Red mass protruding from the vulva	Ensure hands are scrubbed. Lubricate with liquid paraffin and apply gently pressure to replace Prevent self-trauma with the use of an Elizabethan collar
Penis	Paraphimosis – penis is engorged with blood and too big to slide back into the prepuce	Swelling and redness	Apply a cold compress onto the area. This will reduce the blood supply, and the size of the penis Lubricate and replace
	Trauma, e.g. cuts or haemorrhage from an over-amorous dog	Open wounds and haemorrhage	Apply a cold compress onto the area. Pinching the skin in front of the scrotum will reduce the haemorrhage
	Foreign body, e.g. grass/grass seed	Swelling, pain and anuria	Remove if visible. GA/sedation may be required Prepare theatre
Special senses			
Eye	Foreign body, e.g. grass seed	Blepharospasm (eye screwed up), photophobia (fear of light), tears, redness and rubbing	Remove by flushing with sterile saline and/or use a damp cotton bud. GA/sedation or local anaesthetic may be necessary. **Do not** remove a penetrating foreign body
	Prolapse	The eyeball is outside of the patient's head. It will become more inflamed the longer it is out	Replace the eyeball as soon as possible. With scrubbed hands, lubricate the eyeball and lids with 'false tears'. Pull back the eyelids and attempt to replace. Never put any pressure on the eyeball. Advise an owner to keep the eyeball damp with dilute salt water (one teaspoon to one litre of water), before bringing to the surgery
	Chemical splashes	Blepharospasm (eye screwed up), photophobia (fear of light), tears, redness and rubbing	Flush with copious amounts of sterile saline. Dilute vinegar may be used to 'neutralise' alkali splashes and sodium bicarbonate will neutralise acid splashes. Follow with sterile saline
Ear	Trauma	Open wounds or haematoma	Control haemorrhage with a cold compress or pressure bandage. Clean and dress wounds. Apply an ear bandage (refer to Table 8.3, Bandaging techniques). The haematoma may need draining under a GA

(Continued)

Table 9.12 Injuries to the body systems—Cont'd

Area	Possible causes	Symptoms	Treatment
Metabolic disorders			
Hypocalcaemia	Low blood calcium Commonly seen in bitches at the peak of lactation (usually 2–3 weeks). Calcium is depleted from the blood stream to go into the milk. This leaves little calcium for the rest of the body	Restlessness, panting and shivering, progressing into collapse, hyperaesthesia and eventually death	Extra calcium must be provided in the diet. If the patient is already hypocalcaemic then an injection of intravenous calcium 10% must be given under the direction of the veterinary surgeon. Wean the offspring immediately
Hypoglycaemia	Occurs in diagnosed diabetics, where there is an imbalance between the insulin given and glucose available. This can be due to an overdose of insulin, anorexia, strenuous exercise and/or extreme temperatures	Slowed metabolic rate, lethargy, incoordination, and dry mucous membranes, leading to collapse, hyperaesthesia, convulsions and eventually death	If the animal is conscious administer oral glucose solution. Honey or sugar is the best alternative. If the animal is unconscious then an intravenous injection of glucose must be given under the direction of a veterinary surgeon. Glucose can also be given via a stomach tube. This is metabolised at a slower rate
Uraemia	Usually occurs in old dogs and cats with chronic renal failure. The kidneys, which normally excrete toxins, are not working, so the toxins remain in the blood	Polydipsia and polyuria, loss of weight, vomiting, halitosis and mouth ulcers, progressing into epileptiform fits and death	Make the patient comfortable. The use of intravenous fluids can help to alleviate the symptoms; however, there is no cure and euthanasia is often performed
Hyperthermia	Often caused by heatstroke, e.g. dogs left in hot cars. The temperature-regulating centre in the brain is unable to control the body temperature	Restlessness, panting, salivation and distress, progressing into collapse, coma and death. High rectal temperature	Cool the patient as soon as possible. Use a cold shower or hosepipe. Ice packs and wet towels are useful. Monitor rectal temperature every 15 minutes. Cool until normal temperature is reached. Continue to monitor every 30 minutes in case it rises again
Hypothermia	Often seen in young or small animals under anaesthetic. Heat loss is great due to their large surface area compared to body mass	Lethargy, reluctance to move or feed, cold to touch, progressing to collapse and death	Warm the animal as soon as possible. Use a warm environment, blankets, heat pad and/or hot water bottle. Monitor rectal temperature every 15 minutes until normal temperature is reached. Continue to monitor every 30 minutes in case it should fall again

DYSTOCIA – DIFFICULT BIRTH

Procedure: Diagnosis of dystocia

1. **Action:** Ensure that you are familiar with the gestation period and the timings of the stages of parturition for the species with which you are dealing (Table 9.13).

   Rationale: This will enable you to make an accurate assessment of any problems concerning parturition when contacted by the owner.

2. **Action:** Take an accurate history from the owner of the dam – this may be face to face or over the telephone. Make particular note of the breed and age of the bitch or queen, the date of mating, the current behaviour of the dam and the timing of each incident.

   Rationale: This information will help you to assess the stage of parturition (Table 9.13) and whether there is a cause for concern (Tables 9.14 and 9.15). Certain breeds are more prone to dystocia than others.

3. **Action:** Ask the owner if they have done anything to assess or assist the dam, e.g. taking the body temperature at regular intervals, watching behaviour patterns such as restlessness or nesting, administering herbal remedies such as raspberry tea.

   Rationale: Some experienced breeders/owners may have methods by which they assist their animals through parturition and it is important that you are aware of what has been done and at what stage. The information will also help to diagnose the type of dystocia (Table 9.14).

4. **Action:** Make sure that you write down all the details.

   Rationale: You must pass this information to the veterinary surgeon and writing it down will ensure you do not forget any of the important details.

Table 9.13 Stages of parturition

Stage	Symptoms
Preparation	Nesting, restlessness, may seek out the company of the owner. Prepartum hypothermia due to declining levels of plasma progesterone concentration may occur and the body temperature may fall to below 37°C within 24–36 hours of birth. Relaxation and softening of the vulva
Stage 1: Start of contractions until the cervix is fully dilated. May last for 24 hours in the bitch but is difficult to assess as start of contractions is very gradual	Onset of uterine contractions, which push against the dilating cervix. Allantoic fluid may drain from the vulva due to the rupture of the allantochorion (first water bag). The dam may appear uncomfortable and restless. Vomiting, shivering and/or loss of appetite may occur
Stage 2: Full dilation of the cervix until the delivery of the fetus. Puppies may be born every 20–30 minutes while kittens may be born every 30–60 minutes	Stronger uterine contractions push the fetus through the dilated cervix and into the vagina. The fetus may be in anterior or posterior presentation and the amniotic sac surrounding the puppy or kitten may rupture. This is normal and allows the neonate to breathe when born. The dam may break the sac but if not, it must be broken rapidly
Stage 3: Delivery of the placenta. Usually complete within 30–60 minutes	Placenta is expelled from the vulva and may be eaten by the dam. Stages 2 and 3 may be mixed up in multiparous (litter-bearing) species
Puerperium: period during which the uterus involutes (contracts) and returns to normal. It may last for several weeks	A dark discharge known as the lochia may drain from the dam for up to a week after parturition. As long as this odourless and the dam is well there is no need to worry

Table 9.14 Types of dystocia

Type	Comment
Maternal – resulting from factors in the dam	1. Primary uterine inertia – contractions may fail to start or start weakly and then cease. May be due to very large litters, very small litters or may be seen in fat, unfit bitches. This is rare in cats 2. Secondary uterine inertia – contractions may start but then stop. May be due to exhaustion caused by obstruction or during delivery of a large litter. In both cases oxytocin and calcium borogluconate may be given by the veterinary surgeon to strengthen contractions. Caesarean section may be required 3. Obstruction of the birth canal – due to abnormalities such as pelvic deformity, neoplasm or torsion of the uterus. If the obstruction cannot be rectified then a caesarean section is required
Fetal – resulting from factors caused by the fetus	1. Oversized fetuses may result from: (a) Breed conformation, e.g. large head size, brachycephalic breeds (b) Large fetuses as a result of a small litter (c) Abnormalities such as fetal monsters 2. Incorrect presentation – the fetus may be misaligned so that it is unable to progress through the birth canal

Table 9.15 Causes for concern

1. A bitch has passed 70 days of gestation and shows no sign of starting parturition
2. A queen that has passed 65 days of gestation and shows no sign of starting parturition (NB. Persians and Siamese often go up to 70 days' gestation)
3. Dam is restless, strains forcefully but infrequently
4. Straining begins and then ceases
5. Black/green discharge with no sign of parturition beginning
6. Parturition has not started within 48 hours of a drop in body temperature
7. Straining for over an hour with no progress
8. Has produced several fetuses, the last more than 2 hours ago, and the dam is restless
9. Has produced a few fetuses, the last more than 2 hours ago, and a large litter is known to be expected

5. **Action:** If you are concerned, then the owner must be asked to bring the dam into the surgery for the veterinary surgeon to examine.

   Rationale: As a veterinary nurse you may monitor the progress of the dam, but it is the veterinary surgeon that ultimately diagnoses the problem and prescribes the treatment.

6. **Action:** Once the dam has been admitted she may be placed in a quiet kennel to await the veterinary surgeon.

   Rationale: Many parturient dams may cease to make progress when they are in unfamiliar or noisy environments. Try to put her in a quiet area away from other dogs or cats, ensuring that the area is in subdued light and warm.

7. **Action:** The veterinary surgeon will assess the dam to check that she is pregnant. This may be done by ultrasonography or radiography.

   Rationale: An obese bitch or queen may appear to be pregnant, especially if her owner is convinced that she is!

8. **Action:** Wearing gloves and using a water-soluble lubricant, the veterinary surgeon will then gently examine the bitch per vaginam.

    Rationale: This is to check for the presence of a puppy in the birth canal. This is impossible in the queen, although a kitten in the birth canal may be palpable externally.

9. **Action:** Depending on the results of this examination the appropriate treatment will be given (Table 9.14).

    Rationale: In most cases of dystocia, oxytocin will be administered and the dam left for about 30 minutes in a quiet cage to see if this will have an effect on contractions. If progress has still not been made a caesarean section will be performed.

REFERENCES AND FURTHER READING

Aspinall V 2006 The Complete Textbook of Veterinary Nursing. Elsevier, Oxford

British Veterinary Nursing Association – Bandaging Fact Sheets. BVNA, Harlow

Conner J, McKerrel J 1995 A Guide to Animal Bandaging. Millpledge, Retford

Cooper B, Lane DR (eds) 1999 Veterinary Nursing, 2nd edn. Butterworth-Heinemann, Oxford

Hotston-Moore A (ed) 1999 Manual of Advanced Veterinary Nursing. BSAVA, Gloucester

Lane DR, Cooper B (eds) 2003 Veterinary Nursing, 3rd edn. Butterworth-Heinemann, Oxford

Chapter 10

Diagnostic imaging

Suzanne Easton

CHAPTER CONTENTS

Introduction   214

Setting up the X-ray machine   214
Preparing the X-ray room for a radiographic
    examination   214
Preparing the patient for a radiographic
    examination   215

Positioning the patient   215
Thorax   215
Lateral thorax   215
Dorsoventral thorax   217
Abdomen   218
Lateral abdomen   218
Ventrodorsal abdomen   218
Pelvis   219
Lateral pelvis   219
Ventrodorsal pelvis (extended hip position)   219
Skull   221
Ventrodorsal skull   221
Open mouth rostrocaudal view of the tympanic
    bullae   221
Dorsoventral intraoral view of the nasal
    chambers   222
Nasopharynx   222
The limbs   223
Mediolateral view of a distal limb
    extremity   223
Dorsopalmar or dorsoplantar view or
    craniocaudal view of a limb   224
Lateral shoulder   225

Craniocaudal shoulder   225
Spine   226
Lateral spine   226
Ventrodorsal spine   227

Use of contrast media   227
Use of barium in the evaluation of the
    gastrointestinal tract   227
Barium swallow   228
Barium meal or 'follow through'   228
Barium enema   229
Intravenous urography   230
Urethrogram (retrograde urethrography) – male   231
Urethrogram (retrograde vaginourethrography) –
    female   232
Cystography – pneumocystogram, positive contrast
    cystogram, double contrast cystogram   232
Myelography – cisternal and lumbar puncture   233

Techniques for processing radiographs   235
Manual processing   235
Starting up an automatic processor   236
Automatic processing   237
Shutting down the automatic processor   237
Cleaning an automatic processor   238

Maintenance of radiography equipment   239
Care of intensifying screens   239
Checking safelight function   239
Checking for light leakage in a cassette   239
Checking the X-ray tube for leakage of X-rays   240
Checking for the accuracy of the light beam
    diaphragm   240

Checking a cassette for poor film/screen contact 240

Diagnostic ultrasound   241
Preparing the patient for an ultrasound
      examination   241
Care of the ultrasound machine   241

INTRODUCTION

The term radiography covers all the procedures involved in the production and processing of a radiograph. The veterinary nurse is often given the responsibility for positioning the patient, setting up the X-ray machine ready for the exposure and then for processing the radiograph either in an automatic or in a manual processor. It is important that the quality of the resulting radiograph is such that it aids the diagnosis of the veterinary surgeon – if it does not, there is little point in the technique. To achieve a high standard of radiography the nurse must have a clear understanding of the steps involved in each procedure and how each step contributes to the final product. In addition, health and safety considerations are of particular importance when dealing with ionising radiation and the veterinary nurses must always be aware of the danger to themselves and to others in the vicinity of the machine.

Nowadays, radiography is not the only diagnostic imaging technique available in a veterinary practice. Ultrasonography – the use of high frequency sound waves to create an image – is becoming commonplace and the veterinary nurse is likely to be responsible for the preparation of the patient and for setting up and maintaining the machine. The advantage of diagnostic ultrasound is that there is little danger to the patient or to the personnel involved in its use.

This chapter describes the procedures involved in the use of both X-rays and ultrasound and in the care of the equipment associated with both diagnostic techniques.

Procedure: Setting up the X-ray machine

1. **Action:** Place the X-ray machine in the designated room or controlled area.

    Rationale: To ensure that the local rules are followed, the X-ray machine must be used in a specifically designated area as outlined in the rules.

2. **Action:** Make sure that the radiation warning signs are displayed and visible.

    Rationale: Warning signs must be displayed when X-rays are being used. The position of these warning signs will be specified in the local rules.

3. **Action:** Plug the machine into the mains.

    Rationale: Most machines rely on mains electricity to work.

4. **Action:** Switch the X-ray machine on at the console or the main body of the machine.

    Rationale: The machine must be plugged in prior to switching on the machine.

5. **Action:** Check that the mains voltage compensation is accurate.

    Rationale: Mains voltage compensation ensures that the voltage received by the machine remains constant despite fluctuations within the mains voltage.

6. **Action:** Adjust the mains voltage compensation if needed.

    Rationale: Without adjustment of the mains voltage, radiographic exposure factors will not be accurate.

7. **Action:** Set the X-ray tube to the correct height above the film.

    Rationale: The X-ray tube should always be at a standard distance from the film – the film focal distance. This depends on the height of the table and the length of the stand supporting the tube.

8. **Action:** Set the exposure factors suitable for the examination, patient type and the equipment being used.

    Rationale: Exposure factors depend on the type of machine, the film/screen combination, the size of the patient and the region being examined.

Procedure: Preparing the X-ray room for a radiographic examination

1. **Action:** Place the X-ray machine in the room and ensure that the correct exposure factors are set.

Rationale: Setting the exposure factors prior to positioning the patient ensures that once positioned an exposure can be made immediately.

2. **Action:** Place the cassette on the table and centre it under the centre of the X-ray tube.

    Rationale: The cassette should be placed securely on the table to prevent it falling onto the floor and breaking.

3. **Action:** If a stationary grid is being used place this in the correct position over the cassette.

    Rationale: Incorrect use of the grid will result in poor quality/non-diagnostic images.

4. **Action:** Place sandbags, ties and foam pads so that they can be easily reached if needed to position the patient.

    Rationale: Sandbags, ties and foam pads are used to hold the patient in the required position.

5. **Action:** Remove unnecessary equipment from the room.

    Rationale: This includes any objects that may cause an accident or be needed at a later part of the examination.

6. **Action:** Remove any distractions from the room.

    Rationale: Anything that may prevent the animal cooperating or cause unnecessary distress.

Procedure: Preparing the patient for a radiographic examination

1. **Action:** Ensure that there is a valid clinical indication for the examination.

    Rationale: Under the Ionising Radiation Regulations 1999, all examinations must be clinically justified and all exposures must be kept to a minimum.

2. **Action:** Use some form of chemical restraint – either sedation or general anaesthesia – as appropriate to the patient.

    Rationale: Suitable chemical restraint should be used unless the patient is considered to be an anaesthetic risk. Manual restraint should be used only in extreme circumstances as it poses a risk to the health and safety of personnel.

3. **Action:** Remove any artefacts from the patient, e.g. leads, collars, clips, matted or wet hair.

Rationale: Artefacts may distract the attention from and may overlie the main point of interest.

4. **Action:** If required for the procedure, ensure that any preparation of the patient, e.g. fasting, use of an enema or emptying the bladder, has taken place.

    Rationale: In some examinations, the presence of faeces or urine, or food in the stomach may restrict the view of the diagnostic points.

5. **Action:** Position the animal correctly for the radiograph.

    Rationale: If the animal is conscious and/or sedated, it may be necessary to calm the animal while it is positioned.

POSITIONING THE PATIENT (TABLES 10.1, 10.2, FIG. 10.1)

THORAX

Procedure: Lateral thorax (Fig. 10.2A and B)

1. **Action:** Place the patient in right lateral recumbency.

    Rationale: This is the conventional position for a thoracic radiograph.

2. **Action:** Extend the forelegs and secure them using sandbags or ties.

    Rationale: Extending the forelegs prevents the soft tissue mass of the shoulder girdle impeding the view of the thoracic contents.

3. **Action:** Place a pad under the sternum.

    Rationale: This prevents rotation of the chest and ensures that it is in the same horizontal plane as the spine. This prevents distortion of structures in the thorax.

4. **Action:** Place sandbags over the neck and hind legs to hold them in place.

    Rationale: The hind legs should be secure but should not be extended as this rotates the chest.

5. **Action:** Centre the beam (indicated by the cross of the light beam diaphragm) midway between the sternum and spine, level with the caudal border of the scapula.

Table 10.1   Positioning aids

Type	Use	Radiographic density
Troughs – range of sizes	To restrain animal on its back Prevents rotation of the trunk	Radiolucent
Foam wedges – range of shapes and sizes Covered in plastic for ease of cleaning	For lateral views to provide support and prevent rotation of the trunk and for accurate limb positioning. May be useful for supporting the spine and trunk to achieve a horizontal plane	Radiolucent
Sandbags – loose filling allows bending and twisting. Covered in plastic for ease of cleaning	Can be wrapped around to hold limbs in position or placed over the neck	Radio-opaque – do not place in the primary beam
Tapes or ties – range of lengths	Looped around limbs to pull them into position and tie them to cleats on the table	Radiolucent
Wooden blocks	For raising the cassette up to the area of interest	Radio-opaque – do not place in the primary beam

Table 10.2   General principles of positioning

Action	Rationale
Centre the primary beam over the main point of interest	To prevent distortion of the area by an oblique view
Place the area of interest as close as possible to the film	To prevent gross magnification of the part due to an excessive object–film distance. The image may also be blurred
Ensure that the centre of the primary beam is at right angles to the film	To avoid distortion of the image. This is important when examining joint or intervertebral disc spaces
Collimate the beam to as small an area as is realistically possible	To reduce the amount of scattered radiation
Take two views at right angles to each other	To assist in accurate location of a lesion and to visualise the area completely
Try to contain the whole area of interest on a single film	To reduce the number of exposures. If this means that important parts are viewed obliquely, e.g. whole spine, it is better to take views of several smaller areas
When imaging the spine, the body must be supported so that the vertebrae are in the same horizontal plane	To prevent distortion and magnification of individual vertebrae and of the intervertebral disc spaces

Rationale: This ensures that the centre of the primary beam coincides with the base of the heart.

6. **Action:** Collimate the beam to include the front of the shoulder and the edge of the sternum.

Rationale: All regions of the lung field will be included.

7. **Action:** Expose on inspiration.

Rationale: The lungs are fully inflated during inspiration, which provides better contrast between the air and the soft tissues.

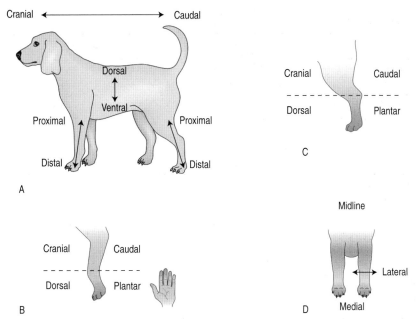

Figure 10.1   Standard nomenclature for body regions. Adapted, with permission, from Masters and Bowden (2001), Butterworth Heinemann.

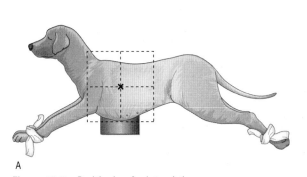

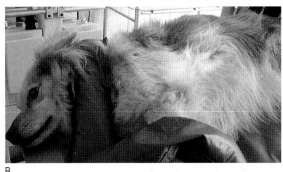

Figure 10.2   Positioning for lateral thorax.

Procedure: Dorsoventral thorax (Fig. 10.3)

1. **Action:** Place the patient in sternal recumbency.

    Rationale: This is particularly used for examination of the heart.

2. **Action:** Support the chin on a pad.

    Rationale: This keeps the head, neck and spine in a horizontal plane. The patient may also be more comfortable.

3. **Action:** Place a sandbag over the neck.

    Rationale: To prevent movement.

4. **Action:** Extend the forelegs and adduct them with the elbows out to the sides.

    Rationale: This prevents the muscle mass of the shoulder girdle overlying the thoracic cavity.

5. **Action:** Centre the beam (indicated by the cross of the light beam diaphragm) in the midline on the caudal border of the scapula.

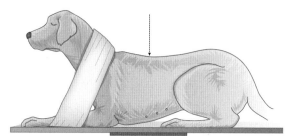

Figure 10.3   Positioning for dorsoventral thorax.

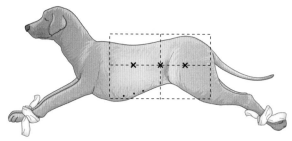

Figure 10.4   Positioning for lateral abdomen.

Rationale: This ensures that the heart base is in the centre of the image.

6. **Action:** Collimate the beam to include the skin surfaces laterally, the thoracic inlet and the diaphragm.

   Rationale: The image will include the cranial and caudal extent of the lung field.

7. **Action:** Expose on inspiration.

   Rationale: The lungs are fully inflated during inspiration, which provides better contrast between the air and the soft tissues.

NB. A ventrodorsal view of the thorax may be used to examine the lungs; however, if the animal is in respiratory distress, this position should be avoided as it may make respiration even more difficult.

ABDOMEN

Procedure: Lateral abdomen (Fig. 10.4)

1. **Action:** Place the patient in right lateral recumbency.

   Rationale: This is the conventional position for viewing the abdomen.

2. **Action:** Place a pad under the sternum.

   Rationale: A pad will support the sternum to keep the body in a horizontal plane.

3. **Action:** Extend the fore- and hindlimbs and secure them with sandbags or ties.

   Rationale: To prevent movement.

4. **Action:** Centre the beam (indicated by the cross of the light beam diaphragm) at the 11/12th intercostal space, just cranial to the last rib.

Rationale: This ensures that the entire abdomen is included.

5. **Action:** Collimate the beam to include the dorsal and lateral skin edges, the diaphragm and pubic symphysis. If the patient is large, then move the beam towards the diaphragm or pubic symphysis depending on the area of interest.

   Rationale: The top of the liver should be included in all radiographs of the complete abdomen.

6. **Action:** Expose on expiration.

   Rationale: During expiration the diaphragm relaxes into its characteristic dome shape and the lungs contract, providing the maximum amount of space for the abdominal contents.

Procedure: Ventrodorsal abdomen (Fig. 10.5)

1. **Action:** Place the patient in dorsal recumbency

   Rationale: Care must be taken if the animal is only lightly anaesthetised.

2. **Action:** Extend each foreleg cranially and secure with a tie or sandbag placed over the carpus.

   Rationale: This prevents rotation of the body. Do not place sandbags over the axillae as this can be uncomfortable.

3. **Action:** Make sure that the body does not rotate so that the sternum and spine are in vertical alignment.

   Rationale: The use of a trough or sandbags placed on either side may help to support this position.

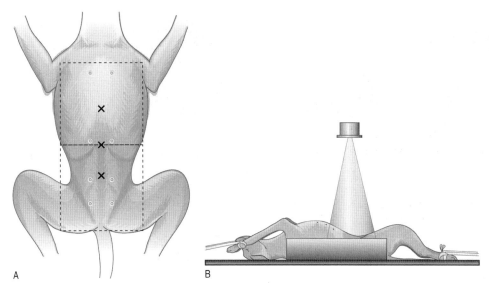

Figure 10.5 Positioning for ventrodorsal abdomen.

4. **Action:** Centre the beam (indicated by the cross of the light beam diaphragm) on the midline at the level of the umbilicus. This point may be adjusted towards the diaphragm or the pubic symphysis in larger breeds of dog.

    Rationale: This ensures that the whole abdominal area is included.

5. **Action:** Collimate the beam to include the lateral skin surfaces, the diaphragm and the pubic symphysis.

    Rationale: The cranial border of the liver must be shown in an abdominal radiograph.

6. **Action:** Expose on expiration.

    Rationale: During expiration the diaphragm relaxes into its characteristic dome shape and the lungs contract, providing the maximum amount of space for the abdominal contents.

PELVIS

Procedure: Lateral pelvis (Fig. 10.6A and B)

1. **Action:** Place the patient in right lateral recumbency.

    Rationale: This is the only way of providing a true lateral projection of the pelvis.

2. **Action:** Place pads between the hind legs.

    Rationale: This ensures that the pelvis does not rotate.

3. **Action:** Centre the beam (indicated by the cross of the light beam diaphragm) over the greater trochanter of the left femur.

    Rationale: The ensures that the wings of the ilium and the acetabulum are visible.

4. **Action:** Collimate the beam to include the entire pelvic area.

Procedure: Ventrodorsal pelvis (extended hip position) (Fig. 10.7A and B)

This is the position required by the BVA/Kennel Club hip dysplasia scheme. It is important to make sure that the radiograph is correctly positioned as those that are not will be returned to the veterinary surgeon. The radiograph must also be labelled with the dog's Kennel Club registration number, the date of radiography and left and/or right markers.

1. **Action:** Place the patient in dorsal recumbency ensuring that the body is straight.

    Rationale: This may be helped by the use of a trough or sandbags placed on either side

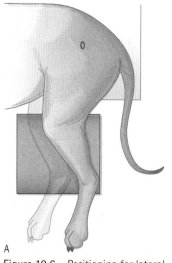

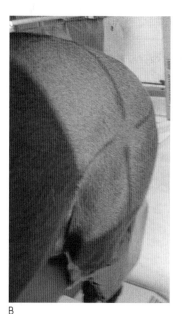

A

Figure 10.6   Positioning for lateral pelvis.

B

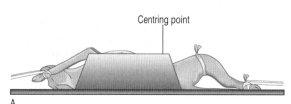

Centring point

A

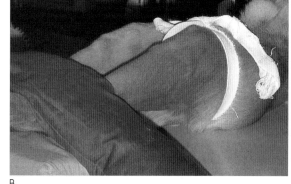

B

Figure 10.7   Positioning (ventrodorsal pelvis) and centring point (arrowed in part A) for assessment of hip dysplasia. Part A redrawn from Lane and Cooper (2003), Butterworth-Heinemann.

of the upper abdomen. If the upper body is straight the pelvis should also be straight. If the pelvis rotates, a foam pad may be placed under the lower hip.

2. **Action:** Extend the hind legs caudally so that the hips and stifles are fully extended. Secure with ties at the hocks.

    Rationale: This will further ensure that the pelvis is straight.

3. **Action:** Rotate the hind legs medially so that the femurs lie parallel to each other and the patellae are centred over the distal femurs.

Rationale: Rotation of the femur places the femoral head into the acetabulum, which gives an indication of the degree of hip dysplasia.

4. **Action:** Hold the femurs together by placing a tie around the level of the mid-femurs. Sticky-tape may be a convenient way of doing this.

    Rationale: The use of ties will ensure that the patient remains in this position.

5. **Action:** Added security may be achieved by placing another tie around the legs at the

level of the mid-tibia. Again sticky-tape may be of use.

6. **Action:** Centre the beam (indicated by the cross on the light beam diaphragm) in the midline over the pubic symphysis.

   Rationale: This should provide equal detail on either side of the pelvic girdle.

7. **Action:** Collimate the beam to include the wings of the ilium and the proximal half of the femurs.

   Rationale: This should demonstrate the entire pelvic girdle and the hip joints. The obturator foramina should be of equal size. Any inequality may be due to tilting of the pelvis and poor positioning.

SKULL

Procedure: Ventrodorsal skull (Fig. 10.8)

1. **Action:** Place the patient in dorsal recumbency.

   Rationale: This ensures that the skull is as close as possible to the film.

2. **Action:** Extend the neck.

   Rationale: Extension makes sure that the head is horizontal.

3. **Action:** Place a foam pad under the neck.

   Rationale: This forces the head back, so that the hard palate is parallel to the table top.

4. **Action:** Centre the beam (indicated by the cross on the light beam diaphragm) in the midline at a point halfway along the interpupillary line.

Rationale: This point may vary with the area to be examined.

5. **Action:** Collimate the beam to include the entire skull.

   Rationale: If necessary collimate more tightly over the area of interest, e.g. tympanic bulla.

Procedure: Open mouth rostrocaudal view of the tympanic bullae (Fig. 10.9)

1. **Action:** Place the animal in dorsal recumbency, with the hard palate perpendicular to the cassette. Tip the nose slightly past the vertical.

   Rationale: This position ensures that the bullae are as close as possible to the cassette. By tilting the head, the skull bones do not obstruct the view of the tympanic bullae.

2. **Action:** Hold the mouth open to form a V-shape, using tapes around each jaw, or place an old needle case (with one end cut off to create a hole) between the teeth of the upper and lower jaws.

   Rationale: In this position, the mandible and the maxilla are removed from the area of interest.

3. **Action:** Orientate the primary beam parallel to the hard palate and centre it (indicated by the cross of the light beam diaphragm) on the base of the tongue.

   Rationale: The tympanic bullae are located directly behind the base of the tongue in this position.

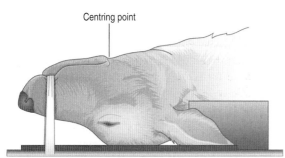

Figure 10.8   Positioning for ventrodorsal skull to show the position of the hard palate.

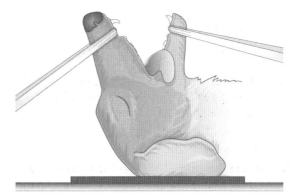

Figure 10.9   Positioning for open mouth rostrocaudal view.

4. **Action:** If the animal is intubated, remove the endotracheal tube before exposure.

   Rationale: The endotracheal tube will be superimposed on the tympanic bullae if not removed.

Procedure: Dorsoventral intraoral view of the nasal chambers (Fig. 10.10)

1. **Action:** The patient must be fully anaesthetised.

   Rationale: The cassette must be placed in the patient's mouth and without anaesthesia the animal will chew on the film.

2. **Action:** Place the animal in sternal recumbency.

   Rationale: This position ensures that the maxilla does not overlie the nasal chambers and provides a comfortable supported position for the animal.

3. **Action:** Extend the neck.

   Rationale: The position of the head is straighter if the neck is extended.

4. **Action:** Place a sandbag over the neck.

   Rationale: This prevents the head from rotating.

5. **Action:** Place a non-screen film into the mouth, corner first, as far into the mouth as possible.

   Rationale: Non-screen film is used as it provides excellent definition.

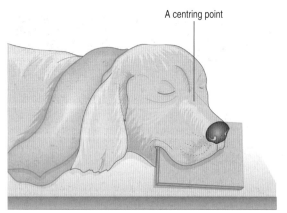

A centring point

Figure 10.10 Positioning for dorsoventral intraoral view of the nasal chambers.

6. **Action:** Centre the beam (indicated by the cross on the light beam diaphragm) on a line midway between the external nares and the interpupillary line.

   Rationale: This allows visualisation of the entire area of the nasal chambers.

7. **Action:** Place a left/right marker on the relevant side.

   Rationale: This ensures that any lesion can be related to the relevant nasal chamber. Most non-screen film cannot be labelled after processing so this must be done prior to exposure.

Procedure: Nasopharynx (Fig. 10.11)

1. **Action:** Place the patient in lateral recumbency.

   Rationale: This will provide radiographic access to the nasopharynx.

2. **Action:** Place pads under the nose and under the neck.

   Rationale: These maintain the skull in a horizontal line and prevent rotation.

3. **Action:** Pull the forelegs caudally to lie against the wall of the thorax using ties.

   Rationale: This pulls the shoulders and associated soft tissue structures away from the area of interest.

4. **Action:** Centre the beam (indicated by the cross on the light beam diaphragm) on the mid-cervical area to include the pharynx and thoracic inlet.

   Rationale: The areas cranial and caudal to the pharynx must be included.

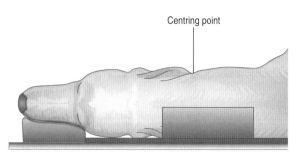

Centring point

Figure 10.11 Positioning for nasopharynx.

5. **Action:** If the animal is intubated, remove the endotracheal tube before exposure.

   Rationale: The endotracheal tube may mask a stricture or a mass.

THE LIMBS

Procedure: Mediolateral view of a distal limb extremity (Figs 10.12A, 10.13B and 10.13C) – general rules

1. **Action:** Place the patient in lateral recumbency, with the limb to be X-rayed closest to the cassette, e.g. right forelimb – place body in right lateral recumbency.

   Rationale: This ensures that the area is in close contact with the film, minimising distortion of the image.

2. **Action:** Extend the uppermost limb caudally (forelimb) or cranially (hindlimb) and support it on the flank using a tie.

   Rationale: The limb and any associated tissue that is not required are pulled out of the area of interest.

3. **Action:** The limb to be X-rayed should lie parallel to the cassette. It may be necessary to prevent rotation of the limb by using a pad.

   Rationale: Rotation of the limb should be avoided as the image should show a true mediolateral view.

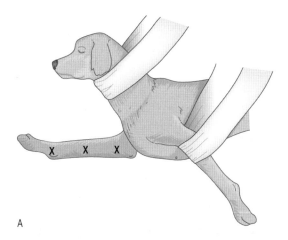
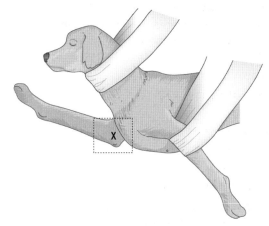

A

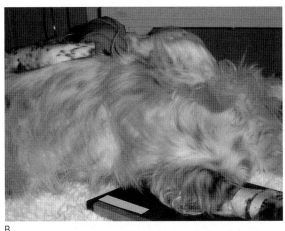
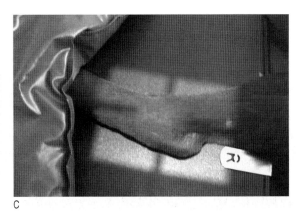

B   C

Figure 10.12   A, Positioning for mediolateral view of a distal extremity. B, Position for mediolateral view of distal left elbow. C, Position for mediolateral view of right hock.

4. **Action:** Stifles and elbow joints should be flexed.

   Rationale: Flexion enables a full examination of the joint.

5. **Action:** Centre the beam (indicated by the cross on the light beam diaphragm) at the level of the joint or mid-shaft.

   Rationale: Accurate centring will avoid distortion.

6. **Action:** Collimate the beam to include the joint above and below the long bone, or a small area above and below the joint in question.

   Rationale: Viewing adjacent structures may aid diagnosis.

Procedure: Dorsopalmar or dorsoplantar view or craniocaudal view of a limb (Fig. 10.13A, B and C) – general rules

1. **Action:** Place the patient in sternal (forelimb) or dorsal (hindlimb) recumbency so that the limb under investigation is parallel to the cassette.

   Rationale: Joints of the hindlimb are better imaged with the patient in dorsal recumbency. This allows the limb to be extended more easily, whilst still keeping the limb in good contact with the film.

2. **Action:** Keep the limb under investigation straight.

   Rationale: On extension, the limb may rotate inwards. To prevent this it may be necessary to lift and rotate the opposing limb.

3. **Action:** Centre the beam (indicated by the cross on the light beam diaphragm) at the level of the joint or the mid-shaft.

   Rationale: This must be accurate to avoid distortion.

4. **Action:** Collimate the beam to include the joint above and below the long bone, or a small area above and below the joint under investigation.

   Rationale: Viewing adjacent structures may aid diagnosis.

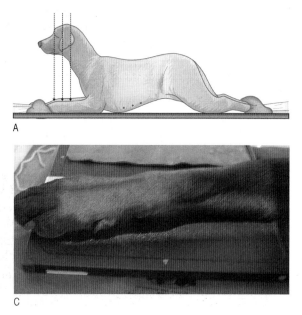

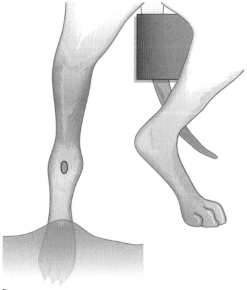

Figure 10.13 Positioning for craniocaudal view of distal forelimb (A), dorsoplantar view of distal hindlimb (B), and dorsopalmar view of distal right forelimb (C).

Procedure: Lateral shoulder (Fig. 10.14A and B)

1. **Action:** Place the patient in lateral recumbency, making sure that the limb to be examined is closest to the cassette.

   Rationale: Lateral recumbency gives adequate access to the shoulder joint.

2. **Action:** Extend the head and neck and secure by placing a sandbag over the neck – be careful to avoid interfering with normal respiration.

   Rationale: This ensures that an endotracheal tube lying in the trachea and larynx is pulled away from the area of the shoulder.

3. **Action:** Pull the affected leg cranially and secure with a tie.

   Rationale: This ensures that the area of the shoulder joint is not overlain by the soft tissues of the other shoulder.

4. **Action:** Pull the opposing limb caudally and secure with a tie.

   Rationale: This draws the soft tissues of the opposing limb away from the shoulder joint to be examined.

5. **Action:** Centre the beam (indicated by the cross on the light beam diaphragm) through the joint space of the shoulder.

   Rationale: Palpating the greater tuberosity of the humerus on the lateral aspect of the bone will provide the correct location.

6. **Action:** Collimate the beam to include the proximal third of the humerus and the distal part of the scapula.

   Rationale: This will cover the complete shoulder joint.

Procedure: Craniocaudal shoulder (Fig. 10.15)

1. **Action:** Place the patient in dorsal recumbency and support in a cradle or with sandbags.

   Rationale: This allows extension of the limb while preventing obstruction by the chest wall.

2. **Action:** Fully extend the limb to be examined cranially and secure with a tie.

   Rationale: Full extension of the limb will demonstrate the joint, without the elbow overlying the area.

3. **Action:** Rotate the thorax until the limb is in the craniocaudal position.

   Rationale: Rotation of the thorax enables the limb to be placed in a true craniocaudal position.

4. **Action:** Centre the beam (indicated by the cross on the light beam diaphragm) over the acromion of the scapula.

   Rationale: The acromion can be palpated on the lateral aspect of the joint, at the distal end of the spine of the scapula. The joint will be in the centre of the radiograph and demonstrated without distortion.

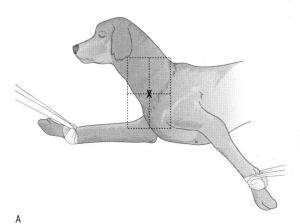

A

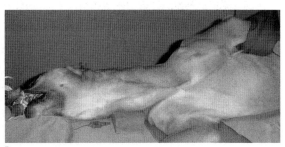

B

Figure 10.14 Positioning for lateral shoulder.

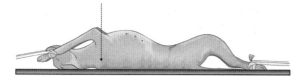

Figure 10.15   Positioning for craniocaudal shoulder.

5. **Action:** Collimate the beam to include the proximal third of the humerus and the distal part of the scapula.

    Rationale: This will cover the complete shoulder joint.

SPINE

Procedure: Lateral spine (Fig. 10.16A and B)

1. **Action:** Place the patient in right lateral recumbency.

Rationale: This will provide an image on which to base a diagnosis.

2. **Action:** Place supporting pads under the natural curves of the spine, i.e. the neck and the lumbar region. Place a pad under the nose.

    Rationale: These supports keep the spine horizontal and parallel with the tabletop. Placing a pad under the nose keeps the head in line.

3. **Action:** Place pads under the sternum and between the limbs.

    Rationale: These prevent rotation, which will pull the spine out of its horizontal position.

4. **Action:** If the cervical spine is to be examined pull the forelimbs caudally.

    Rationale: This ensures that the soft tissues of the shoulder do not overlie the spine.

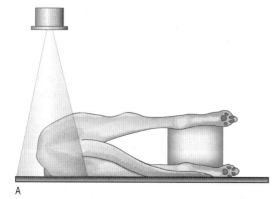
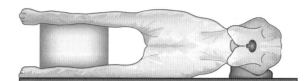
A

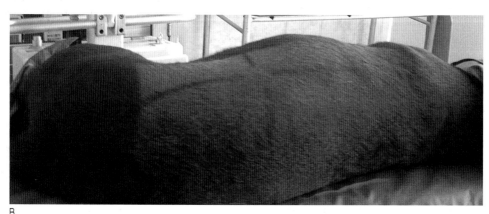
B

Figure 10.16   Positioning for lateral spine.

5. **Action:** Centre the beam (indicated by the cross of the light beam diaphragm) over the area of interest.

   Rationale: Centring must be accurate and care must be taken to avoid trying to cover too large an area at one time – divergence of the beam at the edges of the field will cause artificial narrowing of the joint spaces.

6. **Action:** Collimate the beam to cover about three vertebrae either side of the centre. Include muscle mass but not fat and skin. If the entire spine is to be examined, each image should overlap with the ones on either side.

   Rationale: By ensuring overlap, a complete study of each vertebra can be achieved with a minimum of distortion.

Procedure: Ventrodorsal spine (Fig. 10.17)

1. **Action:** Place the patient in dorsal recumbency supported in a trough or with sandbags.

   Rationale: Support must be provided to prevent rotation. This is even more important if a spinal injury is suspected.

2. **Action:** The spine must be positioned so that the sternum and the spine are in the same vertical plane.

   Rationale: Lack of alignment and rotation will affect the image and may provide an incorrect diagnosis.

3. **Action:** Extend the fore- and hindlimbs and secure with ties.

   Rationale: This provides additional support and prevents rotation of the spine.

4. **Action:** Centre the beam (indicated by the cross of the light beam diaphragm) over the area of interest.

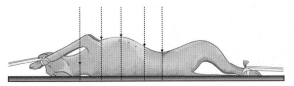

Figure 10.17 Positioning for ventrodorsal spine.

Rationale: Try to select the areas that correspond to those radiographed in the lateral view. In this way you have two planes per area of the spine.

5. **Action:** Collimate the beam to cover about three vertebrae either side of the centre. Include the transverse processes and include muscle mass but not fat and skin. If the entire spine is to be examined, each image should overlap with the ones on either side.

   Rationale: By ensuring overlap, a complete study of each vertebra can be achieved with a minimum of distortion.

USE OF CONTRAST MEDIA

Procedure: Use of barium in the evaluation of the gastrointestinal tract

1. **Action:** Prepare the barium sulphate. It may require mixing with a prescribed amount of water or may be ready-made. This must be done in the preparation room, away from the patient.

   Rationale: Barium should not be prepared near to the X-ray table as it may contaminate the table or the patient.

2. **Action:** Ensure that the patient is prepared as appropriate, e.g. fasted, given an enema. Do not sedate the animal.

   Rationale: Good patient preparation prevents the formation of artefacts on the radiograph, e.g. stomach contents mixed with barium. The use of sedatives will artificially slow gastrointestinal function and may affect the final diagnosis.

3. **Action:** Take plain radiographs before the introduction of contrast material.

   Rationale: These can be used for comparison with the contrast radiographs. Contrast media may mask some diagnostic features.

4. **Action:** If the patient is to be given a barium swallow, mix the barium with a small amount of normal food. Place a small amount of normal food on the top to entice the animal to eat.

Rationale: The use of food allows the processes of eating and swallowing to be seen more clearly.

5.   **Action:** If the patient is to be given a barium 'follow through' or meal, draw up approximately 5 ml/kg of liquid barium into a syringe. The patient may lap up the liquid or be force-fed with it.

Rationale: A larger volume of barium is needed to prevent dilution as it passes down the gastrointestinal tract.

6.   **Action:** If the patient is to be given a barium enema, the barium must be as liquid as possible. Introduce the barium into the rectum using a catheter (retrograde filling). Air may be introduced to provide a double contrast examination (see Fig. 10.18).

Rationale: Barium is used to outline the colon and must be as liquid as possible. Air can be used to enhance the image.

7.   **Action:** Always use the correct volume and consistency of contrast material.

Rationale: If the wrong type and volume of contrast material is used, the radiographs may not be diagnostic.

8.   **Action:** Select the correct patient position and collimate accurately.

Rationale: Incorrect positioning may miss the area of interest and alter the appearance of the pathology present. Collimation will enhance the image.

Procedure: Barium swallow

1.   **Action:** The patient remains conscious, but mild sedation may be needed.

Rationale: The use of general anaesthesia is not recommended, as the animal will be unable to swallow. Sedation should be avoided as this may slow the passage of ingesta down the gastrointestinal tract. If the animal seems likely to object to the taking of serial radiographs, sedation may be necessary.

2.   **Action:** Place the patient in right lateral recumbency and take a plain radiograph.

Rationale: Plain radiographs can be used to compare with the contrast radiographs.

3.   **Action:** Offer the patient food mixed with barium or restrain the patient as described in Chapter 1 and place a syringe full of liquid barium into the corner of the mouth, avoiding spillage. Administer in one bolus.

Rationale: The barium must be given as a bolus to aid visualisation on the radiograph. Any spillage of barium may appear as an artefact on the radiograph.

4.   **Action:** Place the patient in right lateral recumbency and take the X-ray of the oesophageal/thoracic area.

Rationale: Food takes 15–30 seconds to pass down the oesophagus, so the radiograph must be taken quickly. Any barium remaining in the oesophagus will line the mucosa and outline any lesions.

Procedure: Barium meal or 'follow through'

1.   **Action:** The patient should be fasted for 12 hours. Water should be withheld for 2 hours.

Rationale: The presence of food and water will affect stomach function and the appearance and movement of the barium.

2.   **Action:** Moderate sedation may be needed.

Rationale: The patient may object to serial radiographs being taken. Acepromazine has the least effect on gut motility.

3.   **Action:** Take plain radiographs – lateral and ventrodorsal views.

Rationale: These provide a comparison with contrast radiographs. Taking two views allows accurate location of any lesions.

4.   **Action:** Restrain the patient and place a syringe containing barium into the corner of the mouth, avoiding spillage. Administer slowly. It may be necessary to use a stomach tube.

Rationale: The barium must be administered over a short period, so the procedure must be carried out quickly and cleanly. Any spillage of barium may appear as an artefact on the radiograph.

5. **Action:** If fluoroscopy is available, it may be used to observe the movements of the stomach.

   Rationale: Fluoroscopy produces 'live' X-rays and can be used for real-time investigations.

6. **Action:** Take a series of radiographs – right lateral, left lateral, ventrodorsal and dorsoventral centred over the mid-abdomen, immediately after administration of the barium.

   Rationale: These four views ensure that all parts of the stomach are examined.

7. **Action:** Repeat these views 10 minutes later and then at 30-minute intervals until the stomach is empty.

   Rationale: These time intervals allow the movement of barium to be monitored without missing too much detail.

8. **Action:** To demonstrate the small intestine, radiographs should be taken every hour until the stomach is empty.

   Rationale: This ensures that the complete intestinal tract is demonstrated.

Procedure: Barium enema (Fig. 10.18)

1. **Action:** The patient should be fed on a low residue diet for 3 days.

   Rationale: This will ensure that a minimum amount of faeces is present in the colon.

2. **Action:** Prepare the patient by giving a non-irritant enema 2–3 hours before the examination.

   Rationale: This removes the faeces and ensures that barium does not adhere to anything other than the wall of the colon. The presence of faeces may obscure much of the abdominal detail.

3. **Action:** The patient should be given a general anaesthetic or heavy sedation.

   Rationale: This is essential to allow catheterisation of the rectum and the introduction of barium, which can be uncomfortable.

4. **Action:** Place the patient in ventrodorsal and right lateral recumbency and take plain radiographs of the abdomen.

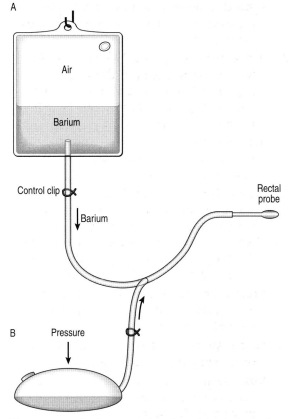

Figure 10.18   Barium enema bag. In position A, the barium flows under gravity into the colon. In position B, barium empties from the colon into the bag and then pressure on the bag will distend the colon with air for the double contrast effect. Adapted, with permission, from Ouster (2000), Butterworth Heinemann.

   Rationale: These will demonstrate any pathology present and may be used for comparison with the contrast radiographs.

5. **Action:** Hang an old drip bag containing a 50–50 mixture of barium and water from a drip stand.

   Rationale: This mixture allows the barium to flow into the colon.

6. **Action:** Insert a Foley catheter into the rectum. This is attached by means of a length of rubber tubing to the drip bag. Attach a clamp to control the flow from the bag.

   Rationale: Control of the barium flow is essential to prevent backflow and overfilling of the colon.

7. **Action:** Adjust the clamp to allow barium to flow slowly into the rectum and colon. Continue until the barium just begins to leak out around the catheter.

   Rationale: Hanging the bag from a drip stand allows the barium to flow into the rectum by gravity.

8. **Action:** Place the patient in right lateral, left lateral and ventrodorsal recumbency – take radiographs.

   Rationale: These views allow the entire colon to be demonstrated.

9. **Action:** kV should be increased above that used for the plain radiographs.

   Rationale: This ensures that the edges of the barium are clearly delineated, which aids interpretation of the radiograph.

10. **Action:** If a double contrast technique is used, lower the drip bag and allow barium to flow back into the bag by gravity.

    Rationale: If the radiograph is taken with both barium and air in the colon, it will not be diagnostic.

11. **Action:** Gently squeeze the bag, forcing air into the rectum and colon.

    Rationale: Air distends the colon while the remains of the barium stick to the colonic mucosa.

12. **Action:** Repeat the radiographs as in step 8.

    Rationale: Reduce the kV as air is of a lower density than barium.

Procedure: Intravenous urography (Fig. 10.19)

1. **Action:** The patient should be starved for 12 hours. Water should be withheld for 2 hours prior to the procedure.

   Rationale: This procedure is performed under a general anaesthetic; starvation ensures that the patient does not vomit and choke.

2. **Action:** Administer an enema.

   Rationale: The presence of faeces in the colon may mask the view of the kidney and ureters.

3. **Action:** Administer a general anaesthetic to the patient.

   Rationale: Intravenous iodine may cause an unpleasant feeling of nausea and may be irritant if perivascular leakage occurs. A large number of radiographs may be needed. If the patient is anaesthetised, these are all made easier.

4. **Action:** Take plain radiographs in right lateral and ventrodorsal recumbency, centred on the umbilicus.

   Rationale: These views will demonstrate all the areas of the urinary tract and can be used for comparison with the later contrast radiographs.

5. **Action:** Introduce a urinary catheter into the bladder and empty it by gentle compression on the bladder or by drawing urine out by syringe. Introduce a small amount of air.

   Rationale: The presence of urine in the bladder will dilute the contrast medium.

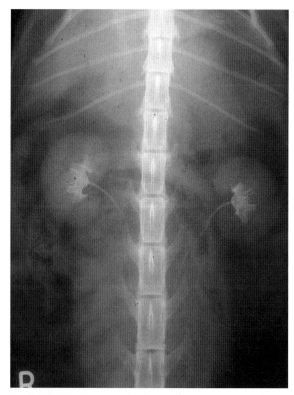

Figure 10.19 Radiograph of a ventrodorsal abdomen to show the effects of intravenous urography.

Air in the bladder enables the ureters passing over the bladder and the position of the neck of the bladder neck to be seen.

6. **Action:** Restrain the patient for an intravenous injection – see Chapter 1.

   Rationale: The cephalic vein is the easiest intravenous route to use in the dog and the cat.

7. **Action:** Inject either:
   - Bolus of warmed contrast medium (iodine 300–400 mg/ml conc.) at a dose of 850 mg iodine/kg bodyweight (approx. 1 ml/kg).
   - Infusion of warmed contrast medium (iodine 150–200 mg/ml conc.) at a dose of 1200 mg iodine/kg bodyweight. May be given using a giving set over a period of 10–15 minutes.

   Rationale: Bolus intravenous urography is recommended for kidney examination. Infusion intravenous urography is used for patients with urinary incontinence and ureteric problems. Warming the iodine solution reduces its viscosity and makes intravenous injection easier.

8. **Action:** As soon as the intravenous injection has been completed, take a ventrodorsal radiograph of the abdomen, centring on the area of the umbilicus.

   Rationale: Clear colourless iodine appears as a radio-opaque material within the urinary system. The kidneys will fill with iodine, demonstrating the size and shape of the kidneys. A ventrodorsal view enables a comparison of both kidneys to be made.

9. **Action:** Take another radiograph after 5 minutes.

   Rationale: The pelvis of each kidney will be outlined by contrast material.

10. **Action:** Place the patient in right lateral recumbency and take another radiograph after 10 minutes.

    Rationale: The ureters will be filled and their size and position can be evaluated.

11. **Action:** Place the patient in right lateral recumbency and take another radiograph after 15 minutes. Centre at the level of the neck of the bladder.

    Rationale: The bladder will be filling and the trigone area should be visible.

12. **Action:** Further radiographs can be taken if abnormalities are detected or if excretion rates are slowed.

    Rationale: Taking additional views can be decided on the basis of individual findings.

Procedure: Urethrogram (retrograde urethrography) – male

1. **Action:** Administer an enema to the patient (but this is not essential).

   Rationale: The presence of faeces may alter the position of the bladder or urethra.

2. **Action:** Administer a sedative to the patient. In some cases a general anaesthetic may be given.

   Rationale: This procedure can be performed with care in a conscious animal but it may cause the urethra to constrict – the interpretation of the radiograph should take this into account.

3. **Action:** Place the patient in right lateral recumbency and take a plain radiograph centred for the neck of the bladder and collimated to include the entire urethra.

   Rationale: This may indicate any lesions that may later be masked by the contrast material.

4. **Action:** Introduce a urinary catheter into the bladder and drain the urine. Remove the catheter.

   Rationale: The presence of urine in the bladder will dilute the contrast medium.

5. **Action:** Select a Foley catheter and flush with contrast material before it is inserted.

   Rationale: This flushes air out of the catheter. If air is present in the catheter when it is inserted into the urethra, the air may appear to be in the urethra and affect the diagnosis.

6. **Action:** Place the patient in right lateral recumbency.

   Rationale: This is the most comfortable position for the patient and provides easy access to the penis and urethra.

7. **Action:** Gently introduce the Foley catheter into the penile urethra and inflate the cuff.

   Rationale: Inflating the cuff prevents backflow of contrast material out of the urethra.

8. **Action:** Inject 5–15 ml of iodine (150 mg/ml) slowly up the catheter.

   Rationale: The addition of KY jelly to the contrast material will increase the degree of urethral distension and may produce a better image.

9. **Action:** Stand back from the patient and take a lateral radiograph. Pull the hind legs cranially to show the ischial arch and pull them caudally to show the penile urethra.

   Rationale: If it is necessary to prevent leakage of the contrast material by occluding the end of the penis manually, your hands and forearms must be protected from scattered radiation by a lead sheet or gloves during the exposure.

Procedure: Urethrogram (retrograde vaginourethrography) – female

1. **Action:** Administer an enema to the patient (but this is not essential).

   Rationale: The presence of faeces may alter the position of the bladder or urethra.

2. **Action:** Administer a general anaesthetic to the patient.

   Rationale: The use of Allis tissue forceps later in the procedure is painful so a general anaesthetic is recommended.

3. **Action:** Place the patient in right lateral recumbency and take a plain radiograph, centred on the neck of the bladder and collimated to include the entire urethra.

   Rationale: This will demonstrate any lesions and provide a comparison with later contrast radiographs.

4. **Action:** Introduce a urinary catheter into the bladder and drain the urine. Remove the catheter.

   Rationale: The presence of urine in the bladder will dilute the contrast medium.

5. **Action:** Select a Foley catheter and flush with contrast material.

   Rationale: This flushes air out of the catheter. If air is present when the catheter is inserted into the vestibule, the air may appear to be in the vestibule and affect the diagnosis.

6. **Action:** Place the animal in right lateral recumbency.

   Rationale: This is the most comfortable position for the patient and provides easy access to the vagina and vestibule.

7. **Action:** Insert the Foley catheter through the vulval lips and into the vestibule, and inflate the cuff.

   Rationale: Inflating the cuff prevents backflow and leakage of contrast material out of the vagina and vestibule.

8. **Action:** Hold the catheter in place and attach a pair of Allis tissue forceps across the vulva.

   Rationale: This procedure prevents further loss of the contrast material, but can be painful in a conscious bitch.

9. **Action:** Inject up to 1 ml/kg bodyweight of iodine (150 mg/ml) slowly up the catheter.

   Rationale: The contrast material enters the vagina under pressure and care must be taken not to overfill the vagina and urethra as rupture can occur.

10. **Action:** Stand back from the patient and take a lateral radiograph.

    Rationale: If it is necessary to prevent leakage of the contrast material by occluding the vulva manually, your hands and forearms must be protected from scattered radiation by a lead sheet or gloves during the exposure.

Procedure: Cystography – pneumocystogram, positive contrast cystogram, double contrast cystogram

1. **Action:** Administer an enema to the patient.

   Rationale: The presence of faeces may alter the position of the bladder.

2. **Action:** Administer a general anaesthetic – although the procedure can be performed under sedation.

Rationale: This is not necessarily a painful procedure, but it may be easier to position the animal if it is sedated or anaesthetised. The urethra may constrict when a fully conscious animal is catheterised and interpretation of the radiograph should take this into account.

3. **Action:** Place the patient in right lateral recumbency and take a plain radiograph centred on the neck of the bladder.

   Rationale: This can be used as a comparison with later contrast radiographs.

4. **Action:** Introduce a urinary catheter into the bladder and drain the urine.

   Rationale: The presence of urine in the bladder will dilute the contrast material.

5. **Action:** With the patient in right lateral recumbency, gently introduce room air into the bladder using a syringe and a three-way tap at a rate of approximately 10 ml/kg bodyweight.

   Rationale: The bladder should feel moderately distended when the abdomen is palpated. Care must be taken to avoid rupturing the bladder.

6. **Action:** Take a lateral radiograph.

   Rationale: This is known as pneumocystogram – the bladder will appear as a dark mass in the caudal abdomen. This is used to detect the presence of calculi in the bladder.

7. **Action:** For a positive contrast cystogram, introduce diluted iodine contrast material at a rate of 10 ml/kg bodyweight after draining the urine from the bladder. Take a lateral radiograph. kV must be increased.

   Rationale: The bladder appears as a radio-opaque mass in the caudal abdomen. kV must be increased as positive contrast is denser than the air in the pneumocystogram.

8. **Action:** For a double contrast cystogram, inject 2–15 ml of iodine (150 mg/ml) into the empty bladder via the catheter and gently roll the patient from side to side.

   Rationale: Rolling the patient ensures that the iodine covers the bladder mucosa.

9. **Action:** Inflate the bladder with air until it feels taut. Take a lateral radiograph.

Rationale: The bladder mucosa appears covered with positive contrast while the lumen appears dark with a shadow of residual contrast material in the centre. This technique is used to evaluate the thickness of the bladder wall, the presence of lesions such as tumours, and the presence of calculi.

10. **Action:** In all cases exposure should be carried out immediately after the contrast material has been injected.

    Rationale: This procedure does not require anyone to remain in the room, so in the interests of radiation safety, normal procedures should be followed.

Procedure: Myelography – cisternal and lumbar puncture (Fig. 10.20)

1. **Action:** Administer a general anaesthetic to the patient.

   Rationale: This procedure is potentially painful and requires accurate placing of a spinal needle in the subarachnoid space. Any sudden movements could have serious consequences.

2. **Action:** Place the patient in lateral recumbency and take plain radiographs of the area under investigation.

   Rationale: This will provide preliminary indications as to the diagnosis and enables exposure factors to be set.

3. **Action:** Clip the neck caudal to the skull (cisternal) or over the lumbar spine (lumbar) and prepare the site as for a surgical procedure.

   Rationale: Care must be taken to prevent the introduction of infection into the spinal cord.

4. **Action:** Select a non-ionic contrast material (200–300 mg/ml iodine) and gently warm it. Dose rate is 0.3–0.45 ml/kg bodyweight depending on size.

   Rationale: Non-ionic iodine provides the least amount of irritation to the spinal cord. Warming reduces the viscosity of the liquid, making it easier to inject.

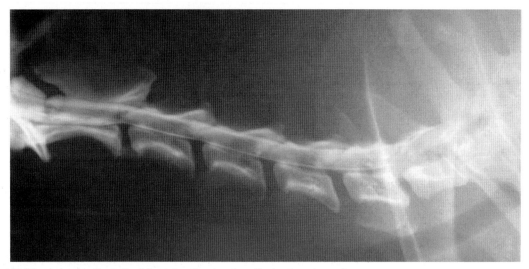

Figure 10.20 Lateral radiograph of the spine showing the effects of myelography.

5. **Action:** For cisternal puncture: raise the table to about 10° tilt with the patient's head at the raised end.

    Rationale: This ensures that contrast material does not flow up into the ventricles of the brain, which could cause pain due to a rise in cerebral pressure and result in fitting.

6. **Action:** Flex the head to an angle of 90° so that the chin touches the sternum.

    Rationale: The needle is to be inserted into the cisterna magna, which is the cranial end of the subarachnoid space just behind the skull. Flexing the neck opens up access to this space.

7. **Action:** Insert a spinal needle of a suitable length, depending on the patient's size, between the skull and the atlas (Fig. 10.21). Advance it until cerebrospinal fluid (CSF) drips from the needle. Collect a sample of CSF.

    Rationale: The presence of CSF indicates that the needle is in the correct position. Analysis of the sample of CSF may be an added diagnostic aid.

8. **Action:** Inject the required amount of contrast material slowly. Remove the needle and extend the neck. Take radiographs.

    Rationale: Slow injection prevents a sudden increase in pressure.

9. **Action:** For lumbar puncture: flex the vertebral column by pulling the hind legs forward.

    Rationale: The site used is at the level of the L4–5 junction or L5–6. This position should not be used if there is any indication of spinal instability.

10. **Action:** Insert a spinal needle of a suitable length into the appropriate junction and note the twitch of the legs and anus.

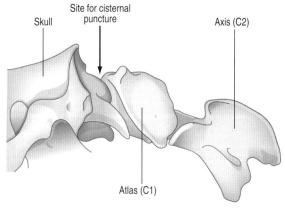

Figure 10.21 Myelography: site for cisternal puncture. Redrawn from Lane and Cooper (2003), Butterworth-Heinemann.

Rationale: This twitch indicates that the needle has passed through the spinal cord.

11. **Action:** Little or no CSF will appear through the needle. If this is the case, inject a small amount of contrast material.

    Rationale: Lack of CSF does not indicate incorrect needle placement. A small amount of contrast material is injected to test for correct needle placement.

12. **Action:** A test radiograph may be taken in lateral recumbency centred over the needle.

    Rationale: This will show whether the small amount of contrast material has reached the correct site.

13. **Action:** Inject the remainder of the contrast material. Remove the needle and straighten the spine. Keep the head raised. Take the radiographs.

    Rationale: If the needle is left in position, it may damage the spinal cord. Keeping the head raised prevents the flow of contrast material towards the brain.

14. **Action:** In either technique, once the contrast material has been introduced, take lateral views of the spine starting at the site of injection and move caudally. In the area of the cervical spine, remove the endotracheal tube from the larynx.

    Rationale: The entire spine should be examined as additional lesions may be found. The endotracheal tube will lie over the spinal cord and make interpretation more difficult.

15. **Action:** When the contrast material has reached the main point of interest, take ventrodorsal and oblique views.

    Rationale: Lateral, ventrodorsal and oblique views allow accurate identification and location of the lesion.

16. **Action:** During recovery, the patient must be placed in its kennel with its head raised.

    Rationale: This prevents flow of contrast material into the ventricles of the brain causing a painful rise in pressure and the risk of fits.

TECHNIQUES FOR PROCESSING RADIOGRAPHS

Procedure: Manual processing (Fig. 10.22)

1. **Action:** Put on a pair of rubber gloves and a plastic apron.

   Rationale: Processing chemicals can be irritant and you should protect your hands and your clothes. Goggles will also protect your eyes from splashes.

2. **Action:** Check that the levels and the temperatures of the developer and fixer tanks are correct. If appropriate check the temperature of the surrounding water bath.

   Rationale: If the levels of chemicals in the tanks are low, the upper parts of the film will not be processed. The temperature of the developer should be 20 °C and the fixer 20–21 °C. Too low temperatures will result in

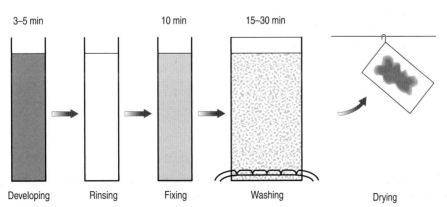

3–5 min   10 min   15–30 min

Developing   Rinsing   Fixing   Washing   Drying

Figure 10.22   Routine for manual processing. Redrawn from Lane and Cooper (2003), Butterworth-Heinemann.

underdevelopment and too high results in overdevelopment (always check the label for accurate temperatures as they may vary).

3. **Action:** Turn off all lights except the safelight.

    Rationale: White light will fog the film. The safelight must have the correct filter for the type of film.

4. **Action:** Lock the door to the darkroom.

    Rationale: Accidental opening of the door will allow light into the room with subsequent fogging of the film.

5. **Action:** Unload the cassette and place the film in a hanger of a suitable design and size.

    Rationale: Hangers minimise handling of the film during processing. There are two designs – channel and clip hangers. The size of the hanger must match that of the film.

6. **Action:** Place the film in the developer tank, moving it gently to remove bubbles and to coat the emulsion evenly. Set the timer and leave in the developer for the recommended time.

    Rationale: Uneven coating of the film will cause uneven development. The recommended time for development is usually 4 minutes. Removing the film too soon causes a pale or underdeveloped film; leaving it for too long causes a dark or over-developed film.

7. **Action:** Take the film out of the developer tank, allowing any excess to drip back into the tank. Replace the lid of the developer tank.

    Rationale: If developer is allowed to mix with the rinse water, the water will become contaminated over a period of time. The lid of the developer tank prevents oxidation of the chemicals by air when it is not in use.

8. **Action:** Place the film in the rinse tank and agitate it gently.

    Rationale: The water stops the action of the developer and rinses the film clean.

9. **Action:** Place the film in the fixer tank and leave for 10 minutes.

    Rationale: Fixer hardens the emulsion and fixes the image so that it can be viewed in white light. You may look at the image after the milky appearance on the film has disappeared (clearing). It must be replaced in the tank for the full time. Timing is not critical but should be a minimum of 8 minutes. If the fixing process is not complete, the film will turn brown when stored.

10. **Action:** Place the film in the wash tank for at least 30 minutes.

    Rationale: The wash tank should be filled with running water and is used to remove any residual chemicals. If chemicals remain on the film, it becomes yellow with time.

11. **Action:** The room light can now be switched on.

    Rationale: The film is no longer sensitive to white light after 30 seconds in the fixer but if you can wait longer there will be no risk of light fogging.

12. **Action:** Hang the film up to dry or place it in a drying cabinet.

    Rationale: The film must be thoroughly dried before storage. Viewing the radiograph for the final interpretation is best done using a dry radiograph as swelling of the emulsion during processing may cause distortion of the image.

13. **Action:** Cassettes should always be reloaded after use in the dry area of the darkroom and stored ready for use. This may be done while you are waiting for the developing process to work.

    Rationale: Loading must be done in the dark or under the safelight to prevent fogging. Avoid any splashing by chemicals in the wet area of the darkroom.

Procedure: Starting up an automatic processor

1. **Action:** Check the levels of water and chemicals in the processor and the replenisher tanks. Check the position of the rollers.

    Rationale: The levels of the chemicals will fall with use. Other users may displace the rollers.

2. **Action:** Turn on the water supply valve.

    Rationale: Water is needed to wash the films and to maintain the constant temperature necessary for processing.

3. **Action:** Turn on the mains supply to the machine and the processor's power switch.

    Rationale: An electricity supply is essential.

4. **Action:** Replace the lid of the processor.

    Rationale: The lid should be removed when not in use, but must be replaced to prevent leakage when in use.

5. **Action:** Check the temperature of the processor.

    Rationale: A low temperature will result in underdevelopment of the films. The machine may take about 20 minutes to reach its recommended temperature.

6. **Action:** Feed two or three old clean films through the processor.

    Rationale: These will remove dried chemicals from the rollers.

7. **Action:** At the same time check that the replenishment pumps are working.

    Rationale: These work whenever a film is in the processor.

Procedure: Automatic processing

1. **Action:** Switch the processor on in the prescribed way and check that the temperature is correct.

    Rationale: If the temperature is too low the films will be underdeveloped. If the recommended set up procedure is not followed, vital stages may be missed, resulting in fogging of the film or a lack of water to the processor.

2. **Action:** Lock the door of the darkroom and switch the lights off.

    Rationale: Accidental opening of the door will allow light in, causing fogging of the film.

3. **Action:** Remove the film from the cassette and place it onto the tray or entry roller of the processor.

    Rationale: The film should be placed in the correct orientation for entry to prevent damage.

4. **Action:** Allow the film to be taken into the processor.

    Rationale: Restricting the movement of the film will cause scratching of the emulsion.

5. **Action:** Wait for the audible or visible indicator before leaving the darkroom, inserting the next film or switching the light back on.

    Rationale: If a second film is put in before the first film has moved into the processor, the two may stick together.

6. **Action:** Reload the cassette and place it in the storage area ready for use.

    Rationale: Loading must be done in the dark or under the safelight to prevent fogging. Avoid any splashing by chemicals or water.

Procedure: Shutting down the automatic processor

1. **Action:** Make sure that there are no films in the processor.

    Rationale: If the processor is switched off with films still passing through, they may be irreparably damaged.

2. **Action:** Turn off the power switch on the processor and the mains isolator switch.

    Rationale: Power should never be left on when the processor is not in use.

3. **Action:** Turn off the water supply.

    Rationale: Water should never be left running unnecessarily.

4. **Action:** Remove the processor cover or lid.

    Rationale: The lid can be removed to give easy access.

5. **Action:** Remove any chemical residue from inside the processor.

    Rationale: Daily removal of any residue reduces damage that may occur if chemicals are left on the working parts for long periods of time.

6. **Action:** Place an antifungal tablet into the wash tank.

Rationale: This reduces the build-up of fungi and algae in the wash water.

7. **Action:** Ensure that the lid or cover is left in a slightly raised position.

    Rationale: Air circulation through the processor reduces the build-up of condensation.

Procedure: Cleaning an automatic processor

1. **Action:** Put on a pair of rubber gloves and a plastic apron.

    Rationale: Processing chemicals can be irritant and you should protect your hands and your clothes. Goggles will also protect your eyes from splashes.

2. **Action:** Switch off the electricity supply to the machine.

    Rationale: The combination of electricity and water could be fatal!

3. **Action:** Drain the water tank by opening the valve.

    Rationale: Draining the water allows proper cleaning to be carried out.

4. **Action:** Remove the cross-over rollers between the tanks and wash them in fresh water.

    Rationale: The cross-over rollers collect chemical residues, which dry on them. At most times these rollers are out of the liquids.

5. **Action:** Place a splashguard between the fixer and the developer tank.

    Rationale: This prevents cross-contamination between the tanks.

6. **Action:** Remove the rollers from the developer tank. Wash in fresh water, remove any residual chemicals and check their movement.

    Rationale: Dried developer on the rollers will scratch the emulsion, giving rise to 'roller marks', and prevent their free movement.

7. **Action:** Replace the developer racks after draining, taking care not to splash developer into the fixer.

    Rationale: This prevents cross-contamination between the tanks.

8. **Action:** Remove the rollers from the fixer tank. Wash in fresh water, remove any residual chemicals and check their movement.

    Rationale: Dried fixer on the rollers will scratch the emulsion, giving rise to 'roller marks', and prevent their free movement.

9. **Action:** Replace the fixer racks after draining, taking care not to splash fixer into the developer.

    Rationale: This prevents cross-contamination between the tanks.

10. **Action:** Remove the rollers from the wash tank and clean in fresh water.

    Rationale: The effect of heat, emulsion residue and water creates a build-up of sludge and algae. This reduces the quality of the image produced and the function of the processor.

11. **Action:** Clean the empty tank with a sponge and fresh water.

    Rationale: Care should be taken to remove any algae that have built up on the tank sides.

12. **Action:** Replace the wash tank racks.

    Rationale: The racks should be replaced carefully and seated in their correct positions.

13. **Action:** Close the valve to the wash tank to allow refilling.

    Rationale: Without water, the processor will not wash the films and may overheat.

14. **Action:** Replace the cross-over racks.

    Rationale: These must be replaced last as they sit over all the other rollers.

15. **Action:** Replace the lid of the processor and switch the power back on.

    Rationale: The lid provides a light-tight seal to prevent fogging of the films.

16. **Action:** Pass a few old clean films through the processor.

    Rationale: These will pick up any residue that has been dislodged during cleaning. It is also a means of checking for correct function before clinical radiographs are processed.

MAINTENANCE OF RADIOGRAPHY EQUIPMENT

Procedure: Care of intensifying screens

1. **Action:** Moisten a soft cloth with a screen cleaning detergent or a small amount of commercial detergent and water.

    Rationale: Intensifying screens are delicate and expensive pieces of equipment – any damage will appear on the radiograph and the screen may be rendered useless. Avoid the use of any material that will scratch the screens. Do not use cotton wool as this leaves small pieces of lint on the screen.

2. **Action:** Wipe the screen gently.

    Rationale: The detergent should be used sparingly and only just touch the screen.

3. **Action:** Do not wet the screen and avoid spilling anything on the back of the screen.

    Rationale: Moisture damages the grains within the screen, affecting their efficiency, and will also cause the cardboard backing to disintegrate.

4. **Action:** Wipe the screen clean with a fresh dry cloth or piece of gauze.

    Rationale: All detergent and moisture must be removed to prevent damage to the screen.

5. **Action:** Stand the cassette upright and leave it slightly open to dry.

    Rationale: This prevents pooling of the detergent and allows air to circulate, reducing condensation.

6. **Action:** Record when the cleaning was done and by whom.

    Rationale: Regular cleaning of the screens improves image quality. Any damage can be traced.

Procedure: Checking safelight function

1. **Action:** Enter the darkroom and switch off the white light.

    Rationale: White light will always fog the film.

2. **Action:** Do not switch on the safelight.

    Rationale: This film will be used to provide a baseline for your assessment.

3. **Action:** Select two films of the type commonly used in the practice but of the smallest size available.

    Rationale: Keep the cost of this assessment to a minimum.

4. **Action:** Take one film (film A) out of any protective covering and place your hand on it for 30 seconds.

    Rationale: If the darkroom is truly lightproof, there will be no image on this film.

5. **Action:** Repeat this process with the other film (B) with the safelight switched on.

    Rationale: If the safelight is leaking light of the wrong wavelength, it will produce an image of the hand. If the safelight is in working order there will be no image on the film.

6. **Action:** Process both films.

    Rationale: The image cannot be seen without processing.

7. **Action:** Compare the two films.

    Rationale: This technique can also be used to assess the degree of lightproofing of the darkroom.

Procedure: Checking for light leakage in a cassette

1. **Action:** Load the cassette to be investigated with a piece of new film and close it securely.

    Rationale: A new film is used to make sure that no fogging is present.

2. **Action:** Expose each edge of the cassette to high intensity light (100 W) for about 15 minutes.

    Rationale: High intensity light simulates the type of light to which the cassette may normally be exposed.

3. **Action:** Process the film and look at it on a viewer.

    Rationale: If the edges of the cassette are leaking light, the processed film will show a dark border. Any border greater than 3 mm wide should be assumed to have resulted from leakage of light.

Procedure: Checking the X-ray tube for leakage of X-rays

1. **Action:** Set up the X-ray machine for a low exposure.

   Rationale: The tube should be set up for normal use to make the test as realistic as possible.

2. **Action:** Close the light beam diaphragm.

   Rationale: This will reduce the exposure of the environment and the risk of scattered radiation.

3. **Action:** Place a series of non-screen films around the X-ray tube head. Make sure each one is labelled with its position in relation to the tube.

   Rationale: Non-screen film is flexible and can be used to cover the entire head.

4. **Action:** Make an exposure.

   Rationale: X-rays will barely escape as the primary beam, but if there is leakage from the head it will affect the films around the head.

5. **Action:** Process the films and look at them on a viewer.

   Rationale: Signs of leakage appear as grey areas on the radiograph and may correspond to joints in the tube head. **The machine should not be used until a further professional assessment has been made**.

Procedure: Checking for the accuracy of the light beam diaphragm

1. **Action:** Place a loaded cassette on the table under the X-ray tube head, keeping the standard film focal distance.

   Rationale: Use a small piece of film to reduce costs.

2. **Action:** Switch on the light beam diaphragm and collimate it to produce an area of approximately 10 cm square.

   Rationale: A small area prevents unnecessary contamination of the immediate environment and reduces the risk of scattered radiation.

3. **Action:** Place a row of paper clips along the perimeter of the illuminated square.

   Rationale: The paper clips mark the edges of the irradiated square once the light beam diaphragm is switched off.

4. **Action:** On each corner place an unfolded paper clip, with one end towards the corner.

   Rationale: The pointed end of the clip accurately delineates the corners.

5. **Action:** Using a low exposure expose the film.

   Rationale: A low exposure reduces the risk of scattered radiation.

6. **Action:** Process and assess the radiograph.

   Rationale: If the light beam indicates the area exposed by the primary beam accurately, the border of paper clips will be on the edge of the exposed film and the points of the unfolded clips will point to the corners. If the light beam diaphragm is inaccurate, an engineer should be called to correct the fault.

Procedure: Checking a cassette for poor film/screen contact

1. **Action:** Place a piece of zinc or copper netting or metallic material with small holes cut out on top of a small loaded cassette.

   Rationale: A specific test tool is available but any metal sheet with holes cut out will do as well. The holes must be present to provide a sharp edge as a means of assessment.

2. **Action:** Collimate the beam to cover most of the cassette, leaving a minimal border around the edge.

   Rationale: All radiographs should have at least a small border around the edge to indicate that the beam has been restricted to some degree.

3. **Action:** Expose the cassette using a low exposure.

   Rationale: A low exposure prevents unnecessary contamination of the immediate environment and reduces the risk of scattered radiation.

4. **Action:** Process and assess the radiograph.

   Rationale: Areas of poor film/screen contact will show as darker blurred areas. Even film/screen contact will produce a sharp uniform image. If the cassette is affected, it will be due to compression and age- ing of the pressure pad underneath the back intensifying screen or warping of the screens. The cassette should be replaced.

DIAGNOSTIC ULTRASOUND

Procedure: Preparing the patient for an ultrasound examination

1. **Action:** Administer a sedative to the patient.

    Rationale: Ultrasonography is a non-invasive painless procedure, which is well tolerated by most animals. In some cases it may be easier to place a sedated patient in the cor- rect position, and procedures such as biopsy or fine needle aspiration may require deeper sedation or a general anaesthetic.

2. **Action:** Place the patient on an examination table in a position that provides sufficient access to the area under examination.

    Rationale: This may mean that the patient can remain standing or lie in lateral or dorsal recumbency. If the patient feels comfortable and secure, it will be unlikely to struggle. Avoid using areas where underlying bone and gas may block the movement of the ultrasound waves.

3. **Action:** Clip the area and apply spirit.

    Rationale: Fur must be removed to provide good contact between the skin and the transducer of the ultrasound machine. Spirit is used to remove any remaining dirt and grease on the skin surface.

4. **Action:** Apply coupling gel to the transducer and the skin.

    Rationale: Coupling gel ensures good con- tact between the skin and the transducer. Trapped air will create an artefact, which may affect the final diagnosis.

5. **Action:** Apply the transducer to the skin within the prepared area.

    Rationale: When the transducer is applied to the skin, high frequency sound waves pass through the patient's soft tissues as pres- sure waves. At interfaces between organs or

between different tissues, some sound waves are reflected and return to the transducer. Here they are detected by the ultrasound equipment, which produces a cross-sectional image of the internal structure of the tissues.

Procedure: Care of the ultrasound machine

1. **Action:** The ultrasound machine should be plugged into the mains and switched on just prior to use. It should be switched off immediately after use.

    Rationale: The machine may overheat if left on for long periods. Where the machine is only used occasionally, leaving it switched on wastes electricity.

2. **Action:** The transducers should be stored in a suitable holder.

    Rationale: All machines are equipped with a holder for the transducers, which will prevent damage. There are two types of transducer – linear array, which pro- duces a rectangular field, and sector transducer, which produces a fan-shaped field.

3. **Action:** The transducer should be attached to the operator throughout the examination.

    Rationale: Transducers are very fragile and should not be dropped or banged. Using a wristband to attach the transducer to the user can prevent this.

4. **Action:** Select the correct mode prior to the examination.

    Rationale: This ensures that the procedure is carried out quickly and efficiently. There are three types of image display modes. Most ultrasonography is performed using B-mode ('brightness' mode); M-mode is used to show movement of structures on the frozen image and is used in echocar- diology; A-mode was the first type and is rarely used.

5. **Action:** Clean the transducer thoroughly after use.

    Rationale: Gel and hair affect the function of the transducer and may be a source of cross-infection.

REFERENCES AND FURTHER READING

Aspinall V 2006 The Complete Textbook of Veterinary Nursing. Elsevier, Oxford

Burns F, Whelehan P, Latham C 1997 Understanding radiography 3. Veterinary Practice Nurse 9(2): 15–21

Bushong S 1997 Radiological Science for Technologists, 6th edn. Mosby, London

Dennis R 1987 Radiographic examination of the canine spine. Veterinary Record 121(2): 31–35

Easton S 2003 Practical Radiography for Veterinary Nurses. Elsevier, Oxford

Ford G 1999 Processing radiographs. Veterinary Nursing 14(5): 187–188

Lane D R, Cooper B (eds) 2003 Veterinary Nursing, 3rd edn. Butterworth-Heinemann, Oxford

Latham C 1996 Radiographic film faults and how to avoid them. Veterinary Practice Nurse 8(3): 17–22

Chapter 11

Diagnostic laboratory techniques

Jennifer Davis

CHAPTER CONTENTS

Introduction 244
Health and safety in the laboratory 244

Care of laboratory equipment 245
Care and use of autoclaves 245
Care and use of the balance 245
Care and cleaning of glassware 246
Care and use of the centrifuge 246
Care and cleaning of the incubator 247
Care and use of the microscope 247
Use of the Vernier scale 249
Care of glass pipettes 250
Use of volumetric and automatic pipettes 250
Decontamination and disposal of laboratory
   waste 251
Care of the water bath 251

Practical laboratory techniques 252
Cytology 252
Preparation of a smear using samples from
   fine needle aspirate (FNA) biopsies, thoracic
   fluid etc. 252
Faecal examination 253
Preparation and storage of faeces for
   examination 253
Worm egg count – modified McMaster method 253
Trypsin digest test – to detect the presence of
   faecal trypsin 254
Iodine stain – to detect the presence of starch
   and muscle fibres in faeces 255

Sudan 3 stain – to detect the presence of fat in
   faeces 255
Haematology 256
Packed cell volume (PCV) 256
Total white blood cell count using a
   haemocytometer 258
Total red cell count using a haemocytometer 260
Preparation of a blood smear 261
Reticulocyte count 262
Giemsa stain – used to demonstrate blood
   parasites 262
Leishman's stain 263
Diff-quik stain 264
Differential white blood cell count 264
Histopathology 265
Preparation of tissue for histological
   examination 265
Microbiology 266
Preparation of bacterial smears 266
Gram's stain – rapid method 266
Methylene blue stain 267
Bacterial culture 267
Parasitology 268
Culture for ringworm fungus 268
Use of a Wood's lamp – to detect *Microsporum
   canis* 269
Collection and examination of coat brushings – to
   demonstrate the presence of surface–living
   ectoparasites 270
Collection of a skin scraping – to demonstrate
   the presence of burrowing ectoparasites 270

Preparation of a smear to identify the presence
    of mites   272
Urine examination   272
Urine preservation   272
Gross examination of urine   273
To test the specific gravity of urine by
    refractometer   273
To test urine for various parameters using a
    dipstick   274
Urine sediment examination   275

INTRODUCTION

Laboratory tests are used to aid or confirm the diagnosis made by the veterinary surgeon. Many of these tests may be sent away to commercial laboratories, but most practices have some form of small laboratory of their own where a range of basic diagnostic tests may be carried out. It is often one of the veterinary nurses who is designated or volunteers to run the laboratory and it is vital that this person is adequately trained to produce consistent good-quality results in which the veterinary surgeon can have confidence. The methods described in this chapter have been in daily use in our practice laboratory. They are simple to carry out, require the minimum of equipment and are easily performed by both student and qualified veterinary nurses.

Biochemical analyses have not been included as most practices use wet or dry biochemical analysers. Although this 'push button' technology is generally reliable, the author strongly recommends the regular throughput of quality control samples with known parameter values to ensure that the machine is reporting correctly.

Haematology analysers allow regular and accurate evaluation of single blood parameters but for complete confidence one should carry out a blood smear (See Differential white blood cell count procedure, p. 264) to assess irregularities in cell morphology and to ascertain whether anaemias are regenerative or non-regenerative etc. I have described no specific methodologies for the range of haematology analysers currently available but it is appropriate to briefly describe the three types of technology employed:

- The QBC Autoread (IDEXX): this utilises qualitative buffy coat analysis. Cells have different densities and the QBC system employs a combination of an oversized haematocrit tube and a float to expand the buffy coat to quantify each type of white cell. In addition, the tube is coated with a fluorescent dye which stains cellular components when subjected to blue violet light.
- Electronic impedance technology: the principle of this type of analyser is that cells are diluted with an isotonic solution, counted and sized by passing them through an aperture on the instrument. Each cell is identified and classified using its resistance to an electrical current.
- Laser flow technology (Lasercyte – IDEXX): this type uses lasers through which a stream of cells is passed. The system counts and identifies cells using the principle that individual types of cell reflect laser light differently depending on their size and granularity.

Enzyme-linked immunosorbent assay (ELISA) tests for feline leukaemia virus (FeLV), feline immunodeficiency virus (FIV), *Giardia*, etc. are now so commonly used and are so simple to perform that specific instructions have not been included. This type of test falls into two groups, the read-by-eye test, which is designed for practice use, and more complex plate ELISA methods, which require a photometer plate reader to assess optical densities and interpretation. The latter is more suited to commercial laboratories.

HEALTH AND SAFETY IN THE LABORATORY

Whilst undertaking laboratory procedures observe the following guidelines:

- Wear a long-sleeved laboratory coat, gloves, mask (where necessary) and eye protection at all times.
- Wear the minimum of jewellery.
- The use of nail varnish is not acceptable and nails must be kept short and clean.

- Do not lick gummed labels, your fingers or suck the ends of pencils, pens, etc.
- A wash basin reserved for hand washing should be available equipped with antibacterial soap and paper towels.
- Hands should be washed on entry to the laboratory and on leaving the room.
- All work surfaces should be cleaned and disinfected daily and after every hazardous procedure.
- As soon as you have finished with equipment, store it away tidily to avoid accidents.
- Samples and contaminated equipment should be disposed of safely and correctly.
- Sharps containers and clinical waste bags must be available in the laboratory at all times.
- If hazardous chemicals are used, take note of warning labels and act accordingly.
- Many bacteria are potential pathogens and should be handled in a contained environment such as a safety cabinet.
- Avoid mouth pipetting.
- Know where the first aid kit is stored, what action to take in an emergency and be familiar with the accident book.
- It is a good idea to list all procedures in a laboratory manual so that all staff members use the same methodologies.
- The use of external quality assurance or quality control schemes ensures confidence in your results.

CARE OF LABORATORY EQUIPMENT

Procedure: Care and use of autoclaves

1. **Action:** Autoclaving is the most reliable method for sterilising culture media and laboratory equipment.

   Rationale: When water is boiled within a closed vessel and at increased pressure, steam is formed and the temperature rises above 100 °C. The high temperature will kill all microorganisms and bacterial spores. (Some spores may survive a 15 minute programme.)

2. **Action:** Before use check that there is sufficient water to cover the element.

   Rationale: Autoclaves must not be allowed to boil dry.

3. **Action:** Load the items.

4. **Action:** Place an indicator strip near to the middle of the load.

   Rationale: These strips change colour to indicate when full sterilisation has taken place.

5. **Action:** Do not overfill the chamber.

   Rationale: Items in the middle of the load may not be completely sterilised if the chamber is overloaded.

6. **Action:** Check that the steam discharge tap is open.

7. **Action:** Adjust the safety valve to the required pressure.

   Rationale: Each type of object has a specific required temperature, e.g. culture media are usually autoclaved at 121 °C for 15 minutes.

8. **Action:** Allow steam and air mixture to escape until all air has been eliminated from the chamber.

   Rationale: You will see the steam escaping.

9. **Action:** Close the discharge tap.

10. **Action:** When pressure reaches the required level, the safety valve will open – at this point start to time the load.

    Rationale: A minute timer is useful.

11. **Action:** When the time is complete, turn off the heater and allow the autoclave to cool.

    Rationale: When cool the gauge should read 0 lb/sq. inch (atmospheric pressure).

12. **Action:** Open the discharge tap.

13. **Action:** Unload the items.

14. **Action:** Pour out any water left in the chamber and wipe clean with a soft cloth.

Procedure: Care and use of the balance

1. **Action:** Always make sure that the balance is placed on an even and stable surface.

   Rationale: Balances are extremely delicate instruments and can be damaged by excessive vibration.

2. **Action:** Items placed on the top pan must be centred for accurate weight distribution.

   Rationale: Use forceps to place items carefully into the middle of the pan.

3. **Action:** Instrument accuracy can be checked using calibrated weights.

   Rationale: Use a suitable weight in the middle of the balance range to check the accuracy. This will depend on the number of decimal places to which your balance measures.

4. **Action:** Before weighing, zero the balance using the 'TARE' button.

   Rationale: If using a balance boat, place the boat on the balance before zeroing the machine.

5. **Action:** Weigh the item under test.

6. **Action:** Record the result.

7. **Action:** Carefully remove the item from the pan.

   Rationale: Use forceps for small items.

8. **Action:** Turn off the power supply to the balance.

9. **Action:** Clean the pan using a damp soft cloth (if spillage has occurred) or a soft clean lint-free tissue.

   Rationale: More detailed maintenance should be carried out by a trained engineer at an annual service.

Procedure: Care and cleaning of glassware

1. **Action:** Important – if the glassware contains hazardous material, autoclave the glassware with the contents intact at 121 °C for 45 minutes prior to discarding the contents.

   Rationale: Health and Safety precautions must be observed when pathogens are likely to be present. Spore-forming organisms may withstand 15 minutes in an autoclave.

2. **Action:** If autoclaving is not required, proceed as follows: rinse the glassware immediately after use and place in a solution of non-toxic commercial laboratory detergent.

   Rationale: Detergents designed for laboratory use are available – harsh detergents are too abrasive and will damage glass.

3. **Action:** Using disposable gloves and a soft brush, remove any material present on the glassware.

   Rationale: Use a test tube brush for narrow tubes – hard brushes scratch the surface of the glass.

4. **Action:** Transfer glassware to a fresh solution of detergent and leave to soak for 20–30 minutes.

   Rationale: Heavy soiling may require a longer soaking.

5. **Action:** Once the glassware is visibly clean, rinse in tap water two or three times.

6. **Action:** Transfer to a container of distilled/deionised water and rinse.

   Rationale: Two or three changes of distilled water are recommended.

7. **Action:** Allow to drain.

   Rationale: Water runs off clean glass evenly. If any dirt remains, areas with a 'greasy' appearance will be visible.

8. **Action:** Dry in drying oven at 160 °C for 1 hour or allow to dry in the air.

   Rationale: If air-drying, the atmosphere must be dust-free.

9. **Action:** If glassware is to be used for sterile procedures, sterilise in an autoclave at 121 °C for 15 minutes.

   Rationale: Bottles should be autoclaved with the lids screwed loosely to allow for the escape of expanding hot air. Tighten the lids after autoclaving, which prevents contaminated air being sucked in by the cooling air. Plug test tubes with cotton wool.

10. **Action:** Always cool glassware slowly. Do not put hot glassware onto a cold surface.

    Rationale: Glass will crack if it is subjected to sudden temperature changes.

11. **Action:** Check for cracks and chips and store in a dust-free atmosphere until use.

    Rationale: Cracks or chips reduce thermal strength leading to sudden breakage.

Procedure: Care and use of the centrifuge

1. **Action:** Always ensure that the centrifuge is placed on an even and stable surface.

   Rationale: Slight vibration occurs when the machine is in motion and an uneven surface may cause the machine to move around.

2. **Action:** Only use tubes recommended by the manufacturer.

   Rationale: Centrifuge tubes often have a tapered bottom and are designed to withstand centrifugal force.

3. **Action:** The top of the centrifuge tube must not protrude above the top of the bucket. When using a microhaematocrit centrifuge, ensure that the plasticine end of the capillary tube is against the outer ring of the instrument.

   Rationale: Centrifugal force pushes material outwards. The plasticine end prevents material escaping from the tube.

4. **Action:** Vacutainer tubes may be spun with their stoppers in place.

   Rationale: If the tube is opened or broken aerosol contamination of the environment could occur.

5. **Action:** Lock the lid of the centrifuge securely.

   Rationale: Most machines will not allow you to use them without locking the lid first. If you do not, the lid may fly open during use.

6. **Action:** Set the spin speed as appropriate.

   Rationale: For example, urine requires a lower speed than heparinised blood for biochemistry.

7. **Action:** After use turn off the power supply.

8. **Action:** Take out the buckets.

9. **Action:** Wipe the rotor and buckets with a soft cloth and mild disinfectant solution.

   Rationale: To prevent contamination of the next sample.

10. **Action:** Replace the buckets and close the lid.

Procedure: Care and cleaning of the incubator

1. **Action:** Remove all media from the incubator.

   Rationale: If you take too long to clean out the incubator, the agar plates have to stand at room temperature, slowing the growth of the bacteria.

2. **Action:** It is sensible to clean the instrument when workload is low but it should be done at least once a week.

   Rationale: Incubators are used to culture bacteria so the risk of contamination of samples is high.

3. **Action:** Remove all the shelves and racks.

   Rationale: These are more easily cleaned when out of the incubator.

4. **Action:** Using a mild detergent and soft cloth, wipe all the incubator surfaces and the shelves.

   Rationale: Take care not to touch any electrical parts. If in doubt, switch off the power supply before cleaning.

5. **Action:** Allow to dry.

6. **Action:** Using a disinfectant solution and fresh cloth, wipe all the incubator surfaces and shelves.

   Rationale: The disinfectant used must be bactericidal and fungicidal to be effective.

7. **Action:** Allow to dry.

8. **Action:** Replace the shelves.

9. **Action:** Place a thermometer in glycerol in the middle of the incubator. Check that the bulb is covered. Switch on the incubator.

   Rationale: The temperature of the glycerol alters slowly and allows the thermometer to be read without rapid fluctuations.

10. **Action:** Read the thermometer after 1 hour.

    Rationale: Most incubators run at $37\,°C \pm 1\,°C$. It is essential to check that the incubator reaches the correct temperature to ensure efficient incubation of the agar plates.

11. **Action:** Every month check on the door seal, electrical wiring and thermostat.

    Rationale: If in doubt about any component inform the practice or laboratory manager.

Procedure: Care and use of the microscope (Fig. 11.1)

1. **Action:** Always ensure that the microscope is placed on an even and stable surface.

   Rationale: Slight vibration will make it difficult to view the object.

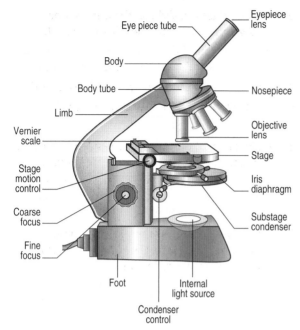

Figure 11.1 A light microscope. Adapted, with permission, from Masters and Bowden (2001), Butterworth-Heinemann.

2. **Action:** Before use, clean the eyepieces, condenser and objective lenses with lens tissue.

   Rationale: Lens tissue is lint-free and prevents bits being left on the surfaces.

3. **Action:** Clean the oil immersion lens with cleaning fluid.

   Rationale: Isopropanol is most commonly used.

4. **Action:** Turn the light control to a minimum.

   Rationale: This prevents a sudden power surge, which may break the bulb when the microscope is switched on.

5. **Action:** Turn on the instrument.

6. **Action:** Adjust the eyepieces.

   Rationale: Use both eyepieces and position them so that both fields converge as one.

7. **Action:** Place the slide on the stage. Some instruments have clips to hold the slide.

   Rationale: The slide should remain firmly in place to avoid unintentional loss of a particular field.

8. **Action:** Move the slide by using the knobs on the mechanical stage.

Rationale: This allows the whole slide to be examined smoothly and accurately without touching the slide with your fingers.

9. **Action:** Examine the slide using the ×10 objective lens.

   Rationale: At this stage the light can be adjusted using the light source knob or by repositioning the condenser.

10. **Action:** Focus first with the coarse and then with the fine adjustment knobs.

    Rationale: Always focus upwards from the slide to prevent accidental damage to the slide.

11. **Action:** If using oil immersion, place a drop of oil onto the slide.

    Rationale: Oil immersion provides increased magnification and is used for examination of bacteria and blood smears.

12. **Action:** Rotate the nosepiece until the ×100 objective lens is above the slide.

13. **Action:** Drop the objective lens into the drop of oil. Always watch what you are doing – do not look at it through the eyepiece, as you will find it impossible to judge distances and may smash through the slide.

    Rationale: The lens must be lying in the oil to avoid distortion of the image. Avoid contaminating the dry lenses.

14. **Action:** Focus using the fine control.

    Rationale: You may need to adjust the light to improve your view.

15. **Action:** After use remove the slide from the stage.

    Rationale: Move the clips before trying to remove the slide.

16. **Action:** Reduce the light and turn off the power.

17. **Action:** Turn the objective lenses on the nosepiece until the lowest power is in position above the stage.

    Rationale: Ready for use next time.

18. **Action:** Remove any oil from the objective lenses using lens tissue and if necessary lens cleaning fluid.

Rationale: Ready for use next time.

19. **Action:** Cover the instrument when not in use.

    Rationale: This will prevent the build-up of dust on the objective and eyepiece lenses.

Procedure: Use of the Vernier scale (Fig. 11.2)

1. **Action:** The Vernier scale is a graduated device attached to the stage of the microscope.

   Rationale: It allows the position of an object on a slide to be accurately recorded so that you can find it again.

2. **Action:** One scale lies along a vertical edge and another along a horizontal edge.

   Rationale: Use both position numbers to give a grid reference similar to that on a map.

3. **Action:** Place the slide on the microscope stage and fix it with the clips if present.

   Rationale: The slide must not move around as this will invalidate your scale references.

4. **Action:** Locate the object you wish to identify.

5. **Action:** Look at the scale on the vertical axis.

   Rationale: See Figure 11.2.

6. **Action:** Record the number where the zero mark on the Vernier plate meets the main scale.

   Rationale: Record the lower number if it falls between two divisions. In Figure 11.2 the zero mark falls between 31 and 32.

7. **Action:** Make a note of which of the marks on the Vernier plate is exactly opposite a division on the main scale.

   Rationale: In Figure 11.2, mark number 6 is exactly opposite a division on the main scale.

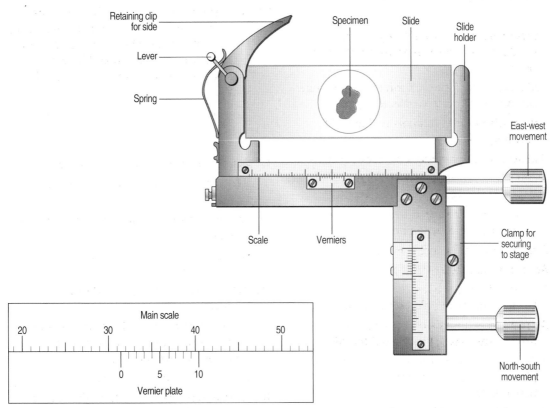

Figure 11.2 The Vernier scale. The zero on the Vernier plate is between 31 and 32 on the main scale, and it is mark number 6 on the Vernier plate that is exactly opposite a division on the main scale. The reading is therefore 31.6.

8. **Action:** Record this reading, placing it after the decimal point.

   Rationale: In Figure 11.2 this will give a reading of 31.6.

9. **Action:** Repeat steps 6–8 using the horizontal axis.

   Rationale: You now have two readings, e.g. 31.6 and 90.1.

10. **Action:** You now have a grid reference for that object on that slide, provided the slide is placed in the same position on the stage.

    Rationale: By tradition, slides are placed on the stage with the label to the right.

11. **Action:** Record your grid reference using the horizontal reading followed by the vertical reading.

    Rationale: In this example, the reference would be 90.1 × 31.6. You may now remove the slide and go back to the same location later on.

Procedure: Care of glass pipettes

1. **Action:** After use, place the pipette in a jar of disinfectant.

   Rationale: Hypochlorite solution containing 1000 mg/l of free chlorine is most commonly used.

2. **Action:** Soak for 1 hour.

   Rationale: This removes bacterial contamination.

3. **Action:** Rinse the pipette several times in tap water.

   Rationale: You may need to use a 'rubber policeman' or pipette filler to fill and empty the pipette. **Do not use your mouth.**

4. **Action:** Rinse the pipette several times in distilled water.

   Rationale: This leaves a clean surface on the glass.

5. **Action:** Rinse the pipette in methylated spirits.

   Rationale: This removes any grease.

6. **Action:** Rinse the pipette in ethanol.

   Rationale: Ethanol evaporates and leaves the inside of the pipette dry.

7. **Action:** Plug the pipettes with non-absorbent cotton wool.

   Rationale: This prevents fluid being sucked up into the pipette filler and reduces cross-contamination.

8. **Action:** Pack into metal pipette canisters for autoclaving at 121 °C for 15 minutes.

   Rationale: The pipettes are sterilised ready for aseptic procedures.

Procedure: Use of volumetric and automatic pipettes

1. **Action:** Using a soft cloth, clean the external parts of the pipette with a weak solution of commercial laboratory detergent.

   Rationale: This removes grime accumulated by daily handling.

2. **Action:** Allow to dry.

3. **Action:** Wipe the barrel end of the pipette (not the plunger) with isopropanol.

   Rationale: Wiping with spirit disinfects the part of the pipette that is attached to the tip.

4. **Action:** Some pipettes require the seals to be greased regularly – refer to the manufacturer's instructions.

   Rationale: Special grease is usually included in the maintenance kit supplied with the pipette.

5. **Action:** When needed for use, attach a disposable tip.

6. **Action:** Depress the plunger, place the tip in the solution and slowly release the plunger.

   Rationale: The fluid will be aspirated into the tip.

7. **Action:** Transfer the tip to your next vessel, e.g. a test tube, and place against the inner side of the vessel. Depress the plunger slowly.

   Rationale: The fluid will run down the side of the vessel.

8. **Action:** Discard the tip.

   Rationale: Tips should not be used more than once to avoid cross-contamination.

9. **Action:** The accuracy of your dispensing may be checked using a weight and balance.

   Rationale: Calibrate the pipette by weight, e.g. 1 ml of distilled water weighs 1 g.

10. **Action:** Pipettes should be stored in a pipette rack or in the box provided when not in use.

    Rationale: If pipettes are not stored properly, the dispensing end may be damaged.

Procedure: Decontamination and disposal of laboratory waste

1. **Action:** If possible, samples and contaminated agar plates should be placed in autoclave bags and autoclaved in a steam autoclave at 121 °C for 45 minutes.

   Rationale: Some spore-forming bacteria will survive a 15 minute run. Make sure that the autoclave has enough water to last a prolonged run. Contaminated laboratory waste should not leave the laboratory in a potentially harmful form.

2. **Action:** It is good practice to include an indicator, e.g. TST strip, to confirm that complete sterilisation has taken place.

   Rationale: If this device fails, the load is still unsafe and it must be reprocessed.

3. **Action:** Once sterilised, place the unopened autoclave bag into yellow hazardous waste bags and send away for incineration by a licensed waste disposal firm.

   Rationale: This further reduces the risk of contaminating the environment with the waste material.

4. **Action:** Sharps and other disposable items must be placed within a yellow commercial sharps bin, which is sealed and sent for incineration.

   Rationale: This ensures that objects such as needles or scalpel blades sticking through will not injure anyone handling the bin.

5. **Action:** Metal items may be cleaned using non-hypochlorite disinfectants.

   Rationale: Hypochlorite disinfectants will react with metal.

6. **Action:** Some equipment may need special cleaning and disinfection.

   Rationale: Always follow the manufacturer's instructions, as there may be delicate parts that could be damaged by incorrect treatment.

7. **Action:** Clean all work surfaces with disinfectant after every procedure.

   Rationale: Disinfectants must contain a bactericide, a fungicide and a virucide to be fully effective.

8. **Action:** At the end of each working day leave the laboratory clean and tidy.

   Rationale: Untidy work areas lead to accidents.

Procedure: Care of the water bath

1. **Action:** Turn off the power supply.

2. **Action:** Remove the thermometer and shelf.

   Rationale: The bath should have a thermometer to monitor the temperature – do not rely entirely on the dial.

3. **Action:** Pour away the water.

4. **Action:** Wipe all the surfaces with detergent.

   Rationale: If there are excessive deposits of calcium, soak the internal surfaces in a solution of Calgon for 2–3 hours.

5. **Action:** Replace the water.

   Rationale: The base tray must be covered – never run a water bath when it is empty.

6. **Action:** Replace the thermometer.

   Rationale: Holders sited on the side of the bath should hold thermometers in place.

7. **Action:** Switch on the power.

8. **Action:** Reduce heat loss by using a lid. This should not be used for open test tube work.

   Rationale: Condensation accumulates on the lid and drips into the fluid in the test tubes.

9. **Action:** Check that the correct temperature has been reached.

   Rationale: Allow 20–30 minutes for the bath to warm up.

10. **Action:** Put the items in a rack inside the bath and set the timer.

    Rationale: Always use the rack – bottles and tubes may float if free-standing.

11. **Action:** After the incubation time is complete, remove the items.

    Rationale: Always use tongs to remove very hot bottles and tubes.

12. **Action:** Turn off the water bath and allow to cool.

PRACTICAL LABORATORY TECHNIQUES

CYTOLOGY

Procedure: Preparation of a smear using samples from fine needle aspirate (FNA) biopsies, thoracic fluid, etc.

Equipment: Microscope slides (degreased in methanol and dried), centrifuge tubes, centrifuge, Pasteur pipette, stains as appropriate.

1. **Action:** Place the sample/fluid in a centrifuge tube and centrifuge at 1500 rpm for 3–5 minutes. Sediment can also be produced in the bottom of the tube by leaving it to stand for about 30 minutes.

    Rationale: Centrifugation is used to spin down the cells and concentrate them at the bottom of the tube. Some samples such as thoracic fluid may contain very few cells.

2. **Action:** A smear may be made by touching a slide against a lesion.

    Rationale: Cells stick to the slide and can be used for the examination. This is known as a 'touch prep'.

3. **Action:** Fine needle aspirates may be prepared without centrifugation if sufficient cells have been harvested. Deposit cells on the slide by pushing the plunger of the syringe.

    Rationale: FNAs are usually rich in cells.

4. **Action:** Decant the supernatant liquid from the centrifuge tube and discard. This leaves the sediment in the bottom of the tube.

    Rationale: The use of a conical tube helps in the separation of the sediment from the supernatant.

5. **Action:** Resuspend the cells by flicking the tube with your finger.

    Rationale: This remixes the cells with any remaining liquid and ensures a more even spread of cells on the slide.

6. **Action:** Using a pipette, place one or two drops onto the centre of a microscope slide.

7. **Action:** Make two smears using the 'squash' method (Fig. 11.3).

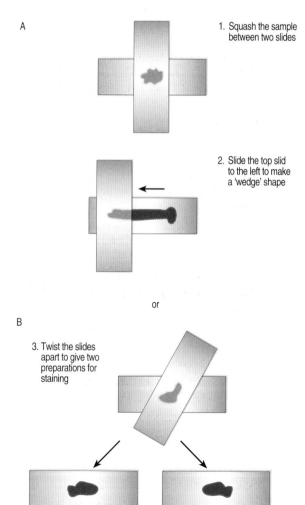

A

1. Squash the sample between two slides

2. Slide the top slid to the left to make a 'wedge' shape

or

B

3. Twist the slides apart to give two preparations for staining

Figure 11.3 'Squash prep' used for cytology.

Rationale: This is used where there are few cells present in the sample. A 'wedge' method will spread the cells too thinly.

8. **Action:** Allow the smears to air-dry.

    Rationale: The use of artificial heat will damage the cells.

9. **Action:** Stain the smear with Leishman's, Gram's or Sudan 3 as appropriate.

    Rationale: Gram's stain is used for bacterial examination, Leishman's stain is used for blood cells and Sudan 3 is used to stain fat in a lipoma.

FAECAL EXAMINATION

Procedure: Preparation and storage of faeces for examination

1. **Action:** Faeces may be collected from the ground immediately after defecation.

    Rationale: Old samples may have deteriorated, parasite eggs may hatch, and larvae may crawl away. Grass, soil or bacteria may contaminate the sample.

2. **Action:** Faeces may be collected using a gloved finger inserted through the anal sphincter into the rectum.

    Rationale: This ensures a fresh uncontaminated sample but care must be taken not to damage the rectal wall.

3. **Action:** Place the sample in a sterile container. There should be sufficient faeces to fill the container.

    Rationale: Too much air in the container encourages parasite eggs to hatch prior to examination.

4. **Action:** Store the faeces in the fridge before examination.

    Rationale: Bacterial growth is slowed down in a cool temperature and the sample is preserved for longer.

5. **Action:** Bacterial tests must be carried out as soon as possible after collection.

    Rationale: More fastidious organisms such as *Campylobacter* spp. may be overgrown by more predominant species such as *Escherichia coli* and will be lost on culture.

Procedure: Worm egg count – modified McMaster method

Equipment: McMaster worm egg counting chamber, measuring cylinder, saturated sugar solution, Pasteur pipette, balance, balance boat, microscope, two glass beakers, tea strainer or sieve, spatula.

1. **Action:** Weigh 3 g of faeces into a beaker.

    Rationale: The faeces should be fresh and moist.

2. **Action:** Measure 45 ml of saturated sugar solution using the measuring cylinder and pour it into the beaker.

3. **Action:** Mix the solution with a spatula.

4. **Action:** Pour the solution through the sieve into a second beaker.

    Rationale: This removes large particles but allows the eggs to go through.

5. **Action:** Discard the debris remaining in the sieve.

6. **Action:** Mix the solution in the beaker gently.

7. **Action:** Allow the solution to stand at room temperature for 5–10 minutes.

    Rationale: This allows the worm eggs to float to the top of the saturated sugar solution.

8. **Action:** If using a single chamber type of McMaster slide, prepare it by placing the coverslip grid-side down.

    Rationale: Some slides have only one chamber and use a coverslip grid, while others have two chambers with integral grids (Fig. 11.4).

9. **Action:** Withdraw approximately 2 ml of the solution using a Pasteur pipette.

    Rationale: Make sure that you have enough liquid to fill the chamber of the slide completely. This stops bubbles forming over the grid.

10. **Action:** Fill the counting chamber and apply the coverslip (Fig. 11.4).

    Rationale: The coverslip must make contact with the solution to avoid inclusion of air bubbles and avoid distortion of the image.

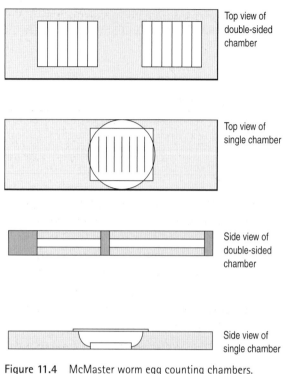

Top view of double-sided chamber

Top view of single chamber

Side view of double-sided chamber

Side view of single chamber

Figure 11.4 McMaster worm egg counting chambers.

11. **Action:** Leave the counting chamber on the bench for 5–10 minutes.

   Rationale: This allows the worm eggs and coccidial oocysts time to float to the top of the chamber. They are then visible when you focus on the grid. NB. tapeworm segments do not float – use a direct smear.

12. **Action:** Examine the counting chamber using the ×10 objective on the microscope.

13. **Action:** Count all the eggs seen over the grid (Fig. 11.5).

   Rationale: Count those on the lines as well as those between the lines.

14. **Action:** Calculate the number of eggs as follows:

- For a single counting chamber, multiply the number of eggs by 100.
- For double-chambered slide, multiply the total number of eggs on the slide by 50.

   This gives the number of eggs per gram of faeces.
   Rationale: This is a quantitative method and is used to evaluate the severity of an infection

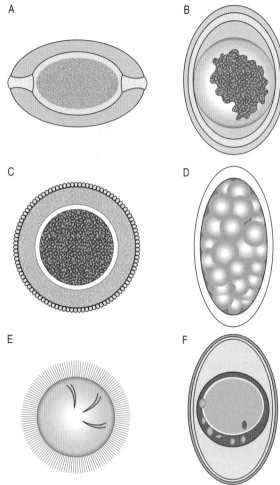

Figure 11.5 Worm eggs and oocysts. A, *Trichuris* spp.; B, *Toxascaris* spp.; C, *Toxocara* spp.; D, *Uncinaria* spp.; E, *Taenia* spp.; F, *Isospora* spp. Redrawn from Lane and Cooper (2003), Butterworth-Heinemann.

by counting the number of eggs in one gram of faeces. (A qualitative analysis tells you whether there are parasites present but does not indicate the severity of the infection.)

Procedure: Trypsin digest test – to detect the presence of faecal trypsin

Equipment: X-ray film (unused), eight test tubes, Pasteur pipettes, incubator at 37 °C, timer, balance, 5% sodium bicarbonate solution, test tube rack.

1. **Action:** Place eight tubes in the test tube rack and add 1 ml of sodium bicarbonate to each – **apart from the first one**.

2. **Action:** Cut a portion of the X-ray film into eight strips.

    Rationale: The strips must be able to fit into the test tubes lengthways.

3. **Action:** Place 9 ml of sodium bicarbonate in the first test tube and add 1 g of faeces.

    Rationale: This gives a dilution of 1:10.

4. **Action:** Take 1 ml of this solution and transfer it to the next tube. Mix well.

    Rationale: This procedure is called a doubling dilution. It gives a dilution of 1:20.

5. **Action:** Take 1 ml of the solution and transfer it to the next test tube. Mix well.

    Rationale: This gives a dilution of 1:40

6. **Action:** Continue in this manner until all the test tubes have a solution in them.

    Rationale: The last one will have a dilution of 1:1280.

7. **Action:** Remove 1 ml from the last tube and discard.

8. **Action:** Place a strip of X-ray film into each tube.

    Rationale: Trypsin, a digestive enzyme that is normally present in the small intestine and acts on protein, will digest the gelatin layer on the film leaving a clear area.

9. **Action:** Incubate the tubes for 35 minutes at 37 °C in an incubator.

    Rationale: This reproduces the conditions in the body.

10. **Action:** When the time is complete, examine each strip in the area which was submerged in the solution.

    Rationale: A clear area indicates the presence of trypsin in the faecal sample. A watermark or an area of partial digestion indicates insufficient trypsin in the sample.

11. **Action:** Record the highest dilution at which digestion has taken place.

    Rationale: If clearing has only occurred in the stronger solutions, e.g. 1:10, but not in the weaker solutions, e.g. 1:320, then the patient may have exocrine pancreatic insufficiency (EPI).

In dogs, this test has been superseded by the serum trypsin-like immunoreactivity test, which is more accurate.

Procedure: Iodine stain – to detect the presence of starch and muscle fibres in faeces

Equipment: Microscope slide, 2% Lugol's iodine or Gram's iodine solution, Pasteur pipettes, coverslip, microscope, staining rack, saline, loop or swab, tap water.

1. **Action:** Using a pipette place 1–2 drops of saline onto the centre of a microscope slide.

    Rationale: Saline emulsifies the faeces and helps to spread it evenly over the slide.

2. **Action:** Dip a swab or loop into the faeces sample and place a little into the saline on the slide. Mix well.

3. **Action:** Allow the mixture to dry for 1 minute.

    Rationale: This fixes the faeces on the slide.

4. **Action:** Place the slide on the staining rack and flood with iodine solution.

5. **Action:** Leave the stain on for 3 minutes.

    Rationale: Iodine binds with the starch in the sample.

6. **Action:** Wash gently with tap water

    Rationale: This stops further staining by the iodine.

7. **Action:** Place a coverslip over the smear.

    Rationale: The smear is best examined when wet. A coverslip prevents the objective lens from becoming contaminated.

8. **Action:** Examine using the ×10 and ×40 objective lenses of the microscope.

    Rationale: Starch granules will be stained black, while muscle fibres have squared ends and stain reddish brown.

Procedure: Sudan 3 stain – to detect the presence of fat in faeces

Equipment: Microscope slide, Sudan 3 stain, normal saline, coverslip, swab or loop, Pasteur pipette, staining rack, microscope.

1. **Action:** Using a pipette, place 1–2 drops of saline onto the centre of the microscope slide.

   Rationale: Saline emulsifies the faeces and helps to spread it evenly over the slide.

2. **Action:** Dip a swab or loop into the faeces sample and place a little into the saline on the slide. Mix well.

3. **Action:** Allow the mixture to dry for 1 minute.

   Rationale: This fixes the faeces on the slide.

4. **Action:** Place the slide on the staining rack and flood the slide with Sudan 3.

5. **Action:** Leave the stain for 3 minutes.

   Rationale: Sudan 3 stain binds with the fat in the sample.

6. **Action:** Wash gently with tap water.

   Rationale: This stops the action of the stain and removes any surplus.

7. **Action:** Place a coverslip over the smear.

   Rationale: The smear is best examined when wet. A coverslip prevents the objective lens from becoming contaminated.

8. **Action:** Examine using the ×10 and ×40 objective lenses of the microscope.

   Rationale: Fat globules will stain orange red.

HAEMATOLOGY

Procedure: Packed cell volume (PCV)

Equipment: Blood sample in EDTA tube, capillary tube (plain), microhaematocrit reader, microhaematocrit centrifuge, soft plasticine or Cristoseal.

1. **Action:** Collect a blood sample in an EDTA tube.

   Rationale: Sodium ethylene diamine tetra-acetic acid (EDTA) is an anticoagulant and prevents the blood from clotting. It is used to preserve most blood samples used for haematology.

2. **Action:** Gently agitate the sample and place the end of a capillary tube in the blood.

3. **Action:** Hold the tube at a 45° angle and allow the tube to fill until it is ¾ full.

   Rationale: Blood will be drawn up the tube by capillary action.

4. **Action:** Place the opposite end of the tube into the plasticine pad.

   Rationale: If you use the end containing the blood, you will contaminate the plasticine.

5. **Action:** Twist the capillary tube two or three times and take it out of the plasticine.

   Rationale: This creates a plug which will prevent blood running out of the tube.

6. **Action:** Wipe the tube with soft tissue.

   Rationale: To remove excess blood which could be a source of infection.

7. **Action:** Place the tube in one groove of the centrifuge with the plasticine plug facing outwards against the outer rim.

   Rationale: Centrifugal force causes the fluids to spin outwards. The sealed end prevents blood escaping as it is forced towards the perimeter.

8. **Action:** Place a similar tube on the opposite side of the centrifuge.

   Rationale: This balances the tube under test and reduces vibration and subsequent damage to the centrifuge.

9. **Action:** Screw the safety plate down over the tubes and close the lid.

   Rationale: The safety plate prevents the tubes spinning out of position. Both plate and lid are essential for safety.

10. **Action:** Centrifuge for 5 minutes at 10 000 rpm.

11. **Action:** When the machine stops, remove the lid, safety plate and tube.

    Rationale: Never attempt to open the centrifuge while it is still running.

12. **Action:** Place the tube into the groove on the microhaematocrit reader.

    Rationale: The blood will have separated into three layers (Fig. 11.6) – from the top downwards:

- plasma
- buffy coat – white blood cells
- red blood cells.

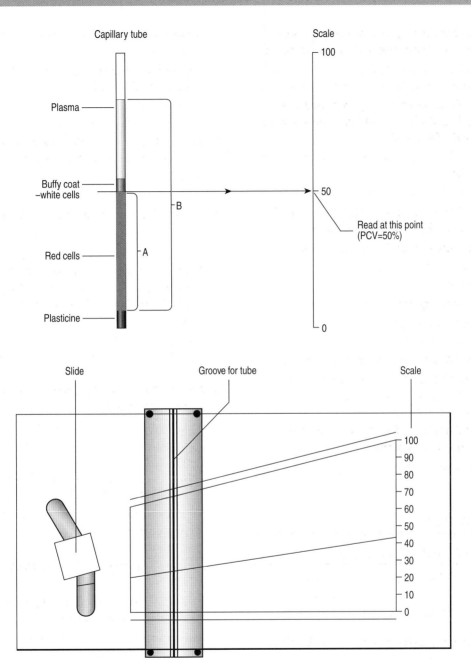

Figure 11.6 Measuring packed cell volume. A is the length of the tube occupied by red cells; B is the total length of the column of blood.

13. **Action:** Line up the top of the plasticine plug with the line on the bottom of the reader (Fig. 11.6).

    Rationale: The top of the plug marks the lowest point of the blood column.

14. **Action:** Line up the top of the plasma with the diagonal line at the top of the reader (Fig. 11.6).

    Rationale: The bottom of the plasma meniscus is used as the measuring point.

15. **Action:** Move the slide so that the middle line is level with the top of the red cells (Fig. 11.6).

16. **Action:** Read the measurement from the scale on the right side of the reader.

    Rationale: The scale is marked 1 to 100 – the reading can be expressed as a percentage, i.e. 45 becomes 45% etc.

17. **Action:** The PCV is the percentage of whole blood that consists of red blood cells.

    Rationale: PCV can also be calculated by measuring the length of tube occupied by red cells (A) and the total length of the blood column (B) (Table 11.1).

    $$PCV\% = A/B \times 100.$$

Procedure: Total white blood cell count using a haemocytometer

Equipment: Blood sample in EDTA tube, haemocytometer and coverslip (Fig. 11.7), 2000 μl (2 ml) and 100 μl (0.1 ml) volumetric pipettes and tips, sterile container, tissue, white cell counting fluid (glacial acetic acid – Table 11.2), microscope.

1. **Action:** Using a 2 ml volumetric pipette, place 2 ml of white cell counting fluid (glacial acetic acid) in a sterile container.

   Rationale: Particles of dust from a dirty container may be mistaken for cells when counting.

2. **Action:** Mix the blood in an EDTA tube by gentle agitation. Add 0.1 ml of the blood to the white cell counting fluid and mix well.

   Rationale: This is a 1 in 20 dilution.

3. **Action:** Leave to stand at room temperature for 5–10 minutes.

   Rationale: The addition of glacial acetic acid to whole blood results in lysis of the red cells, leaving only the white cells to be counted.

Table 11.1 Haematology ranges for the dog and the cat

Blood parameter	Dog	Cat
Red blood cells ($\times 10^{12}$/litre)	5.0–8.5	5.5–10.0
Packed cell volume (% of whole blood)	37–57	27–50
Total white blood cells ($\times 10^9$/litre)	6–15	4–15
Mature neutrophils ($\times 10^9$/litre)	3.6–10.5	2.5–12.5
(% of all blood cells)	60–70	45–75
Band neutrophils ($\times 10^9$/litre)	0–0.3	0–0.45
(% of all blood cells)	0–2	0–3
Eosinophils (% of all blood cells)	2–10	4–12
Basophils (% of all blood cells)	Rare	Rare
Monocytes (% of all blood cells)	3–10	0–4
Lymphocytes – small (% of all blood cells)	12–30	20–55
Lymphocytes – large (% of all blood cells)	Approx. 8%	Variable
Platelets ($\times 10^9$/litre)	200–500	200–600

A

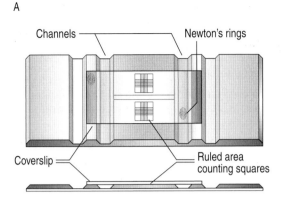

Improved Neubauer haemocytometer

B

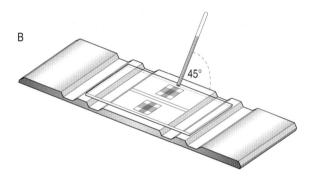

To fill the counting chamber

Figure 11.7   To prepare a red or white cell count.

4. **Action:** Place the coverslip on the
    haemocytometer and press firmly until
    Newton's rings can be seen.

    Rationale: Newton's rings appear as coloured
    rings and indicate that close contact has

been made between the coverslip and the
counting slide. Close contact ensures that
the area filled with blood is an accurate
volume.

5. **Action:** Using a capillary tube, draw up some
    of the treated blood and fill one side of the
    counting chamber. Do not allow fluid to
    flow into the well surrounding the plinth
    on which the grid is situated (Fig. 11.7).

    Rationale: If the end of the capillary tube is
    placed at the outside edge of the cover-
    slip, fluid will run under the coverslip and
    across the grid. Removing the capillary tube
    just before the fluid reaches the end of the
    grid will halt the flow.

6. **Action:** Wait for 2 minutes.

    Rationale: At first the white blood cells float
    around and are impossible to count. Wait
    for 2 minutes and they will settle.

7. **Action:** Place the counting chamber on the
    microscope stage, being careful to keep it
    horizontal. Using the ×10 objective lens,
    count the white cells in all four large corner
    squares (Fig. 11.8 – marked W).

    Rationale: Each large corner square is made
    of 16 smaller squares. You will count the
    white cells in (16 × 4) 64 small squares
    (Fig. 11.8).

8. **Action:** Count only the white cells in the
    spaces and those on the top and right hand
    lines of each square.

    Rationale: If you count all the cells on all the
    lines, you will count some cells twice.

Table 11.2   Leucocyte and erythrocyte counting fluids

	Leucocyte counting fluid	Erythrocyte counting fluid (Gowers' solution)
Contents	2 ml glacial acetic acid	12.5 g anhydrous sodium sulphate
	1 ml gentian violet (1% aqueous)	33.3 g glacial acetic acid
	100 ml distilled water	200 ml distilled water
Method	Filter through filter paper before use and shake well until mixed. Store in a dark glass bottle	Filter through filter paper before use and shake well until mixed. Store in a dark glass bottle
Use	Destroys red cells, leaving only white cells in the blood sample. Used for total white cell count by means of a haemocytometer	Destroys white cells, leaving only red cells in the blood sample. Used for red cell count by means of a haemocytometer

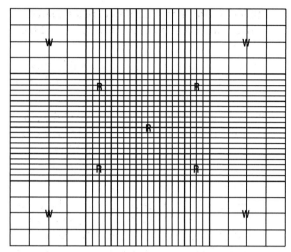

Figure 11.8 Image of haemocytometer viewed under the microscope. Count the squares labelled R to calculate a red blood cell count. Count the squares labelled W to calculate a white blood cell count.

9. **Action:** To calculate the number of white cells:

Total number of white cells in all 4 large squares = A.

The number of cells per litre of blood = $A/20 \times 10^9$.

Procedure: Total red cell count using a haemocytometer

Equipment: Blood sample in EDTA tube, haemocytometer and coverslip (Fig. 11.7), 20 ml and 0.1 ml (100 µl) volumetric pipettes and tips, sterile container, tissue, red cell counting fluid (Gowers' solution – Table 11.2) microscope.

1. **Action:** Using a pipette dispense 20 ml of red blood cell solution into a clean sterile container.

    Rationale: Particles of dust in a dirty container may be mistaken for cells when counting.

2. **Action:** Mix the blood in an EDTA tube by gentle agitation. Add 0.1 ml of the blood to the red cell counting fluid and mix well.

    Rationale: This gives a dilution of 1:200

3. **Action:** Leave to stand at room temperature for 5–10 minutes.

    Rationale: Red cell solution (Gowers' solution) destroys white cells so that only the red cells remain.

4. **Action:** Place the coverslip on the haemocytometer and press gently until Newton's rings appear.

    Rationale: Newton's rings appear as coloured rings and indicate that close contact has been made between the coverslip and the counting slide. Close contact ensures that the area filled with blood is an accurate volume.

5. **Action:** Using a capillary tube, draw up some of the treated blood and fill one side of the counting chamber. Do not allow fluid to flow into the well surrounding the plinth on which the grid is situated (Fig. 11.7).

    Rationale: If the end of the capillary tube is placed at the outside edge of the coverslip, fluid will run under the coverslip and across the grid. Removing the capillary tube just before the fluid reaches the end of the grid will halt the flow.

6. **Action:** Wait for 2 minutes.

    Rationale: At first the red blood cells float around and are impossible to count. Wait for 2 minutes and they will settle.

7. **Action:** Place the counting chamber on the microscope stage, being careful to keep it horizontal. Using the ×10 objective lens locate the central square of the nine large squares (Fig. 11.8).

8. **Action:** Change to the ×40 objective lens.

9. **Action:** Count all the cells in 5 of the 25 small squares in the central area (Fig. 11.8 – marked R).

    Rationale: Each small square is divided into 16 smaller squares – a total of 80 (16 × 5) small squares are counted.

10. **Action:** Count only the cells in the spaces and those resting on the top and the right hand lines of each square.

    Rationale: If you count the cells on all the lines you will count some cells twice.

11. **Action:** To calculate the number of red cells:

$$\text{Total number of cells} = A$$

$$A/100 = \text{no. of red cells} \times 10^{12}/l.$$

Procedure: Preparation of a blood smear

Equipment: Blood sample in EDTA tube, microscope slides previously soaked in methanol and dried, capillary tube, glass cutter, marker pen.

1. **Action:** Keep EDTA blood sample at room temperature. If it has been previously refrigerated, allow time for it to warm up.
2. **Action:** Mix the sample thoroughly by gently rolling it between your hands for about a minute.

   Rationale: This suspends the cells evenly. Over-vigorous mixing will damage the cells.
3. **Action:** Prepare a spreader by chipping one corner off a glass slide. If necessary use a glass cutter.

   Rationale: The use of a spreader stops the smear overlapping the edges of the slide.
4. **Action:** Take a clean microscope slide which has been soaked in methanol and dried.

   Rationale: Methanol removes grease from the slide and stops gaps appearing in your smear.

5. **Action:** Using a capillary tube, place a small drop of blood on the right hand end of the slide.

   Rationale: Too large a drop makes the smear too thick; too small a drop gives too short a smear and/or hesitation lines.
6. **Action:** Place the spreader to the left of the blood drop at an angle of 45° to the horizontal and draw backwards to 'pick up' the blood.

   Rationale: The blood will run along the spreader as it makes contact.
7. **Action:** Push the spreader forward with even pressure towards the left hand end of the slide. The sides of the smear should be parallel and there should be a 'feathery tail' (Fig. 11.9).

   Rationale: The smear should take up two-thirds of the slide and should be bullet-shaped. Straight edges are needed for the 'battlement' technique of counting cells.
8. **Action:** Label the slide with a marker pen.

   Rationale: This is important because if you make several slides at once, they will all look the same.
9. **Action:** Dry the smear in the air.

   Rationale: The use of heat will damage the cells.
10. **Action:** Stain the smear with an appropriate stain.

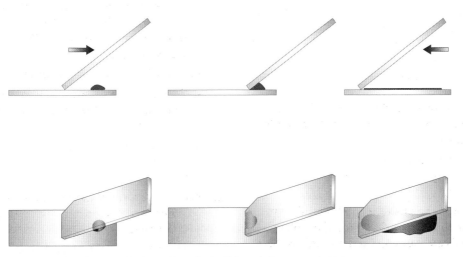

Figure 11.9 Preparing a blood smear. Redrawn from Aspinall (2006), Butterworth-Heinemann.

Procedure: Reticulocyte count (Fig. 11.10)

Equipment: Blood sample in EDTA tube, new methylene blue stain, centrifuge, centrifuge tube, Pasteur pipettes or volumetric pipette, incubator at 37°C, microscope.

1. **Action:** Using a pipette dispense 2 ml of methylene blue stain into a centrifuge tube.

   Rationale: Check that the stain is new methylene blue – you should not use McFadyean's methylene blue as this is used for identification of anthrax bacilli.

2. **Action:** Using a pipette add 4–5 drops of well-mixed EDTA blood.

   Rationale: A heparinised sample is not suitable for haematology.

3. **Action:** Mix gently and place in the incubator at 37°C for 30 minutes.

   Rationale: The sample can be incubated at room temperature if no incubator is available.

4. **Action:** Remove from the incubator and place in the centrifuge.

   Rationale: Make sure that you balance the centrifuge with a tube of a similar weight to avoid vibration and damage to the machine.

5. **Action:** Spin at 1000 rpm for one minute.

   Rationale: Spinning for faster or for longer will damage the cells.

6. **Action:** Remove and discard the supernatant fluid using a pipette.

7. **Action:** Gently flick the tube with your fingers.

Rationale: This resuspends the cells in any remaining fluid.

8. **Action:** Use this material to prepare a blood smear as previously described.

9. **Action:** Place the slide under the microscope and using first the ×10 and then ×40 objective lens, look for red blood cells with dark-blue-stained strands in them.

   Rationale: These cells are the immature red blood cells known as reticulocytes (Fig. 11.10). The dark blue strands are remains of the endoplasmic reticulum in the cytoplasm. The presence of reticulocytes indicates that new red blood cells are being formed by the bone marrow to replace those lost, e.g. by old age or haemorrhage.

10. **Action:** Count a total of 500 cells, noting the number of reticulocytes.

    Rationale: Select an area where individual cells can be seen – this indicates that the smear is one cell thick – known as a mono-layer.

11. **Action:** Calculate the number of reticulocytes as follows:

$$\text{Reticulocyte count} = \frac{\text{no. of reticulocytes} \times 100\%}{\text{total no. of cells counted}}$$

12. **Action:** A correction factor is now applied to this number.

    Rationale: In order to measure accurately the responsiveness of the bone marrow, the count takes the PCV of the patient into consideration.

13. **Action:** To calculate:

$$\text{Corrected reticulocyte count} = \frac{\text{reticulocyte count} \times \text{patient's PCV}}{\text{normal PCV for the species}}$$

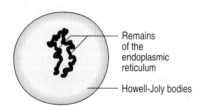

Figure 11.10   A reticulocyte. An immature circulating red cell, it can be stained with a supravital stain, e.g. new methylene blue.

Remains of the endoplasmic reticulum

Howell-Joly bodies

Procedure: Giemsa stain – used to demonstrate blood parasites

Equipment: Prepared blood smear, Coplin staining jar, Giemsa stain – neat, Giemsa stain – diluted 1:3 with buffered water (pH 6.8), filter paper, distilled water (pH 6.8), Pasteur pipettes, staining rack, methanol, forceps, microscope, microscope oil.

1. **Action:** Prepare a blood smear as previously described and air-dry. Place on the staining rack.

   Rationale: Do not use heat to dry the smear as this will damage the cells.

2. **Action:** Using a pipette, flood the smear with methanol.

3. **Action:** Leave for 3–5 minutes.

   Rationale: This fixes the smear.

4. **Action:** Drain off the methanol and allow the slide to dry in the air.

5. **Action:** Flood the slide with neat Giemsa stain pouring it through filter paper onto the slide. Leave it for 30 seconds.

   Rationale: Filtering the stain removes sediment, which may be mistaken for blood parasites.

6. **Action:** Using forceps, transfer the slide to the Coplin jar containing Giemsa stain diluted 1 part to 3 parts with buffered water (pH 6.8). Leave for 15–20 minutes.

   Rationale: The slide is held vertically in the Coplin jar to prevent a build-up of stain sediment on the smear.

7. **Action:** Remove the slide from the Coplin jar with forceps and rinse with buffered water.

   Rationale: Avoid using tap water – an incorrect pH will alter the staining characteristics of the cells.

8. **Action:** Wipe the underside of the slide and allow to dry.

   Rationale: Do not touch the top of the slide – you will remove the blood smear!

9. **Action:** Place the smear on the microscope stage and examine under oil immersion (×100).

   Rationale: This stain is used to identify the presence of blood parasites such as *Haemobartonella felis*. It is also useful for differential white cell counts.

Giemsa is a Romanowsky stain – one that uses a combination of two dyes, haematoxylin and eosin.

Procedure: Leishman's stain

Equipment: Prepared blood smear, Leishman's stain – neat, Leishman's stain – diluted 1:3 with buffered water (pH 6.8), buffered distilled water pH 6.8, Coplin jar, tissues or blotting paper, staining rack, filter paper, forceps, microscope, microscope oil.

1. **Action:** Prepare a blood smear as previously described and air-dry. Place on the staining rack.

   Rationale: Do not use heat to dry the smear, as this will damage the cells.

2. **Action:** Flood the slide with neat Leishman's stain, pouring it through a piece of filter paper. Leave for 1 minute.

   Rationale: Filtering the stain removes sediment, which may be mistaken for blood parasites.

3. **Action:** Using forceps, transfer the slide to the Coplin jar containing Leishman's stain diluted with buffered distilled water to a pH of 6.8. A gold film should be visible on the top of the liquid. Leave for 5 minutes.

   Rationale: The Coplin jar holds the slide in a vertical position to prevent the build-up of sediment. The gold film indicates that the stain is at the correct pH.

4. **Action:** Using forceps, remove the slide and rinse with buffered water.

   Rationale: Do not use tap water – if the pH is incorrect it may change the staining characteristics of the cells.

5. **Action:** Wipe the underside of the slide and air-dry.

   Rationale: Do not touch the top of the slide – you will remove the blood smear!

6. **Action:** Examine under the microscope using oil immersion (×100).

   Rationale: Leishman's is the stain most commonly used for differential white cell counts because it provides good cellular definition.

Leishman's stain is a Romanowsky stain – one that uses a combination of two dyes, haematoxylin and eosin.

Procedure: Diff–quik stain

Equipment: Prepared blood smear, Diff-quik stain, Coplin jars, forceps, distilled water buffered to pH 7.2, tissue, microscope, immersion oil.

1. **Action:** Prepare a blood smear as previously described and air-dry.

   Rationale: Do not use heat to dry the smear, as this will damage the cells.

2. **Action:** Dispense the staining solutions into Coplin jars.

   Rationale: These glass jars with lids will prevent dust from falling into the stains.

3. **Action:** Dip the slide into the fixative solution for 1 second, five times. Allow excess to drip back into the jar.

   Rationale: Leaving the slide in the fixative for too long results in unsatisfactory staining.

4. **Action:** Dip the slide into stain solution 1 for 1 second, five times. Allow excess to drip back into the jar.

   Rationale: This solution stains the cellular components red.

5. **Action:** Dip the slide into stain solution 2 for 1 second, five times. Allow excess to drip back into the jar.

   Rationale: This solution stains the cellular components blue.

6. **Action:** Rinse the slide with buffered water.

7. **Action:** Wipe the underside of the slide.

   Rationale: If you always keep the smear side facing towards you while staining, you will not be tempted to wipe the wrong side and lose your smear.

8. **Action:** Allow the smear to air-dry.

   Rationale: Do not use heat to dry the smear as this will damage the cells.

9. **Action:** Place the slide on the microscope stage and examine using oil immersion (×100).

Rationale: Stains must be renewed once a week to maintain their effectiveness.

Diff-quik is a Romanowsky stain – one which uses a combination of two dyes. Although it is quick and easy to use, it gives poor cellular definition.

Procedure: Differential white blood cell count

Equipment: Prepared blood smear, Leishman's or Giemsa stain, microscope, immersion oil.

1. **Action:** Prepare a blood smear and air-dry as described previously.

2. **Action:** Stain using either Leishman's or Giemsa stain as described previously.

   Rationale: Leishman's stain provides good cellular definition and is quicker to do than Giemsa.

3. **Action:** Place the slide on the microscope stage and examine under ×10 objective lens.

   Rationale: This enables you to select an area at least one-third from the end of the smear on the side edge.

4. **Action:** Move out the ×10 objective and place a drop of oil on the slide. Move the ×100 objective into position, making contact with the drop of oil.

   Rationale: Watch what you are doing from the side not through the lens – this may damage the slide. The use of oil immersion provides increased magnification.

5. **Action:** Carefully focus on the selected field using the fine adjustment knob.

   Rationale: Do not use the coarse focus as the incremental movements mean your view goes out of focus very quickly.

6. **Action:** Move the slide following the line of a 'battlement' (Fig. 11.11) as follows: move 2 fields along the edge of the smear, 2 fields up, 2 fields along, 2 fields down. While you are doing this count 100 white blood cells.

   Rationale: This enables you to cover a reasonable area of the smear and overcomes biased cell distribution on the slide. You may count more than 100 – the greater the number of cells counted the greater the accuracy of the sample.

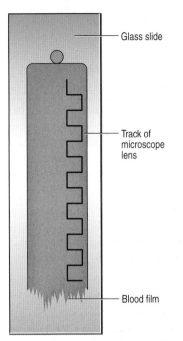

Figure 11.11 The battlement technique for differential blood films. Redrawn from Lane and Cooper (2003), Butterworth-Heinemann.

7. **Action:** As you count, record the numbers of each cell type (Fig. 11.12).

   Rationale: You may record your results manually on paper or by using some form of commercial differential counter.

8. **Action:** Calculate the percentage of each cell type using these figures (Table 11.1).

   Rationale: For example, suppose you have counted 72 neutrophils among your 100 cells, then the percentage of neutrophils in the blood is $72/100 = 72\%$.

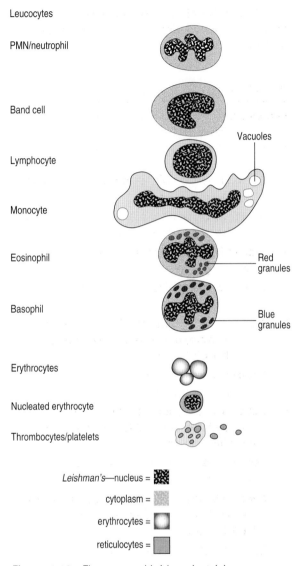

Figure 11.12 The range and Leishman's staining characteristics of blood cells visible in a blood smear. PMN, polymorphonuclear leucocyte. Redrawn from Lane and Cooper (1994), Butterworth-Heinemann.

HISTOPATHOLOGY

Procedure: Preparation of tissue for histological examination

Equipment: Formol saline, wide-mouthed sample container, scissors or scalpel.

1. **Action:** Make up 10% formol saline by diluting one part of formalin with nine parts of normal saline.

   Rationale: 10% formol saline is the most commonly used fixative.

2. **Action:** Select a wide-mouthed container.

   Rationale: Tissue is soft when taken from a patient and hardens as it becomes fixed. Removing hardened tissue from a narrow-mouthed container is very difficult.

3. **Action:** Select a piece of tissue, no more than 1–2 cm thick. If the tissue sample is large slice it into two or three pieces.

   Rationale: Diffusion through the tissue takes too long if the tissue is too thick.

4. **Action:** Add approximately 10 times the volume of the sample of formol saline.

   Rationale: The sample must be completely submerged in the formol saline.

5. **Action:** If the sample is to be posted, avoid using any more than 60 ml of formol saline. If the sample will not be adequately fixed in 60 ml, fix it in a large pot, remove it and wrap it in formalin-soaked gauze and post in a plastic bag.

   Rationale: Always check the postal regulations before sending samples through the post. Formalin is toxic and must not be allowed to leak out of the package.

6. **Action:** Wrap the sample in absorbent material and place in a leak-proof polypropylene transport box.

   Rationale: Glass bottles should not be sent through the post.

7. **Action:** Send it to the laboratory using 'next day' delivery.

   Rationale: Samples may deteriorate if left too long.

MICROBIOLOGY

Procedure: Preparation of bacterial smears

Equipment: Platinum loop (may use a single use/disposable loop), Bunsen burner, glass microscope slide, sterile normal saline, agar plate containing bacterial growth.

1. **Action:** Heat the platinum loop in the flame of a Bunsen burner. Allow it to cool. (Disposable loops do not require heating – they are supplied sterile. Each disposable loop will allow one action, after which it must be discarded into clinical waste.)

   Rationale: Flaming the platinum loop will sterilise it. Cooling prevents damaging the bacteria.

2. **Action:** Using the loop place 2–3 drops of saline onto the centre of the microscope slide.

   Rationale: This is used to dilute and spread the bacterial colony.

3. **Action:** Flame and cool the loop again.

4. **Action:** Using the loop, select an isolated bacterial colony and carefully remove it from the agar plate.

   Rationale: If there is more than one type of organism on the plate, you will need to make a smear for each type.

5. **Action:** Mix the colony with the saline on the slide, spreading out the fluid to cover 1–2 cm.

   Rationale: Mixing with saline results in a single layer of cells, allowing you to identify the shape of the cells.

6. **Action:** Flame and cool the loop. Discard in the appropriate way.

   Rationale: The loop has been contaminated and must be sterilised before it is discarded to prevent the spread of disease.

7. **Action:** Pass the smear gently over the Bunsen burner flame until it is dry.

   Rationale: This fixes the slide. If the smear is still wet when it is stained, some bacteria may float off, contaminating the stain and causing the loss of some areas of the smear.

8. **Action:** Stain the smear using Gram's or methylene blue.

Procedure: Gram's stain – rapid method

Equipment: Prepared bacterial smear, crystal violet stain, Gram's or Lugol's iodine, acetone, carbol fuchsin (dilute) or safranine, staining rack, wash bottle containing tap water, blotting paper or tissue, microscope, timer, Pasteur pipettes.

1. **Action:** Place the prepared smear on the staining rack with the smear facing upwards.

   Rationale: You can also stain smears in Coplin jars.

2. **Action:** Using a pipette, flood the slide with crystal violet for 30 seconds.

Rationale: At this stage the cell walls of Gram-positive organisms absorb the stain and become purple.

3. **Action:** Wash the slide with tap water.

   Rationale: To remove the crystal violet stain.

4. **Action:** Flood the slide with iodine for 60 seconds.

   Rationale: This fixes the smear.

5. **Action:** Flood the slide with acetone for 2–3 seconds.

   Rationale: This decolorises the smear and is a rapid stage.

6. **Action:** Wash the slide with water.

   Rationale: To remove the stain.

7. **Action:** Flood the slide with carbol fuchsin for 30 seconds.

   Rationale: This counterstains the bacteria – Gram-negative bacteria stain pink at this stage.

8. **Action:** Wash the slide with tap water.

   Rationale: To remove the stain.

9. **Action:** Wipe the back of the slide.

   Rationale: Do not wipe the front of the slide and lose the smear.

10. **Action:** Pass the slide rapidly over the flame of the Bunsen burner to dry it.

    Rationale: Do not overheat as the slide may shatter.

11. **Action:** Place the slide under the microscope and examine using oil immersion (×100).

    Rationale: Bacteria range in size from 0.5 µm to 5 µm in length and are best viewed under high magnification. Gram-positive bacteria, e.g. *Clostridia* spp., *Staphylococcus* spp., *Streptococcus* spp., stain purple; Gram-negative bacteria, e.g. *Escherichia coli*, *Salmonella* spp., stain pink. Gram's stain is used to identify the shape of bacteria and to classify them into Gram-positive or Gram-negative groups.

Procedure: Methylene blue stain

Equipment: Prepared bacterial smear, staining rack, Löffler's methylene blue, tissue or blotting paper, Pasteur pipette, wash bottle containing tap water, microscope.

1. **Action:** Place the prepared smear on the staining rack with the smear facing upwards.

   Rationale: You can also stain in Coplin jars.

2. **Action:** Using a pipette, flood the slide with methylene blue stain and leave for 3 minutes.

   Rationale: This stains the bacterial cells.

3. **Action:** Wash the slide with tap water.

   Rationale: To remove the stain.

4. **Action:** Pass the slide rapidly over the flame of the Bunsen burner to dry it.

   Rationale: Do not overheat as the slide may shatter.

5. **Action:** Place the slide under the microscope and examine using oil immersion (×100).

   Rationale: Bacteria range in size from 0.5 µm to 5 µm in length and are best viewed under high magnification. The bacteria stain blue. Methylene blue stain is used to identify the shape of the bacteria.

Procedure: Bacterial culture

Equipment: Sample material, Petri dish containing agar gel, platinum loop (may use a single use/disposable loop), Bunsen burner, incubator, marker pen.

1. **Action:** Label the Petri dish with an appropriate laboratory code.

   Rationale: Use the client's name, a number or the animal's name – develop your own system. It is important not to mix up samples – all agar plates look alike in the incubator.

2. **Action:** Flame the platinum loop in the Bunsen flame – heat until red hot from the handle end towards the loop and then bring up through the flame.

   Rationale: This sterilises the loop and kills all bacteria, making it safe to use.

3. **Action:** Cool the loop by waving it in the air for a few seconds.

Rationale: If the loop is too hot, it will kill bacterial cells and produce no growth on the plate.

4. **Action:** Dip the loop into the sample.

    Rationale: If it sizzles, it is too hot!

5. **Action:** Pick up the half of the Petri dish containing the agar and turn it over so that the surface of the agar is uppermost.

    Rationale: Petri dishes have a base into which the agar is poured and allowed to set, and a lid – they look similar.

6. **Action:** Smear the material on the loop over a small area on the left of the agar (Fig. 11.13).

    Rationale: This is known as the 'well' and is the start of your inoculation area.

7. **Action:** Replace the Petri dish into its lid.

    Rationale: Do not leave agar plates open to the air for too long as they may become contaminated.

8. **Action:** Flame and cool the loop as before. Remove the lid of the dish and check that the loop has cooled by placing it on a piece of the agar on one side of the plate.

    Rationale: If it sizzles it is too hot.

9. **Action:** Pick up the Petri dish and, using the loop, make 3–4 short streaks all in the same direction from the 'edge' of the well (Fig. 11.13). Take care not to tear the agar.

    Rationale: This action begins to spread the contents of the sample evenly over the plate.

10. **Action:** Continue to spread the sample over the plate as shown in Figure 11.13.

    Rationale: The aim is to dilute the sample and so form single colonies of bacteria on the final stroke.

11. **Action:** Place the lid on the dish and put it in the incubator with the agar side on top.

    Rationale: If the lid is uppermost, condensation will occur. The water droplets will drip down onto the surface of the agar, causing the bacterial colonies to spread.

12. **Action:** Do not stack plates more than two or three high inside the incubator.

    Rationale: Air must be able to circulate freely and overcrowding will prevent this.

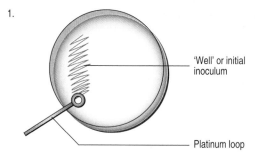

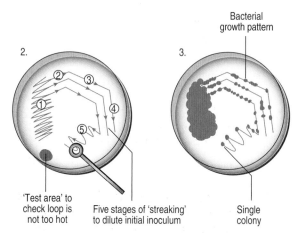

Figure 11.13 Technique for the inoculation of an agar plate.

13. **Action:** Incubate at 37°C for 18–24 hours.

    Rationale: Most pathogenic bacteria are described as normothermic and will grow at normal body temperature.

14. **Action:** Remove from the incubator and examine for signs of bacterial growth.

    Rationale: Colonies of bacteria appear as round often slightly raised 'lumps' – the colour may be characteristic of the species. They are distributed along the streak lines.

15. **Action:** If there is no visible growth, incubate the plate for another 18–24 hours.

    Rationale: Some bacteria take longer to grow than others.

PARASITOLOGY

Procedure: Culture for ringworm fungus

Equipment: Sabouraud's agar or commercial ringworm agar, e.g. Dermatofyt, forceps, Bunsen burner, marker pen, microscope slide, coverslip, inoculation loop, lactophenol cotton blue stain, Pasteur pipette.

Remember ringworm fungi are zoonotic – always wear gloves when handling samples!

1. **Action:** Place the forceps in the flame of the Bunsen burner for a few seconds. Remove and allow to cool to room temperature.

   Rationale: The forceps must be sterilised before use to reduce the risk of bacterial contamination.

2. **Action:** Remove the lid of the Petri dish containing the Sabouraud's agar or peel off the cover of the commercial agar.

   Rationale: Avoid contaminating the agar with your fingers.

3. **Action:** Using the forceps, take six to eight hairs from the sample to be examined and place them in the centre of the agar. Replace the lid or seal the cover of the commercial agar.

   Rationale: Avoid contamination by micro-organisms in the atmosphere.

4. **Action:** Incubate at room temperature for up to 28 days.

   Rationale: Ringworm fungus grows very slowly, although some species may grow within 4 days.

5. **Action:** When fungal growth is visible, examine and identify.

   Rationale: On Sabouraud's medium, growth appears as a white fluffy colony. On a commercial agar, an indicator placed in the agar results in a red coloration. Some contaminants may also create a colour change – it is important to identify the fungus under the microscope.

6. **Action:** To make a smear of the fungus, use a pipette to place 2–3 drops of lactophenol cotton blue stain in the centre of a glass microscope slide.

   Rationale: The stain helps to spread the colony over the slide. The phenol in the stain inactivates spores and the blue stain aids visualisation of the fungal spores and mycelia.

7. **Action:** Sterilise a platinum loop by passing it through the flame of the Bunsen burner and allow to cool.

   Rationale: To prevent contamination of the fungus.

8. **Action:** Using the loop, pick up a small amount of the fungal colony and mix with the stain on the slide. Sterilise and discard the platinum loop.

   Rationale: To prevent contamination by any remaining fungus on the loop.

9. **Action:** Place a coverslip over the material.

   Rationale: The use of a coverslip provides a uniform layer for examination.

10. **Action:** Place the slide under the microscope and examine using the ×10 objective and then the ×40 objective lenses.

    Rationale: Ringworm is caused by dermatophytes such as *Trichophyton* and *Microsporum* spp. Look for the typical micro- and macroconidia (Fig. 11.14). Lactophenol cotton blue is used to stain the background and the spores to aid visualisation of the fungus.

Procedure: Use of a Wood's lamp – to detect *Microsporum canis*

Equipment: Wood's lamp, eye protection.

Remember ringworm fungi are zoonotic – always wear gloves when handling samples or suspected cases!

1. **Action:** This is best performed in a darkened room.

   Rationale: A darkened room will intensify the fluorescent effect.

2. **Action:** Put on the eye protectors.

   Rationale: Ultraviolet light is potentially dangerous and can damage the conjunctiva and the retina.

3. **Action:** Switch on the lamp and allow it to warm up for 5 minutes.

A

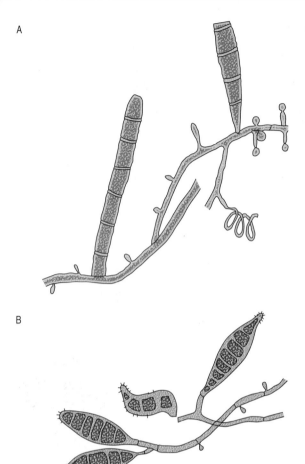

B

Figure 11.14 Microscopic appearance of ringworm fungus. A, *Trichophyton* spp.: look for septate hyphae, micro- and macroconidia; the latter are thin-walled and cylindrical. B, *Microsporum* spp.: look for septate hyphae, micro- and macroconidia; the latter are thick-walled, long, spindle-shaped or distorted. Redrawn from Lane and Cooper (1994), Butterworth-Heinemann.

4. **Action:** Ask an assistant (also wearing eye protectors) to restrain the patient on a non-slip examination table.

    Rationale: If the animal feels secure, it will be less likely to try to escape.

5. **Action:** Hold the lamp over the affected areas and look for signs of apple green fluorescence.

    Rationale: Only 60% of cases of *Microsporum canis* infection show this fluorescence. Lack of fluorescent areas does not rule out ringworm infection. Other particles in the

coat, e.g. skin flakes, dirt, detergent and paraffin oil may fluoresce a non-specific blue–white.

6. **Action:** Turn off the lamp immediately after use.

    Rationale: Long exposure to ultraviolet rays will burn the skin.

Procedure: Collection and examination of coat brushings – to demonstrate the presence of surface-living ectoparasites

Equipment: Toothbrush, flea or nit comb, Petri dish.

1. **Action:** Comb or brush through the patient's fur and collect the superficial debris and hairs in a Petri dish.

    Rationale: The fur may contain parasites, eggs, and faeces as well as skin scales and dirt.

2. **Action:** Examine with a hand lens or low powered microscope.

    Rationale: This is used to demonstrate the presence of surface-living ectoparasites such as *Cheyletiella* spp., fleas and lice (Fig. 11.15).

3. **Action:** If the presence of fleas is suspected, take a sample of hair containing black specks and cover with a few drops of water.

    Rationale: Flea dirt appears as gritty black specks in the coat. These are made of partially digested blood, which forms a pink-stained solution when dissolved in water.

Procedure: Collection of a skin scraping – to demonstrate the presence of burrowing ectoparasites

Equipment: Sterile sharp scalpel blade, clippers, clean collecting pot, suitable antiseptic powder or ointment.

1. **Action:** Select a suitable area of the patient for sampling and gently clip. If many areas are affected, take samples from several of them.

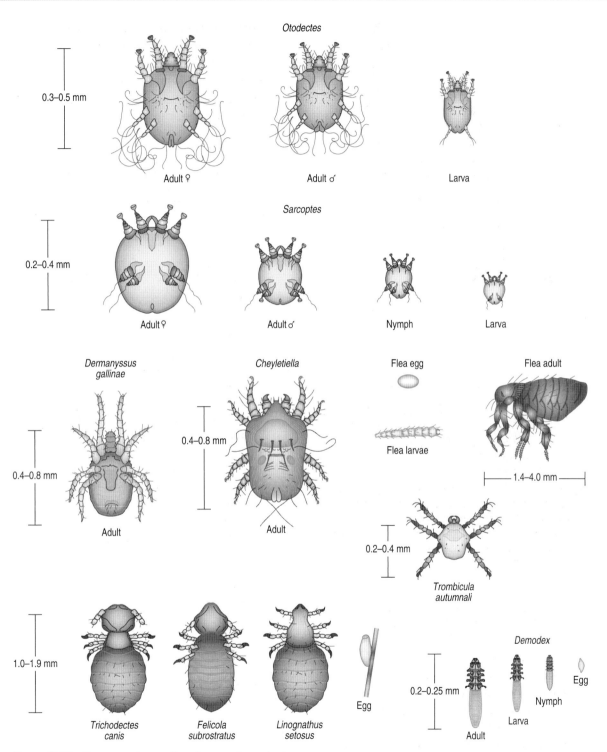

Figure 11.15 Common ectoparasites of companion animals.

Rationale: This reduces the amount of hair in the sample. The technique is used to demonstrate the presence of burrowing mites such as *Sarcoptes* and *Demodex*, which will not be present on superficial hair (Fig 11.15).

2. **Action:** Hold a sharp sterile scalpel blade at right angles to the skin and draw repeatedly across the area until it bleeds.

   Rationale: The presence of blood indicates that the deeper layers of the skin have been reached. Use of a sharp blade makes the whole procedure easier and less painful for the patient.

3. **Action:** Place the scalpel blade and all the skin debris into a clean collecting pot.

   Rationale: This need not be sterile as identification of mites will not be confused with the appearance of contaminating micro-organisms.

4. **Action:** Dress the scraped area with a suitable antiseptic.

   Rationale: This prevents the development of secondary bacterial infection.

Procedure: Preparation of a smear to identify the presence of mites

Equipment: Scraped skin sample, 10% potassium hydroxide, glass slide, coverslip, Pasteur pipette, microscope, Bunsen burner, forceps.

1. **Action:** Place some of the material collected by skin scraping onto the centre of a microscope slide.

   Rationale: Do not use too much material as the parasites may be masked by skin debris.

2. **Action:** With a pipette add 2–3 drops of 10% potassium hydroxide.

   Rationale: This solution is caustic – take care!

3. **Action:** Place a coverslip over the sample.

   Rationale: This provides a uniform layer to examine and prevents the lens from becoming contaminated.

4. **Action:** Holding the slide with forceps, warm it gently over a Bunsen burner – do not boil it.

Rationale: Warming breaks down and clears the debris, making the parasites easier to see.

5. **Action:** Allow the slide to cool.

6. **Action:** Place the slide under the microscope and examine under the ×4 objective and then the ×10.

   Rationale: Larger parasites such as *Sarcoptes* may be seen under ×4 magnification, but *Demodex* will only be seen under a higher magnification (Fig. 11.15).

7. **Action:** You may have to prepare several slides from your sample to be certain of the result.

   Rationale: Parasites may only be present in low numbers and may easily be missed if only one smear is made.

This technique may be used to demonstrate the presence of ear mites – *Otodectes cynotis* (Fig. 11.15). Brown coloured discharge is collected from the ear and treated in the same way before microscopic examination.

URINE EXAMINATION

Procedure: Urine preservation

Equipment: Collecting containers.

1. **Action:** Samples may be collected by catheterisation, midstream free flow or cystocentesis. (For catheterisation techniques, see Chapter 3.)

   Rationale: Free flow samples can be collected by the owner and are the most commonly used. A midstream sample is more representative of the bladder contents as the first part of the stream may contain contaminants from the urethra.

2. **Action:** Collect the sample into a clean, preferably sterile, container.

   Rationale: Owners may use clean jam jars, plastic containers or commercially designed collecting equipment. Cats may use any empty, clean litter tray or commercially prepared urine-collecting litter. If the sample is to be used for bacteriology, the container must be sterile

3. **Action:** Transfer the urine into a boric acid tube and a plain sample tube.

    Rationale: Boric acid is used to preserve samples for bacteriology. The bacterial numbers remain unchanged in the boric acid solution until it is tested. Plain tubes are used for specific gravity estimation, dipstick tests, and sediment examination. They may also be used for bacterial examination if used within 20 minutes of collection.

4. **Action:** If the sample cannot be despatched or tested immediately, store it in the fridge.

    Rationale: Refrigerated urine should be tested within 24 hours of collection.

Procedure: Gross examination of urine

Equipment: Urine sample in clean sample pot.

1. **Action:** Collect sample in clean transparent pot as described previously.

    Rationale: You must be able to examine the urine easily.

2. **Action:** Look at the colour of the sample.

    Rationale: Normal urine is yellow but it may vary in intensity. Deep yellow urine will be more concentrated than pale yellow urine; brown-yellow colour may indicate the presence of bilirubin; red colour may indicate the presence of blood or haemoglobin. Some drugs may change the colour of urine.

3. **Action:** Hold the sample up to the light and examine its clarity.

    Rationale: Normal urine is clear. Increased turbidity indicates the presence of sediment, e.g. crystals, bacteria, pus or blood cells.

4. **Action:** Remove the lid of the container and smell the sample.

    Rationale: Normal urine has a smell that is characteristic of the species, e.g. tomcat urine is instantly recognisable and is different from that of the queen. The smell of ammonia

may be caused by stale urine; the smell of peardrops is due to the presence of ketones.

Procedure: To test the specific gravity of urine by refractometer

Equipment: Urine sample, refractometer, Pasteur pipettes, distilled water, lint-free tissue.

1. **Action:** To calibrate the refractometer, wipe the glass prism (Fig. 11.16) with a piece of lint-free tissue and using a pipette, place 2 drops of distilled water onto the prism. Place the plastic cover over the prism.

    Rationale: The refractometer must be calibrated before use to ensure that it measures accurately.

2. **Action:** Hold the refractometer up to the light and look at the scale through the eyepiece. Note the point on the scale that marks the boundary between the light and dark areas.

    Rationale: For distilled water, this should read 1.000.

3. **Action:** If the reading is not exactly 1.000, adjust the refractometer using the screw on the top of the instrument until the reading is 1.000.

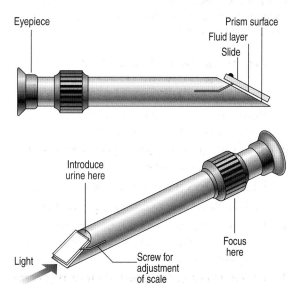

Figure 11.16   Refractometer – for measuring the specific gravity of urine.

Rationale: NB: some refractometers may have a different method of adjustment – check the instructions. The refractometer will now read accurately.

4. Action: Wipe off the distilled water with a piece of dry tissue.

5. Action: Using a fresh pipette, place 2 drops of the test urine onto the prism. Close the plastic cover.

Rationale: If you use the same pipette, you may dilute the urine sample with water remaining in the pipette.

6. Action: Hold the refractometer up to the light and read the scale as before. Record your result.

Rationale: Normal specific gravity of dog urine is 1.018–1.045. Normal specific gravity of cat urine is 1.020–1.040. Urine shows a higher specific gravity in cases of dehydration, reduced water intake and shock and a lower specific gravity where water intake is increased as is seen in cases of pyometra and chronic renal failure.

7. Action: Rinse off the urine with distilled water and wipe with lint-free tissue.

Rationale: Do not leave the urine sample to dry on the prism.

8. Action: Replace in the case.

Rationale: The refractometer must be stored in its case to prevent accidental damage and keep it dust-free.

Procedure: To test urine for various parameters using a dipstick

Equipment: Fresh urine sample, minute timer, dipstick test.

1. Action: Select the correct type of dipstick test. The sticks are presented in a screw-top container containing large numbers of sticks. The instructions are printed on the label.

Rationale: Commercial reagent dipsticks consist of a series of test reagent pads mounted on a plastic strip. The tests vary in number and in type, e.g. some may test only glucose, while others may have as many as 10 tests including those for pH, protein, blood and bilirubin. Make sure that the tests you need are included on the stick and that the tests are validated for animals – some are validated for humans and may give irrelevant results.

2. Action: Check the expiry date.

Rationale: Out-of-date dipsticks may give unreliable results.

3. Action: Remove the lid of the dipstick container and take out one stick. Replace the lid.

Rationale: Do not contaminate the remaining dipsticks with urine.

4. Action: Dip the stick in the fresh urine sample until all the pads are wet.

Rationale: Results are more accurate if the sample is fresh. Never use on a preserved sample. Stale samples may have bacterial growth or be contaminated by faeces or blood, which may affect the results.

5. Action: Remove the stick from the urine and tap gently on the side of the sample pot.

Rationale: To remove any surplus urine.

6. Action: Using the timer, make sure that you keep to the time intervals stated on the side of the bottle.

Rationale: Each test pad requires a specific time in contact with the urine before it reacts appropriately.

7. Action: Check that you read the results from the correct end of the stick.

Rationale: If you read from the wrong end, you will get results that are incorrect for that test pad.

8. Action: Hold the dipstick container in one hand and the dipstick in the other and compare the colour of each pad with the correct one on the side of the container.

Rationale: Each reagent pad will change colour and the range of colour changes is illustrated on the label accompanied by the appropriate result.

9. Action: Record your results.

Rationale: Do not rely on your memory – the results may need to be kept for some time.

10. **Action:** Dispose of the dipstick in the clinical waste.

    Rationale: Pathogens may be present on the stick.

Procedure: Urine sediment examination

Equipment: Fresh urine sample, microscope, glass slide, coverslip, Pasteur pipettes, urine centrifuge tube, centrifuge, Sedistain (optional).

1. **Action:** Using a pipette place 3–5 ml of urine in a centrifuge tube.

   Rationale: A conical tube helps to separate the sediment from the supernatant.

2. **Action:** Place the tube in the centrifuge.

3. **Action:** Place a similar tube on the opposite side of the centrifuge.

   Rationale: The machine must be balanced to prevent vibration and damage.

4. **Action:** Spin at 1000–2000 rpm for 2–3 minutes.

   Rationale: Spinning for a longer time will damage any cells present in the urine.

5. **Action:** Using a pipette, remove and discard most of the supernatant, being careful not to disturb the sediment.

   Rationale: Only the sediment is required for this procedure.

6. **Action:** Flick the test tube with your fingers.

   Rationale: This resuspends the sediment in any remaining liquid and makes a more even smear on the slide.

7. **Action:** If you wish, add 1–2 drops of Sedistain to the sediment in the tube, but this is optional.

   Rationale: Sedistain may make the material in the sediment easier to identify. Follow manufacturer's instructions for identification of cells, etc.

8. **Action:** Using a pipette, place 1–2 drops of the sediment onto the centre of a glass slide and add a coverslip.

   Rationale: This provides a uniform layer for examination and protects the lens from contamination.

9. **Action:** Place the slide under the microscope and examine using the ×10 and ×40 objective lens.

   Rationale: Look for evidence of casts, red and white blood cells, epithelial cells, spermatozoa, mucin threads, bacteria and crystals (Fig. 11.17).

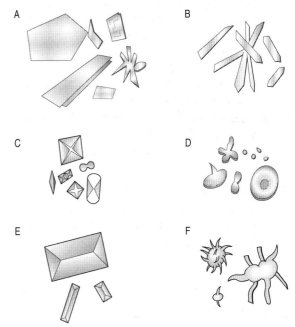

Figure 11.17 Urine crystals: A, urates; B, hippuric acid; C, calcium oxalate; D, calcium carbonate; E, struvite; F, ammonium urate. Redrawn from Lane and Cooper (2003), Butterworth-Heinemann.

REFERENCES AND FURTHER READING

Aspinall V (ed) 2006 The Complete Textbook of Veterinary Nursing. Elsevier, Oxford

Benjamin M 1974 Outline of Veterinary Clinical Pathology, 2nd edn. Iowa State University Press, Iowa

Cooper B, Lane D R (eds) 1999 Veterinary Nursing. Butterworth-Heinemann, Oxford

Davidson M, Else R, Lumsden J 1998 Manual of Laboratory Techniques. BSAVA, Gloucester

Kerr M 2002 Veterinary Laboratory Medicine, 2nd edn. Blackwell Science, Oxford

Lane D R, Cooper B (eds) 1994 Veterinary Nursing. Butterworth-Heinemann, Oxford

Lane D R, Cooper B (eds) 2003 Veterinary Nursing, 3rd edn. Butterworth-Heinemann, Oxford

Pinches M 2006 Getting results in clinical pathology 2. Pros and cons of in-clinic haematological testing. In Practice 28: 144–146

Simpson G (ed) 1996 Practical Veterinary Nursing. BSAVA, Gloucester

Chapter 12

Treatment of exotic species

Rachel Mowbray

CHAPTER CONTENTS

Introduction   278

The rabbit   278
Handling and restraint   278
To restrain a rabbit   278
To sex a rabbit   281
Administration of medicines   281
To administer fluids or liquid medication   281
To place a naso-oesophageal feeding tube   282
Subcutaneous injection   282
Intramuscular injection   283
Intravenous injection   283
Intraperitoneal injection   284
To place an intraosseous catheter   285
General anaesthesia   285
Induction of anaesthesia   285
Maintenance and monitoring
   of anaesthesia   287
Postoperative care   287

Small rodents   288
Handling and restraint   288
To restrain a chinchilla   288
To sex a chinchilla   289
To restrain a gerbil   289
To sex a gerbil   290
To restrain a guinea pig   290
To sex a guinea pig   291
To restrain a hamster   291
To sex a hamster   291

To restrain a mouse   292
To sex a mouse   293
To restrain a rat   293
To sex a rat   294
Administration of medicines   294
To administer fluids or liquid medication   294
To administer medication by parenteral
   routes   295
To collect a blood sample   296
General anaesthesia   297
Induction of anaesthesia   297
Maintenance and monitoring of anaesthesia   298
Postoperative care   298

The ferret   299
Handling and restraint   299
To restrain a ferret   299
To sex a ferret   300
Administration of medicines   300
To administer fluids or liquid medication   300
Subcutaneous injection   301
Intramuscular injection   301
Intraperitoneal injection   301
Intravenous injection   302
General anaesthesia   302
Induction of anaesthesia   302
Maintenance and monitoring of anaesthesia   303
Postoperative care   303

Cage and aviary birds   304
Handling and restraint   304

To capture and restrain a bird   304
To capture a bird using the towel method   305
To clip the wings   306
Administration of medicines   307
To administer fluid via a crop tube   307
Intramuscular injection   308
Intravenous injection   308
Intraosseous injection   309
To collect a blood sample   310
General anaesthesia   310
Induction of anaesthesia   310
Maintenance and monitoring of anaesthesia   311
Postoperative care   312

Reptiles   312
To restrain a snake   312
To administer fluids or liquid medication   313
Intravenous injection or blood sampling   314
To restrain a tortoise or terrapin   315
To administer fluids or liquid medication   316
Intravenous injection or blood sampling   317
To restrain a lizard   318
To administer fluids or liquid medication   318
Intravenous injection or blood sampling   319
General anaesthesia   320
Induction of anaesthesia   320
Maintenance and monitoring of anaesthesia   320
Postoperative care   321

INTRODUCTION

The presentation of various exotic species of animal to the veterinary surgeon for treatment is now an everyday occurrence. The care and handling needed by these animal differs from that required by dogs and cats in the following ways:

- Response to human contact – most exotic species have an innate fear of humans and any form of human contact is likely to induce a degree of distress. Certain individual animals, e.g. some rabbits, guinea pigs and ferrets, may tolerate or actively seek human company but to most the instinct is to run, or in some cases, to attack. This must be taken into consideration when providing nursing care – observe the patient unobtrusively, avoid unnecessary physical contact and be aware that most 'exotics' do not appreciate the sound of the human voice.

- Methods of restraint – some species are small and agile and can be easily injured by inept handling while others have wings, providing a different means of escape. Reptiles are cold-blooded, depending on their environment for heat and energy – they may suddenly become very active in the warmth of your hands. All are capable of causing injury to the ill-prepared handler.

- Reaction to anaesthesia – the term 'exotics' covers a wide range of species showing an equally wide range of differing responses to anaesthetic agents. It is not the brief of this chapter to describe the action of each anaesthetic agent but veterinary nurses must ensure that they are familiar with the clinical parameters and the reflexes that can be used to monitor the level of anaesthesia.

By understanding that the nursing care required by exotic species is different from that normally given to dogs and cats, the veterinary nurse can significantly increase the chances of recovery and survival of the exotic patient.

THE RABBIT – *ORYCTOLAGUS CUNICULUS*

For biological data – see Table 12.1.

HANDLING AND RESTRAINT

Procedure: To restrain a rabbit

1. **Action:** Observe the rabbit before handling.

    Rationale: To assess the nature and condition of the rabbit – if it is aggressive you may need to ask for assistance. Restraint may cause respiratory arrest in dyspnoeic animals. Severe stress and fear may lead to cardiac arrest.

2. **Action:** Rabbits should be handled gently but firmly.

    Rationale: Rabbits have an innate fear of humans, whom they perceive as predators.

Table 12.1   Biological data relating to rabbits and small rodents

	Chinchilla	Gerbil	Guinea pig	Golden hamster	Mouse	Rat	Rabbit
Lifespan (years)	10–12	3–4	4–8	2–3	2–3	3–4	5–12
Adult weight	400–600 g	50–60 g	750–1000 g	80–120 g	20–40 g	400–800 g	1–8 kg
Body temperature (°C)	38–39	37.4–39	38.6	36.2–37.5	37.5	38.0	38.3–39.4
Respiratory rate (breaths/min)	40–80	90–140	90–150	70–80	100–250	70–150	35–60
Pulse rate (beats/min)	100–150	250–500	130–190	280–412	500–600	260–450	130–325
Oestrus cycle (days)	41 Seasonally polyoestrous	4–6	15–17	4	4–5	4–5	No regular cycle. Induced ovulator
Age at puberty	8 months	10 weeks	M 8–10 weeks F 4–5 weeks	6–10 weeks	6–7 weeks	8–10 weeks	4–6 months
Gestation period (days)	111	24–26	63	16	19–21	20–22	28–32
Development of young at birth	Precocial	Altricial	Precocial	Altricial	Altricial	Altricial	Altricial
Weaning age	6–8 weeks	24–27 days	2–3 weeks	3–4 weeks	3–4 weeks	3–4 weeks	4–6 weeks
Type of diet	Herbivorous Coprophagic	Omnivorous Coprophagic	Herbivorous Need vitamin C	Omnivorous Coprophagic	Omnivorous Coprophagic	Omnivorous Coprophagic	Herbivorous Coprophagic
Natural behaviour	Nocturnal Social	Nocturnal Monogamous	Diurnal Social	Nocturnal Solitary	Nocturnal Social	Nocturnal Social	Crepuscular Social

3. **Action:** Talk quietly to the rabbit and approach from behind the head.

   Rationale: The eyes of the rabbit are placed on each side of the head, providing good lateral vision, but very poor backwards vision. There is no need to offer a hand for the rabbit to sniff – it may be mistaken for food.

4. **Action:** If the animal is fractious, grasp by the scruff and support the weight with one hand under the hindquarters (Fig. 12.1).

   Rationale: Never pick a rabbit up by the ears! The hind legs must be supported at all times. Rabbits have a fragile skeleton and large lumbar muscles. By struggling or kicking, rabbits can easily break their hind legs or dislocate or fracture their spines,

resulting in paralysis. They also have large claws, which may injure you.

5. **Action:** More docile rabbits may be restrained by placing one hand under the thorax, gripping the forelegs between the thumb and forefingers of that hand. Support the hind end with your other hand.

   Rationale: Some rabbits may resent being scruffed. The back should be kept in a normal curved position to avoid spinal fracture.

6. **Action:** To carry the rabbit, tuck the head and front feet under your upper arm and support the body along your forearm (Fig. 12.2).

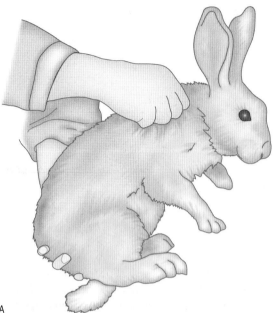

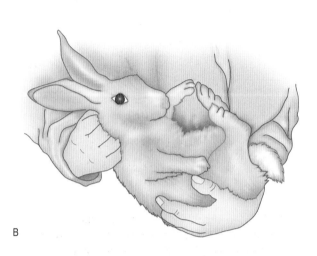

B

A

Figure 12.1 Restraining a rabbit.

Rationale: Keeping the rabbit close to your body avoids the risk of it kicking and scratching you. Keeping its head in the dark makes the rabbit relax.

7. **Action:** A large towel can be used as an additional means of restraint. Place the rabbit on the opened towel with its head projecting from one side. Wrap the towel around the body, covering the feet and leaving the head exposed (Fig. 12.3).

Rationale: Covering the feet protects the handler from injury while the head is available for examination and administration of medicines.

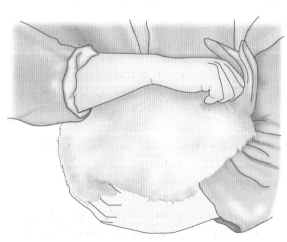

Figure 12.2 Carrying a rabbit with the head tucked under your arm.

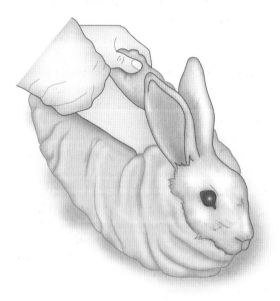

Figure 12.3 A large towel wrapped securely around the rabbit can be very helpful for restraint.

A   B

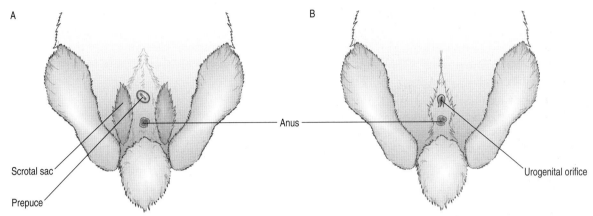

Scrotal sac

Prepuce

Anus

Urogenital orifice

Figure 12.4   Sexing a rabbit. Redrawn from O'Malley (2005), Saunders.

8. **Action:** An excessively aggressive rabbit may be removed from a cage by throwing a towel over the animal and covering it completely. The rabbit can be unwrapped when it is safely on the examination table.

    Rationale: Care must be taken to avoid injuring the rabbit or being injured yourself.

Procedure: To sex a rabbit

1. **Action:** Hold the scruff of the rabbit and support its weight by placing one hand under its hindquarters.

    Rationale: The rabbit must be held firmly to avoid possible injury to itself or to you.

2. **Action:** Gently lower the rabbit onto an examination table so that it lies in dorsal recumbency. Maintain your hold on the scruff and tilt the animal so that it is almost upside down.

    Rationale: In this position the rabbit is almost 'hypnotised' and is easier to examine.

3. **Action:** Using your forefinger and middle finger, apply pressure to the vent area just in front of the anus. It may be easier for the examination to be carried out by an assistant while you maintain a firm hold on the rabbit (Fig. 12.4).

    Rationale: In both sexes the area will protrude. Bucks (male) under 5 weeks old will show a blunt white tube without a central line while older bucks will show a pink tube with a pointed end that resembles a bullet; the doe (female) has a central slit-like opening to the vulva with a band of pink tissue on either side.

NB. Young rabbits are difficult to sex up to the age of about 3 weeks. Adult bucks have large scrotal sacs which are visible lateral and cranial to the penis. The testes can be retracted. Adult does often have a prominent fur-covered dewlap under the chin.

ADMINISTRATION OF MEDICINES

Procedure: To administer fluids or liquid medication

1. **Action:** Place the rabbit in sternal recumbency on an examination table and wrap it in a towel as previously described.

    Rationale: Using this method the legs are restrained but the head is exposed, providing access to the mouth.

2. **Action:** Take the head in one hand and tilt slightly to one side.

    Rationale: In this position, one corner of the mouth is uppermost.

3. **Action:** Using a syringe of an appropriate size containing the liquid medication, place the nozzle into the uppermost corner of the mouth.

Rationale: Avoid using large syringes as they are difficult to control.

4. **Action:** Apply gentle pressure to the syringe and give the medication. Allow time for the rabbit to swallow.

   Rationale: Give fluid in boluses of 0.25–0.5 ml. If the fluid is given too fast, the rabbit will choke or the liquid may escape out of the mouth.

Procedure: To place a naso–oesophageal feeding tube

Rabbits always breathe through their noses, so this procedure is not recommended for rabbits showing signs of respiratory distress.

1. **Action:** Select a 5–8F (French gauge) feeding tube.

   Rationale: The size depends on the size of the rabbit.

2. **Action:** Lay the tube along the outside of the rabbit's body, from the external nares to the caudal end of the sternum. Mark the point of the external nares with a tape or ballpoint pen.

   Rationale: As the tube is passed through the nasal cavity and down the oesophagus, the pen or tape mark will reach the opening to the nasal cavity and indicates that the end of the tube has reached the distal oesophagus, close to the entrance to the stomach.

3. **Action:** Restrain the rabbit in sternal recumbency and wrap in a towel as previously described.

   Rationale: In this position the body is restrained but there is access to the head.

4. **Action:** Apply local anaesthetic spray to one of the rabbit's nostrils. Wait for 3–5 minutes.

   Rationale: This desensitises the opening to the nasal cavity and facilitates tube placement.

5. **Action:** Apply Xylocaine gel to the end of the tube.

   Rationale: This lubricates the passage of the tube so that it can be inserted without resistance.

6. **Action:** Raise the rabbit's head and place the tip of the tube into the selected nostril at the ventral meatus. Gently advance the

tube medially and ventrally. Return the head to a normal position as the pharynx is approached. Continue until the mark on the tube lies at the entrance to the nasal cavity.

   Rationale: This ensures that the tube passes down into the distal oesophagus.

7. **Action:** Take a radiograph of the lateral thorax and abdomen.

   Rationale: It is important to check that the tube is in the oesophagus and not in the trachea. Introducing a small volume of saline down the tube is a simple means of monitoring, but rabbits do not always cough when this is done. The use of a lateral radiograph is a more reliable method. The rabbit will be conscious and must be restrained – make sure that correct radiological protection measures are carried out.

8. **Action:** Pass the external part of the tube over the bridge of the nose and between the ears. Fix in place using superglue, tape or sutures at the external nares and at the base of one ear.

   Rationale: It is important that the tube is not dislodged by patient interference.

9. **Action:** If necessary, use a Buster collar.

   NB. This technique can be used to administer liquid oral medication or for feeding hospitalised rabbits.

Procedure: Subcutaneous injection

1. **Action:** Place the rabbit in sternal recumbency on a suitable examination table with a non-slip surface.

   Rationale: If the rabbit feels secure it will be less likely to struggle and injure itself. Minimal restraint is needed but the rabbit must be prevented from leaping off the table.

2. **Action:** Select a sterile 21G or 23G needle and a syringe of an appropriate size. Draw up the drug to be administered.

   Rationale: Large volumes can be given by subcutaneous injection.

3. **Action:** Grasp the loose skin of the scruff and inject the drug into the subcuticular space.

    Rationale: You may draw back on the syringe prior to injection of the drug to check that a vein has not been penetrated, but this is not usually necessary with a subcutaneous injection.

4. **Action:** Withdraw the needle and gently massage the site.

    Rationale: To aid dispersion of the drug. Absorption of a drug from this area takes about 30–40 minutes.

Procedure: Intramuscular injection

1. **Action:** Place the rabbit in sternal recumbency on a suitable examination table with a non-slip surface.

    Rationale: If the rabbit feels secure it will be less likely to struggle and injure itself.

2. **Action:** Select a 23G needle and a syringe of appropriate size. Draw up the drug to be administered.

    Rationale: 0.5–1.00 ml can be given by this route. Large volumes will cause pain and damage to muscle tissue.

3. **Action:** Grasp the scruff of the rabbit with one hand.

    Rationale: This prevents the rabbit from moving or leaping off the table.

4. **Action:** Inject into the lumbar muscles.

    Rationale: This is a large muscle mass, which is easily accessible. The procedure can be performed single-handedly in docile rabbits. Assistance may be required if the patient is more active.

5. **Action:** Alternatively the quadriceps group of muscles on the cranial aspect of the thigh may be used. Restrain the rabbit in sternal recumbency and extend a hind leg towards the veterinary surgeon.

    Rationale: This position provides easy access to the muscle group.

6. **Action:** The veterinary surgeon will hold the muscle between the finger and thumb of the left hand and introduce the needle into the muscle with the right hand.

    Rationale: Assuming that the veterinary surgeon is right-handed.

7. **Action:** Draw back on the syringe to check that a vein has not been penetrated.

    Rationale: Muscle tissue is well supplied with blood vessels and there is a danger of accidental venepuncture. Care must also be taken to avoid the sciatic nerve, which runs behind the femur.

8. **Action:** If no blood appears in the hub of the needle, inject the drug into the muscle.

9. **Action:** Withdraw the needle, applying gentle pressure over the site.

    Rationale: To aid dispersion of the drug. Absorption from this area takes approximately 15–20 minutes.

Procedure: Intravenous injection

1. **Action:** Place the rabbit in sternal recumbency on an examination table with a non-slip surface.

    Rationale: If the rabbit feels secure it will be less likely to struggle and injure itself.

2. **Action:** Wrap the rabbit in a towel with the head uncovered as previously described.

    Rationale: This restrains the body while providing access to the head.

3. **Action:** Clip the fur lying over the marginal ear vein of one ear. Clean the site but avoid the use of spirit.

    Rationale: The marginal ear vein runs down the side of each ear. The use of spirit can collapse the vein, making sampling and injection more difficult.

4. **Action:** Apply local anaesthetic cream to the site. Wait for 10 minutes.

    Rationale: This desensitises the area so that the rabbit is less likely to shake its head when the needle is introduced.

5. **Action:** Place a ball of cotton wool soaked in hot water under the ear.

    Rationale: This causes the vein to dilate, making it easier to visualise.

6. **Action:** Apply pressure to the base of the selected ear.

    Rationale: This pressure acts as a tourniquet preventing blood returning from the ear pinna to the heart, so dilating or 'raising the vein' and making it more visible.

7. **Action:** Maintain the pressure while the veterinary surgeon inserts a 23G needle through the overlying skin into the marginal ear vein.

    Rationale: The vein should be clearly visible.

8. **Action:** The veterinary surgeon will draw back on the syringe.

    Rationale: If blood appears in the hub of the needle, the vein has been penetrated.

9. **Action:** If blood appears in the hub of the needle, release the pressure on the vein a little, while the veterinary surgeon injects the drug to be given.

    Rationale: Do not inject more than 1.5 ml as larger volumes may cause damage to the vein.

10. **Action:** When the procedure is complete, the veterinary surgeon will slowly withdraw the needle while you apply pressure over the injection site for a few seconds.

    Rationale: This prevents haemorrhage into the surrounding tissues.

NB. If repeated injections are to be given, use an intravenous or a butterfly catheter held firmly in place with superglue or tape. If collecting a blood sample, use the saphenous, the cephalic or the jugular veins. The maximum volume that can be collected at one time is 2.5 ml.

Procedure: Intraperitoneal injection

1. **Action:** Place the rabbit in sternal recumbency on an examination table with a non-slip surface.

    Rationale: If the rabbit feels secure it will be less likely to struggle and injure itself.

2. **Action:** Grasp the scruff with one hand and the hind legs with the other hand.

    Rationale: The rabbit must be held firmly to prevent it struggling during the procedure.

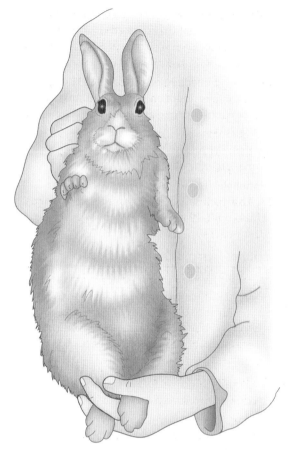

Figure 12.5   Restraining a rabbit for an intraperitoneal injection.

3. **Action:** Pick the rabbit up and hold it in dorsal recumbency with its spine against your chest (Fig. 12.5).

    Rationale: This position exposes the abdomen for injection, but care must be taken with dyspnoeic patients.

4. **Action:** The veterinary surgeon will introduce a short needle at a point midway between the xiphisternum and the pubis.

    Rationale: This position should avoid accidental penetration of the bladder or stomach. Rabbit skin is thin and a short needle easily penetrates the abdominal wall.

5. **Action:** Draw back on the syringe and examine the contents.

Rationale: If blood, urine or gut contents appear, reposition the needle. If nothing appears in the hub of the needle, it is safe to proceed with the injection.

6. **Action:** If there is nothing in the syringe, gently inject the contents of the syringe.

   Rationale: Up to 50 ml of fluid can be given by this route.

7. **Action:** When the procedure is complete, withdraw the needle.

NB. This technique can be used to collect samples of fluid from the peritoneal cavity and of urine from the bladder.

Procedure: To place an intraosseous catheter

1. **Action:** Select an appropriate site.

   Rationale: In the rabbit the proximal femur and the proximal tibia provide ease of access and a medullary cavity from which fluid can be rapidly absorbed.

2. **Action:** Prepare the site aseptically.

   Rationale: To prevent the introduction of infection.

3. **Action:** Infiltrate the area with local anaesthetic.

   Rationale: To desensitise the tissues. The rabbit may be under a general anaesthetic but this depends on the nature and condition of the individual patient.

4. **Action:** Select a spinal needle or plain needle of an appropriate size and insert it into the bone.

   Rationale: The needle must be of a size that will enter the medullary cavity – use a radiograph of the leg or previous experience to assess the size.

5. **Action:** Flush the needle with heparinised saline.

   Rationale: The needle may become blocked with tissue fragments. Heparinised saline will ensure that it is patent.

6. **Action:** Fix the needle in place with tissue glue or by suturing.

   Rationale: It is important that the needle does not become dislodged.

7. **Action:** Attach a short length of tubing and a syringe or attach a fluid giving set to the needle.

   Rationale: This procedure may be used to give a bolus of fluid or a slow infusion. Absorption from this site is as rapid as the intravenous route.

8. **Action:** If the needle is to be left in situ, bandage the area. You may need to use a Buster collar.

   Rationale: To prevent the risk of infection, to reduce limb mobility and to prevent patient interference. A Buster collar will also prevent interference but intraosseous catheters are usually well tolerated.

9. **Action:** When giving further fluid or drugs through the needle maintain an aseptic technique.

   Rationale: To prevent the introduction of infection.

10. **Action:** Flush with heparinised saline before each use.

    Rationale: To flush out any blood clots.

11. **Action:** Keep the needle patent by flushing with heparinised saline at least three times daily even if it is not being used.

    Rationale: To maintain patency.

NB. This route is useful for small animals whose veins are often fragile and easily damaged by needles and catheters. If the needle is dislodged, haemorrhage from the site is unlikely to occur.

GENERAL ANAESTHESIA

For general considerations see Table 12.2.

Procedure: Induction of anaesthesia

1. **Action:** Weigh the rabbit.

   Rationale: To calculate the correct dose of anaesthetic. It is important not to overdose the patient.

2. **Action:** During the induction process the rabbit must be handled gently and calmly.

Table 12.2   Points to be considered during anaesthesia of the rabbit

Action	Rationale
1. There is no need for preoperative starvation of rabbits.	1. Rabbits are unable to vomit. Starvation may cause a fatal hypoglycaemia, especially in smaller individuals. The stomach is never completely empty as rabbits exhibit coprophagia.
2. Avoid dehydration by giving fluids intravenously, subcutaneously, intraperitoneally or intraosseously.	2. This is not usually necessary in routine operations but can be particularly important in rabbits that are in a poor state of health or anorexic.
3. Keep the patient warm at all times using a heat pad or by wrapping in 'bubblewrap' but check regularly for signs of hyperthermia.	3. Hypothermia may be a problem in small animals, particularly during anaesthesia and postoperatively, as they have a large surface area in relation to their bodyweight. Anaesthetics depress temperature regulation and may cause vasodilation. If viscera are exposed during surgery, heat loss will be increased.
4. Apply an ophthalmic lubricant to protect the eyes.	4. Rabbits have bulging eyes, which are prone to drying out during anaesthesia. If ketamine is used in any anaesthetic combination, the eyes will remain central and fixed.
5. Make sure that the tongue is pulled forward if the patient is not intubated.	5. A rabbit's tongue is large and may obstruct the airway.

Rationale: This process easily distresses a rabbit and it may contribute to cardiac or respiratory arrest.

3. Action: If using an injectable agent, e.g. fentanyl/fluanisone or ketamine/medetomidine, give by the appropriate route, restrain the patient as described previously (Table 12.3).

Rationale: Injectable agents provide a rapid and stress-free induction. Use small syringes for more accurate dosing.

4. Action: Supplement with oxygen by mask or by intubating the patient.

Rationale: This should be done even when using injectable agents.

5. Action: If using inhalation anaesthesia, e.g. isoflurane, induce using a mask or an induction chamber.

Rationale: Using a mask is easier if the rabbit has been given a premedicant. An induction chamber of a suitable size for the patient may take several minutes to fill. Induction by either of these methods is not recommended as the rabbit may hold its breath or may struggle violently, injuring its back. The most commonly used anaesthetic, isoflurane, is irritant to mucous membranes.

6. Action: Give 100% oxygen for 1–2 minutes before attempting to intubate the rabbit.

Rationale: To increase the oxygen concentration in the anaesthetic mixture. Intubation is more difficult than in the dog and the cat and may take longer as the glottis and larynx are not visible.

7. Action: Intubate the rabbit by placing it in sternal or dorsal recumbency with the head and neck extended. Use a laryngoscope to illuminate the area and an 'introducer', such as that found inside a cat urinary catheter, to stiffen the endotracheal tube. Slide the tube over the 'introducer' into the trachea and remove the 'introducer'.

Rationale: The glottis of the rabbit is small and obscured by the tongue. A fatal laryngospasm may occur if care is not taken.

8. Action: Alternatively intubation may be performed 'blind'. Estimate the position

Table 12.3 Anaesthetic agents used in small rodents and rabbits

Drug	Species, dose rate and route of administration				Duration of anaesthesia
	Mouse	Rat	Guinea pig	Rabbit	
Fentanyl/fluanisone (Hypnorm)	0.2–0.5 ml IM 0.3–0.6 mg/ml IP	As mouse	–	0.2–0.4 ml	Sedation only 30–45 min
Fentanyl/fluanisone (Hypnorm)/diazepam	0.4 ml/kg 5 mg/kg	0.3 ml/kg 2.5 mg/kg	1 ml/kg IM 2.5 ml/kg	0.3 ml/kg IM 2 mg/kg IP	45–60 min
Fentanyl/fluanisone (Hypnorm)/midazolam*	10 ml/kg*	2.7 ml/kg*	8 ml/kg*	0.3 ml/kg IM 0.5–1 ml/kg IV	45–60 min
Ketamine/medetomidine	200 mg/kg 0.5 mg/kg	90 mg/kg 0.5 mg/kg	40 mg/kg 0.5 mg/kg	35 mg/kg 0.5 mg/kg	20–30 min
Propofol	26 mg/kg IV	10 mg/kg IV	–	10 mg/kg IV	5 min
Atipamezole	1 mg/kg IM, IP, SC, IV to reverse any combination using medetomidine				

*One part fentanyl/fluanisone (Hypnorm) to one part midazolam (5 mg/ml) to two parts water.
IM, intramuscular; IP, intraperitoneal; IV, intravenous; SC, subcutaneous.
Source: Hotston-Moore (1999).

of the larynx externally and advance the endotracheal tube until it lies in the correct position. Check for correct positioning.

Rationale: The larynx may be palpated externally. Listen for respiratory sounds through the tube to check positioning. A transparent tube may show evidence of condensation from the moisture in the exhaled breath.

9. **Action:** Attach the endotracheal tube to the anaesthetic circuit.

Rationale: Circuit must be appropriate to the species, e.g. Ayer's or Jackson Rees modified T-piece.

10. **Action:** Take appropriate steps to keep the rabbit warm at all times.

Rationale: Heat loss can be reduced by wrapping in 'bubblewrap' or a 'space blanket' or by use of a heat pad.

Procedure: Maintenance and monitoring of anaesthesia

1. **Action:** Make sure that you are familiar with the reactions of the rabbit under general anaesthesia.

Rationale: Rabbits are not as relaxed as dogs and cats.

2. **Action:** Pay particular attention to the rate and depth of respiration.

Rationale: This is the most reliable method of monitoring the depth of anaesthesia. Laboured breathing and pauses between breaths indicate deep anaesthesia.

3. **Action:** Monitor the tension of the jaw.

4. **Action:** Pinch the ear.

Rationale: Absence of a headshake indicates an acceptable level of surgical anaesthesia.

5. **Action:** Assess the pedal reflex.

Rationale: This reflex remains for longer than in the dog and cat and is only lost under deep anaesthesia.

6. **Action:** The corneal and palpebral reflexes can also be used to assess depth of anaesthesia.

Rationale: These are similar to those in the dog and cat.

Procedure: Postoperative care

1. **Action:** The rabbit must be monitored until it is completely conscious and behaving normally.

Rationale: Avoid too much direct attention, e.g. talking to the rabbit, as this will increase the levels of stress. Observe from a discreet distance.

2. **Action:** Place the rabbit in a cage in a room which is warm, quiet and dimly lit.

   Rationale: Bright lights and noise will distress the rabbit during recovery.

3. **Action:** Ensure that the rabbit is kept warm using a heatpad or Vetbed, or blankets or towels placed under and over the body. Avoid the use of shavings or hay etc.

   Rationale: Hypothermia can be fatal or will prolong the recovery period. Loose bedding such as shavings may clog the mouth and nose.

4. **Action:** Monitor the core temperature until completely conscious.

   Rationale: Use a rectal thermometer but try to avoid excessive manipulation of the recovering rabbit.

5. **Action:** If necessary be prepared to give oxygen.

   Rationale: This will increase the rate of recovery.

6. **Action:** If the rabbit shows signs of pain, e.g. tooth grinding, grunting, lack of appetite, or if the condition warrants it, provide analgesia.

   Rationale: Any procedure that would cause pain in any other species should be considered to cause pain in the rabbit and would warrant the use of analgesics. Correct use of analgesics, e.g. carprofen or buprenorphine, will do no harm.

7. **Action:** If the rabbit does not eat or drink soon after recovery, consider providing fluid therapy – either intravenously or intraperitoneally; this should include glucose.

   Rationale: Lack of fluid may rapidly cause serious dehydration. Lack of food may lead to a fatal hypoglycaemia. Both will compromise recovery.

8. **Action:** Monitor urine and faeces output.

   Rationale: General anaesthesia and surgery may impair both kidney and intestinal function. Overhandling of the intestine may cause paralytic ileus, which is indicated by a lack of faeces.

SMALL RODENTS

For biological data see Table 12.1.

HANDLING AND RESTRAINT

It is the natural response of a frightened rodent to bite. This can be avoided by knowing how to handle each species correctly, but if you are bitten:

- Replace the rodent in its cage with your finger still in its mouth. As the rodent feels its feet on a firm surface it should let go!
- Do not attempt to pull your finger from the rodent's mouth, as the injury will be made worse by the backward-pointing curved teeth.
- Do not shake the rodent off your finger, as this will cause serious injury to the rodent.
- Wash the bite thoroughly under running water, apply antiseptic ointment and cover for as long as you are working with the animals.
- Consult your doctor if it becomes excessively painful or swollen.
- Keep your tetanus vaccination up to date.

The chinchilla – *Chinchilla lanigera*

Procedure: To restrain a chinchilla

1. **Action:** If the chinchilla is tame, pick it up by placing one hand around its shoulders.

   Rationale: Chinchillas are relatively easy to handle; most are not aggressive and rarely bite. Be aware of the pressure you are putting on the chest as this can restrict normal breathing.

2. **Action:** Avoid grasping hold of the fur.

   Rationale: Rough handling can cause patches of fur to come away in your hand – a condition known as 'fur slip'. In the wild this mechanism enables the chinchilla to escape from predators. New fur may take several months to grow back and may be of a different shade.

3. **Action:** Once removed from the cage, most chinchillas will sit quietly on your forearm gently restrained by the base of the tail.

   Rationale: If the animal feels supported and secure it will be unlikely to try to escape.

4. **Action:** More nervous or active animals can be lifted by the base of the tail, with your other hand supporting the body.

    Rationale: Only lift by the base of the tail as further down may injure the tail. Do not leave the animal unsupported for any longer than is necessary.

5. **Action:** To restrain for any clinical procedure, hold the base of the tail with one hand and place the other around the shoulder and chest.

    Rationale: This can be used to hold the animal firmly for such procedures as injection and examination.

Procedure: To sex a chinchilla

1. **Action:** Grasp the base of the tail with one hand and support the body around the shoulders.

    Rationale: If the animal feels supported and secure it will be unlikely to try to escape.

2. **Action:** Hold the chinchilla in dorsal recumbency, moving the tail to expose the genital area.

    Rationale: This can be done single-handedly unless the chinchilla struggles.

3. **Action:** Examine the genital area and measure the anogenital distance.

    Rationale: This is the distance between the anus and the opening of the vulva (female) or the penis (male) and is longer in the male than in the female (Fig. 12.6).

The female chinchilla has a large cone-shaped clitoris, which may be mistaken for the penis of the male. Adult male chinchillas have a pair of large testes which are very obvious during the breeding season of November–March.

The gerbil – *Meriones unguicularis*

For biological data see Table 12.1.

Procedure: To restrain a gerbil

1. **Action:** If the gerbil is tame and used to being handled, scoop it into your cupped hands.

Rationale: Gerbils are extremely active creatures and can jump horizontally and vertically.

2. **Action:** If the gerbil is less tame, immobilise it by placing your hand over it.

    Rationale: This will prevent it escaping. The darkness will temporarily calm it.

3. **Action:** Move your hand to grasp the scruff and lift the animal clear of the cage.

    Rationale: Most gerbils are not aggressive, but some will try to bite – make sure that you grasp enough scruff to prevent it turning around to bite.

4. **Action:** Further restraint can be achieved by using your other hand to hold the base of the tail.

    Rationale: Do not hold the tip of the tail as the skin may be shed, leaving a raw and painful tail.

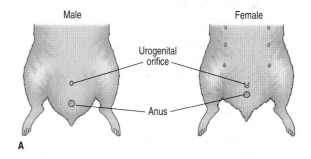

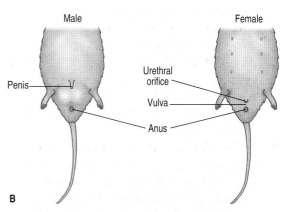

Figure 12.6   General method of sexing rodents: A, hamsters; B, mice.

Procedure: To sex a gerbil

1. **Action:** Restrain the gerbil by grasping the scruff as described previously.

   Rationale: If the gerbil feels secure and comfortable it will be less likely to struggle or to attempt to bite you.

2. **Action:** Examine the ventral surface of the gerbil.

   Rationale: Male gerbils have no teats; females have four pairs of teats arranged along the ventral body wall of the thorax and the abdomen.

3. **Action:** Examine the genital area and measure the anogenital distance (Fig. 12.6).

   Rationale: The anogenital distance is the distance between the anus and the opening of the vulva (female) or the penis (male) and is longer in the male than in the female (Fig. 12.6). Adult male gerbils have a pair of testes lying in the inguinal region.

The guinea pig – *Cavia porcellus*

For biological data see Table 12.1.

Procedure: To restrain a guinea pig

1. **Action:** Guinea pigs should be brought to the surgery in small covered boxes.

   Rationale: Guinea pigs are nervous animals and a box provides security and darkness, which will calm them.

2. **Action:** Open the box in a dim light if possible.

   Rationale: This will reduce stress, but you must be able to examine the patient.

3. **Action:** Pick up the animal by placing one hand around its shoulders and chest (Fig. 12.7).

   Rationale: Guinea pigs are generally non-aggressive and can be handled gently but firmly.

4. **Action:** Lift the guinea pig clear of the cage or box, supporting its weight with your other hand.

   Rationale: This is important if the animal is pregnant or heavy.

5. **Action:** Move your thumb from around the shoulders and place it under the mandible (Fig. 12.7).

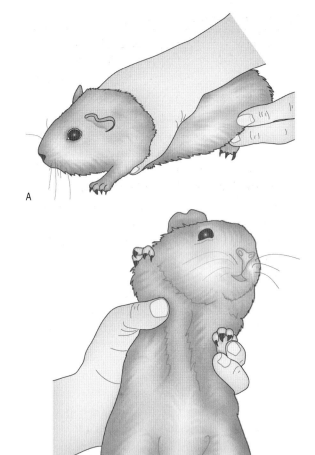

Figure 12.7 Restraining the guinea pig for examination. A, Initial restraint is achieved by grasping the animal around the shoulders. B, The hindquarters should be supported if the animal weighs more than 200–300 g.

   Rationale: This prevents the animal from lowering its head to bite.

6. **Action:** If further restraint is needed, place the guinea pig in dorsal recumbency and extend the hind legs.

   Rationale: The animal will be unable to move.

Procedure: To sex a guinea pig

1. **Action:** Restrain the guinea pig in dorsal recumbency as previously described.

   Rationale: This provides good exposure of the genital area.

2. **Action:** Examine the inguinal region.

   Rationale: Both male (boar) and female (sow) have a single pair of nipples in the inguinal region. Adult males have a pair of large testes.

3. **Action:** Examine the genital opening.

   Rationale: Females have a Y-shaped opening; males have a slit-shaped opening.

4. **Action:** Apply gentle pressure on either side of the genital opening.

   Rationale: In the male, the penis will extend and protrude. Female guinea pigs have a pale coloured clitoris, which may protrude, but it is much less obvious than the male penis.

   NB. Guinea pigs can be sexed as early as 1–2 days old.

Hamster – *Mesocricetus auratus* (Syrian or golden hamster)

Procedure: To restrain a hamster

For biological data see Table 12.1.

1. **Action:** Waking a sleeping hamster can provoke an aggressive response.

   Rationale: Allow the hamster time to wake up before attempting to pick it up.

2. **Action:** As the hamster runs around on the floor of the cage or box, grasp a large section of the scruff (Fig. 12.8).

   Rationale: Hamsters are unpredictable and often aggressive. It is important to take a large area of scruff to prevent the animal turning around to bite you.

3. **Action:** Lift the hamster upwards.

   Rationale: Hamsters are not very heavy and can be lifted with one hand.

4. **Action:** Draw the scruff tight to prevent the hamster from moving around.

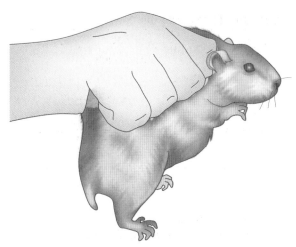

Figure 12.8   Picking a hamster up by the scruff of the neck.

   Rationale: In this position you can inject the animal, and examine the teeth and the oral pouches. If the scruff is too tight the eyes will bulge.

5. **Action:** If the hamster does not need to be examined or injected, you can pick it up in your cupped hands or allow it to run into a small cup or jug.

   Rationale: The hamster can be moved from cage or box to an induction chamber but is not sufficiently restrained for any clinical procedure.

Procedure: To sex a hamster

1. **Action:** Restrain the hamster in one hand using the scruff as previously described.

   Rationale: Make sure you are holding enough of the scruff to prevent the hamster turning around and biting you.

2. **Action:** Examine the genital area and measure the anogenital distance (Fig. 12.6).

   Rationale: Adult males have a pair of large testes. These are visible from the dorsal surface as the hamster runs around. The anogenital distance is the distance between the anus and the opening of the vulva (female) or the penis (male) and is longer in the male than in the female. (Fig. 12.6).

3. **Action:** Examine the ventral surface of the hamster.

Rationale: The male hamster has no teats; the female has six pairs arranged along the ventral body wall of the thorax and abdomen.

4. **Action:** If the hamster is mature, examine the region of the hips.

   Rationale: Male hamsters have a scent gland over each hip. This becomes pigmented as the animal ages. The gland is not present in the female.

NB. The much smaller Chinese and Russian hamsters are also popular children's pets. The techniques for handling and sexing these species are exactly the same as described for the Syrian hamster.

The mouse – *Mus musculus*

For biological data see Table 12.1.

Procedure: To restrain a mouse

1. **Action:** If the mouse is tame and used to being handled, scoop it into your cupped hands.

   Rationale: This works well for tame mice, but many mice are very nervous and may attempt to bite – a careful approach is essential.

2. **Action:** If the mouse is not used to being handled, pick it up by the base of the tail.

   Rationale: Do not pick it up by the tip of the tail as the outer skin may be shed, leaving the tail raw and painful.

3. **Action:** Lift the mouse clear of the cage and place it on a rough surface such as a towel, your sleeve or the top of the wire cage.

   Rationale: Mice are light enough to be lifted by the tail without the need to support the body.

4. **Action:** Pull the mouse gently backwards (Fig. 12.9).

   Rationale: The mouse will grip the surface and is sufficiently restrained for an initial examination.

5. **Action:** With your other hand grasp a large amount of scruff between your finger and the base of your thumb while keeping control of the tail.

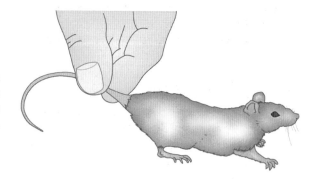

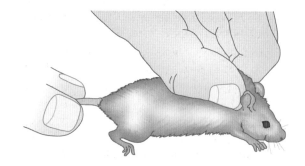

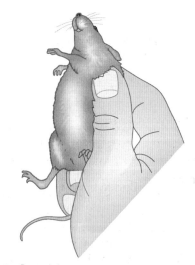

Figure 12.9   Restraining a mouse.

Rationale: If you do not take enough of the scruff, the mouse will be able to turn round and bite you.

6. **Action:** Lift the mouse up and transfer your hold on the tail to between the third and fourth fingers of that hand (Fig. 12.9).

   Rationale: The mouse is restrained securely and as it is held in one hand only your other hand is free to examine or inject it.

Procedure: To sex a mouse

1. **Action:** Restrain the mouse by the scruff and tail as previously described.

   Rationale: Mice can easily struggle and escape if not held securely.

2. **Action:** Examine the ventral surface of the body.

   Rationale: Male mice do not have teats; females have seven pairs arranged along the ventral body wall of the thorax and abdomen.

3. **Action:** Examine the genital region and measure the anogenital distance (Fig. 12.6).

   Rationale: The anogenital distance is the distance between the anus and the opening of the vulva (female) or the penis (male) and is longer in the male than in the female (Fig. 12.6). Adult males have a pair of large testes lying in the inguinal region.

The rat – *Rattus norvegicus*

For biological data see Table 12.1.

Procedure: To restrain a rat

1. **Action:** With one hand, grasp the body around the shoulders and lift clear of the cage.

   Rationale: Rats are intelligent, docile animals which rarely bite unless they are frightened or in pain. Be aware of how much pressure you are applying to the chest – too little will allow the animal to escape; too much will compress the chest and may make the animal bite you.

2. **Action:** Position your thumb so that it lies under the lower jaw (Fig. 12.10).

   Rationale: Use your thumb to apply pressure and to push the jaw up. This will prevent the animal from biting.

3. **Action:** Alternatively, if the rat is aggressive or unused to being handled, pick it up by the base of the tail.

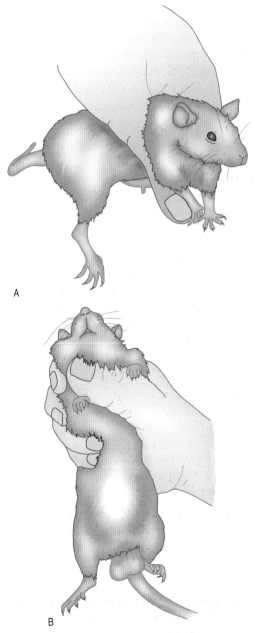

A

B

Figure 12.10   Restraining a rat.

Rationale: Do not pick up by the tip of the tail as the outer skin may be shed, leaving a raw and painful tail.

4. **Action:** Place the rat on the cage lid, or on a rough surface, maintaining your grip on the tail.

    Rationale: This provides something to which the rat can grip.

5. **Action:** As the rat moves forward, place your other hand over the shoulders and chest.

    Rationale: Do not hold too tightly, as this will affect the rat's respiration and may cause distress.

6. **Action:** Move your thumb and forefinger to lie behind the rat's elbows so that the forelegs are pushed forward to cross under the chin.

    Rationale: The rat is held securely and it can be examined without the risk of being bitten.

7. **Action:** If the rat struggles when first restrained, allow it to rest on your sleeve with a minimum of restraint.

    Rationale: After a short time, the rat will relax.

NB. Rats do not like being picked up by the scruff and this may cause the animal to bite.

Procedure: To sex a rat

1. **Action:** Restrain the rat by picking it up around the shoulders.

    Rationale: If the rat feels secure it will be less likely to struggle or to bite.

2. **Action:** Lift it clear of the cage and hold it in dorsal recumbency.

    Rationale: In this position you have access to the relevant parts of the animal.

3. **Action:** Examine the ventral surface of the body.

    Rationale: Male rats do not have teats; females have five pairs arranged along the ventral body wall of the thorax and abdomen.

4. **Action:** Examine the genital area and measure the anogenital distance (Fig. 12.6).

    Rationale: The anogenital distance is the distance between the anus and the opening of the vulva (female) or the penis (male) and

is longer in the male than in the female (Fig. 12.6). Adult males have a pair of large testes lying in the inguinal region.

ADMINISTRATION OF MEDICINES

Procedure: To administer fluids or liquid medication

1. **Action:** Medication such as antibiotics can be given to small rodents in the drinking water or in food.

    Rationale: Withhold all other sources of water or food, so that the animal has to take in the medication. However, this is not recommended as the animal may not be eating or drinking normal amounts – the precise dose is unknown.

2. **Action:** If the animal is not drinking, liquid medication or replacement fluids can be given by inserting a syringe or pipette into the side of the mouth at the level of the diastema (space between the incisors and molar teeth).

    Rationale: Use an unbreakable syringe to prevent the animal biting through the nozzle. Sweeten the liquid with fruit juice to increase acceptability.

3. **Action:** The chinchilla, guinea pig and rat can be given liquid through a 3–4F catheter inserted into the pharynx, oesophagus or stomach. Make a mouth gag by drilling a hole crossways through a 1 ml syringe case. Place the 'gag' across the mouth of the patient and pass the catheter through the hole and down the pharynx. Ensure that the catheter is correctly placed before injecting any fluids by listening for respiratory sounds in the tube or by taking a lateral radiograph of the animal.

    Rationale: This technique enables you to give volumes of up to 5 ml. The use of the gag prevents the patient biting through the catheter. It is vital to check that the catheter is not in the trachea as the administration of fluid into the lungs may 'drown' the animal or cause aspiration pneumonia.

Procedure: To administer medication by parenteral routes

For details of injection sites see Table 12.4. General points to be considered:

1. **Action:** For most procedures, use a 23G or 25G needle.

   Rationale: Small needles cause less damage to the tissues.

2. **Action:** If giving small volumes of drugs use small syringes.

   Rationale: Larger sizes are more difficult to handle when restraining small, struggling rodents.

3. **Action:** When using the intramuscular route, give small volumes.

   Rationale: Large volumes may cause tissue damage, pain, irritation and possible

Table 12.4 Parenteral routes for the administration of medicines in small rodents

Species of rodent	Subcutaneous	Intramuscular	Intraperitoneal	Intravenous
Chinchilla	Scruff or the flank Avoid rough handling as this causes 'fur slip'	Quadriceps group on cranial thigh or semimembranosus/ semitendinosus on caudal thigh. No more than 0.3 ml	Restrain with head lower than hindquarters. Insert needle in posterior quadrant to the right of the midline 2.5 cm in front of pubis	Use the cephalic, saphenous or jugular veins
Gerbil	Scruff. Up to 2 ml	Quadriceps group No more than 0.3 ml Not recommended	Restrain with head downwards Insert needle into lower left quadrant. Give 3–4 ml	Not recommended
Guinea pig	Lift the skin between the scapulae. Up to 10 ml	Quadriceps group. No more than 0.3 ml	Restrain with head lower than hindquarters. Insert needle in posterior quadrant to the right of the midline 2.5 cm in front of pubis at 45°	Ear veins, but these are very small and fragile. Apply local anaesthetic cream to prevent head shaking when needle is introduced
Hamster	Scruff. Up to 3–4 ml	Quadriceps group No more than 0.1 ml. Not recommended	Restrain with head downwards. Insert needle either side of midline in inguinal region, caudal to umbilicus which avoids the caecum, at angle of 45°. Aspirate before injecting	Not recommended
Mouse	Scruff. Up to 2 ml	Quadriceps group No more than 0.05 ml Not recommended	Insert needle into lower right quadrant to avoid caecum on the left at angle of 20°. Aspirate before injecting – should be a vacuum. Give 2–3 ml	Lateral tail veins Warm complete mouse or tail to dilate the veins; 0.2 ml can be injected
Rat	Scruff or flank Up to 5–10 ml	Quadriceps group. No more than 0.3 ml	Insert needle into lower right quadrant to avoid caecum on the left at angle of 20°. Aspirate before injecting – should be a vacuum. Give 10–15 ml	Lateral tail veins. Warm complete rat or the tail to dilate the veins; 0.5 ml can be injected

self-mutilation at the site. This route is not recommended in very small rodents, e.g. mice.

4. **Action:** When restraining an animal for an intraperitoneal injection, hold the animal with its head downwards.

   Rationale: This allows the intestines to fall cranially, making them less likely to be punctured by the needle. This is not recommended for debilitated or dyspnoeic animals – restrain them vertically.

Procedure: To collect a blood sample

1. **Action:** The sample required may be as small as a drop of blood or a larger volume.

   Rationale: A drop of blood can be used to make a smear to examine the red or white cells. Larger volumes may be used for biochemical analysis.

2. **Action:** In any species no more than 10% of the total blood volume may be taken at any one time.

   Rationale: For details of blood volumes see Table 12.5.

3. **Action:** Select the appropriate site for the species (Table 12.5).

   Rationale: In all the small rodents clipping a nail may yield a small volume of blood, but this is not recommended unless really necessary as it causes pain and distress.

4. **Action:** Prepare the site aseptically.

   Rationale: To prevent the introduction of infection.

5. **Action:** Select a suitably sized needle and a 1 ml syringe.

   Rationale: Choose a size that is as large as is practicable for the species. The needle must be able to enter the vein and must not be so small that it impedes the flow of blood and damages the red cells, leading to haemolysis of the sample.

6. **Action:** Ask an assistant to restrain the animal appropriately and to apply pressure to the selected vein – known as 'raising the vein'.

Table 12.5 Blood sampling in small rodents

Species	Adult blood volume (ml/kg)	Total adult blood volume (ml)	Maximum sample volume (ml)	Site for venepuncture	Comments
Rabbit	57–65	58.5–585	5–50	Cephalic, jugular	Large variation in size
Chinchilla	100	40–60	5	Cephalic, jugular	
Gerbil	66–78	8	0.5	Jugular, cardiac puncture	Cardiac puncture must only be performed under a general anaesthetic (GA). Risk of permanent heart damage
Guinea pig	69–75	50–60	5	Ear vein, cardiac puncture	Cardiac puncture must only be performed under a GA Risk of permanent heart damage
Hamster	78	8	0.5	Cardiac puncture	Cardiac puncture must only be performed under a GA Risk of permanent heart damage
Mouse	58.5	2	0.25	Lateral tail vein	Dilate the vein by warming the tail
Rat	54–70	30	3	Lateral tail vein, jugular	Dilate the vein by warming the tail

Rationale: When collecting blood it will be necessary for an assistant to restrain the animal to avoid injury to the animal and causing it distress. Pressure should be applied to the vein to dilate it, making it more obvious for venepuncture.

7. **Action:** Introduce the needle into the vein at an angle to the skin with the bevel uppermost. Once the needle is in the vein, advance it parallel to the skin.

    Rationale: The body of the needle now lies within the lumen of the vein.

8. **Action:** Either allow blood to drip from the hub of the needle into a collecting pot, or attach the syringe and gently pull back the plunger.

    Rationale: Larger volumes can be collected by using a syringe. The vein will collapse around the needle if you try to withdraw the blood too quickly. The blood sample may also be haemolysed as a result of red cell damage.

9. **Action:** Empty the syringe into an appropriate collecting pot and rotate gently.

    Rationale: If the sample is to be analysed the pot must contain an appropriate anticoagulant, e.g. EDTA, lithium heparin. Gentle rotation will mix the blood with the anticoagulant; over-enthusiastic mixing will damage the blood cells.

10. **Action:** Ask your assistant to apply pressure over the site of venepuncture while you slowly withdraw the needle from the vein.

    Rationale: To prevent haemorrhage into the surrounding tissues and encourage clotting.

11. **Action:** Dress the site appropriately.

    Rationale: To prevent infection and to prevent self-mutilation at the site.

GENERAL ANAESTHESIA

Procedure: Induction of anaesthesia

1. **Action:** Many patients to be anaesthetised are geriatric.

    Rationale: Small rodents have a short lifespan, which must be considered when undertaking anaesthesia.

2. **Action:** The patient may already be debilitated, in poor condition or obese before it is presented to the veterinary surgeon.

    Rationale: These all increase the risks of anaesthesia.

3. **Action:** The patient may be affected by a pre-existing illness.

    Rationale: Make a careful clinical examination to identify any risk factors, e.g. chronic respiratory disease.

4. **Action:** The patient may be anorexic and dehydrated. Always assess the level of dehydration and delay anaesthesia until it has been corrected.

    Rationale: Provide replacement fluid therapy by the appropriate route.

5. **Action:** There is no need for preoperative fasting in small rodents.

    Rationale: Fasting may lead to a fatal hypoglycaemia. Many species exhibit coprophagia so the stomach and intestines are rarely completely empty.

6. **Action:** Weigh the patient.

    Rationale: This enables accurate anaesthetic doses to be calculated and provides a baseline for clinical assessment during recovery, e.g. whether the animal is eating or drinking.

7. **Action:** Anaesthetic induction may be performed in an induction chamber or by mask using an inhalation anaesthetic agent such as 4% isoflurane.

    Rationale: Induction chambers are preferred, as masks are often too big for small rodents. Induction by inhalation is stressful to the patient and there is a risk of injury as the patient may struggle during the procedure. The advantage is rapid recovery, which reduces the risk of hypothermia.

8. **Action:** Induction can be performed using injectable agents (see Table 12.3).

    Rationale: These provide a smooth, stress-free induction but recovery rates may be longer depending on the choice of drug.

Procedure: Maintenance and monitoring of anaesthesia

1. **Action:** Once the patient is anaesthetised, maintain using an inhalation anaesthetic agent, e.g. 2% isoflurane delivered by mask, or supplement injectable drugs with oxygen by mask.

   Rationale: Small rodents are difficult to intubate. Inhalation anaesthesia delivered by mask may lead to fluctuations in depth.

2. **Action:** Monitor body temperature and keep the patient warm at all times by using a heat pad, or wrapping in 'bubblewrap' or a 'space blanket'.

   Rationale: Small rodents have a large surface area to bodyweight ratio, which means that they lose heat rapidly. Under anaesthesia the body's ability to regulate the core temperature is impaired, adding to the problem of hypothermia.

3. **Action:** Prepare the surgical site carefully.

   Rationale: Rodent skin is thin and can be easily nicked by clippers. Avoid the use of spirit to sterilise the site as this will further cool the patient.

4. **Action:** Apply ophthalmic ointment to the eyes.

   Rationale: Rodents have prominent eyes, which can be dried by the heat of the operating light and the lack of a blink reflex, leading to keratitis and corneal ulceration.

5. **Action:** Monitor the depth of anaesthesia using reflexes and monitoring equipment.

   Rationale: Each species varies in its response to anaesthesia and it is important to become familiar with these variations. The use of electronic monitoring equipment may be difficult as it is designed and calibrated for use in larger animals such as the cat and the dog.

6. **Action:** Monitor respiration.

   Rationale: Respiratory depression or arrest can be overcome by oxygen delivered by mask or by the use of respiratory stimulants such as doxapram.

Procedure: Postoperative care

1. **Action:** After the surgical procedure is complete, place the patient in a secure, warm cage in a quiet, warm and darkened room and cover with a towel, blanket, 'bubblewrap' or a 'space blanket' as appropriate.

   Rationale: Hypothermia during recovery can be fatal. Initially the temperature of the cage should be kept at 35 °C falling to 26–28 °C as the animal regains consciousness. Any noise or bright light will overstimulate a recovering animal.

2. **Action:** Observe the patient quietly and unobtrusively.

   Rationale: Rodents do not appreciate being touched or talked to as a dog would. Look at the animal from a distance and only interfere if it is really necessary.

3. **Action:** Monitor the core temperature.

   Rationale: To be aware of hypothermia before it becomes critical.

4. **Action:** Monitor respiration.

   Rationale: Respiratory depression or arrest may also occur during the recovery period.

5. **Action:** If the patient shows signs of pain, e.g. tooth grinding, vocalisation, aggression, hunched position, provide analgesia.

   Rationale: Any procedure that would cause pain in any other species should be considered to cause pain in the rodent and would warrant the use of analgesics. Correct use of analgesics, e.g. carprofen or buprenorphine, will do no harm.

6. **Action:** Continue to monitor the patient after it has regained consciousness.

   Rationale: Observe whether the animal is eating or drinking. Note the production of faeces and urine.

7. **Action:** Instruct the owner of the warning signs to watch out for when the patient is taken home.

   Rationale: The owner should monitor the patient for at least 24 hours after the surgical procedure.

Table 12.6   Ferrets – biological data

Parameter	Measurement	Comment
Lifespan	5–11 years	
Adult weight	Jill: 600–900 g Hob: 1–2 kg	Weight fluctuates with the time of year – heavier in the winter
Body temperature	38.8 °C (37.8–40 °C)	Rises to 40 °C when the ferret is excited
Respiratory rate	33–36 breaths/min	
Pulse rate	200–400 beats/min	
Oestrous cycle	Seasonally polyoestrous Induced ovulator	Season starts in March and continues until September. Female remains in oestrus until she is mated. Ovulation occurs 30–40 hours after mating
Age at puberty	Jill: 7–10 months Hob: 5–14 months	Puberty occurs in the spring after birth, so age varies
Gestation period	38–44 days	Young are altricial. May be eaten by the jill if disturbed
Litter size	2–6	
Weaning age	6–8 weeks	
Diet	Carnivorous	Require 30% protein; 30% fat. Can be fed on tinned or dry cat food

THE FERRET – *MUSTELA PUTORIUS FURO*

For biological data see Table 12.6.

HANDLING AND RESTRAINT

Procedure: To restrain a ferret

1. **Action:** Place one hand around the shoulders and the neck.

    Rationale: Ferrets vary in temperament – some are quite tame and relax when handled while others may be aggressive. The ferret has a well-muscled neck which must be held firmly.

2. **Action:** Lift the ferret clear of the cage and support the hind end with your other hand (Fig. 12.11).

    Rationale: Ferrets can be quite heavy and need to be supported. The body should not be stretched as this causes them to struggle. Some ferrets like to be dangled

by the front end while their knuckles are rubbed!

3. **Action:** Move your thumb so that it lies under the lower jaw. Place your forefinger around the neck, leaving the other fingers under the forelegs (Fig. 12.11).

    Rationale: This prevents the ferret from moving its head to bite you.

4. **Action:** Hold the ferret gently but firmly.

    Rationale: Ferrets are very agile creatures designed for going down holes and they can wriggle free if not held firmly.

5. **Action:** Tame ferrets may rest along the handler's forearm.

    Rationale: Gentle restraint is usually adequate for a physical examination. Handle ferrets that may be in pain with caution as they may bite.

6. **Action:** If a more secure hold is required, grasp a large portion of scruff and suspend the body.

    Rationale: The ferret has a large area of scruff. Suspending the animal induces relaxation.

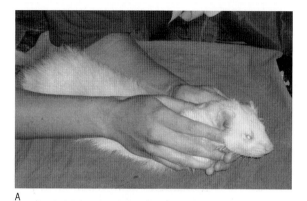

A

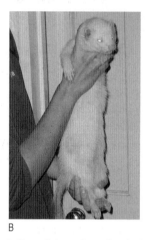

B

Figure 12.11 A, Restraining a ferret by placing it on a towel on a table. B, Lifting a ferret and supporting the hind end with the other hand.

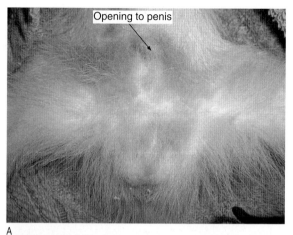

A

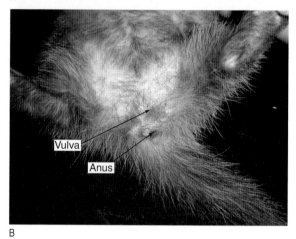

B

Figure 12.12 A, Male (hob) ferret. B, Female (jill) ferret.

Procedure: To sex a ferret

1. **Action:** Restrain the ferret by the scruff or by holding around the shoulders as previously described.

   Rationale: This position leaves one hand free to examine the ferret.

2. **Action:** Examine the genital area.

   Rationale: In the male (hob), the opening to the penis is situated on the ventral abdomen just caudal to the umbilicus, giving a long anogenital distance (Fig. 12.12A). Male ferrets have a pair of testes that enlarge during the breeding season. In the female (jill) the vulva lies close to the anus and becomes swollen when the female is in oestrus (Fig. 12.12B).

ADMINISTRATION OF MEDICINES

Procedure: To administer fluids or liquid medication

1. **Action:** Restrain the ferret by the neck and shoulders and support the hind end on a table or allow it to dangle.

   Rationale: In this position you have control of the head. Supporting the hind end on a table may encourage the ferret to struggle. This will depend on the weight, temperament and condition of the ferret.

2. **Action:** Using a small syringe filled with the liquid, place the nozzle into the side of the mouth.

Rationale: Avoid using large syringes, as they are difficult to manipulate while holding the patient. This procedure may be used to give liquid medication or replacement fluid.

3. **Action:** Slowly deposit the liquid towards the back of the tongue.

   Rationale: Do not give the medication too fast as the ferret lacks a cough reflex and may aspirate the liquid.

Procedure: Subcutaneous injection

1. **Action:** Grasp a large section of the scruff of the ferret.

   Rationale: Ferrets have a large scruff and this position both restrains the ferret and provides a suitable site for the injection.

2. **Action:** Select a sterile 23G needle and a syringe of an appropriate size, fill with the medication and introduce the needle into the scruff.

   Rationale: A maximum of 5–10 ml can be given at this site.

3. **Action:** Apply pressure to the plunger and inject the drug.

   Rationale: There is no need to draw back on the syringe in a subcutaneous injection as the risk of penetrating a blood capillary is low.

4. **Action:** Remove the needle from the scruff.

   Rationale: Absorption of the drug from this site takes about 30 minutes.

Procedure: Intramuscular injection

1. **Action:** Ask an assistant to restrain the ferret in sternal recumbency on the examination table, placing one hand behind the head and the other pinning the lumbar region to the table.

   Rationale: This restrains the body firmly, preventing struggling and possible injury to the ferret and to the handler.

2. **Action:** Locate either the quadriceps group on the cranial aspect of the thigh or the semimembranosus/semitendinosus group on the caudal aspect of the thigh.

   Rationale: These muscles are relatively large and can be easily located between the finger and thumb. Do not use the lumbar muscles as these are thin and penetration of a kidney is a risk if the ferret struggles.

3. **Action:** Select a sterile 23G needle and a syringe of an appropriate size, fill with the drug and introduce the needle into the muscle.

   Rationale: The muscle mass is small so only small volumes can be given by this route – maximum of 0.5 ml.

4. **Action:** Draw back on the syringe.

   Rationale: Muscle tissue has a good blood supply and there is a risk of penetrating a blood vessel.

5. **Action:** If no blood appears in the hub of the needle, gently inject the drug.

   Rationale: Do not inject too rapidly as the pressure may cause the drug to spurt out of the hub.

6. **Action:** Apply gentle pressure over the injection site and withdraw the needle.

   Rationale: This aids dispersion of the drug. The rate of absorption from this site is 15–20 minutes.

Procedure: Intraperitoneal injection

1. **Action:** Ask an assistant to restrain the ferret by holding it around the shoulders and chest with the thumb under the chin and the fingers under the forelegs as previously described (Fig. 12.11).

   Rationale: This restrains the body firmly, preventing struggling and possible injury to the ferret and to the handler.

2. **Action:** Use the other hand to support the hind end.

   Rationale: The hind end must be held firmly to prevent the ferret moving around and injuring itself during the procedure.

3. **Action:** In this position the assistant should rest the body against his or her chest, presenting the ventral abdomen towards you.

Rationale: The ventral abdomen is the site of the injection.

4. **Action:** Select a 21–23G needle and a small syringe and fill it with the drug to be administered.

   Rationale: This procedure may also be used to administer fluid therapy. A maximum of 8 ml can be given at any one time.

5. **Action:** Introduce the needle to one side of the midline and into one of the lower quadrants of the abdomen. The needle should be pointing cranially.

   Rationale: This will decrease the risk of entering one of the abdominal organs.

6. **Action:** Draw back on the syringe.

   Rationale: To check that you have not penetrated an organ. If urine, intestinal contents or blood appear in the syringe, reposition the needle.

7. **Action:** If the hub of the needle is empty, inject the drug into the peritoneal cavity and withdraw slowly.

Procedure: Intravenous injection

1. **Action:** Restrain the ferret in sternal recumbency by grasping a large section of the scruff and placing the legs firmly on a table.

   Rationale: If the ferret feels secure it will be less likely to try and escape.

2. **Action:** Extend one of the forelegs towards the veterinary surgeon with the elbow in the palm of your hand.

   Rationale: This is the same position as is used in the dog or the cat.

3. **Action:** Place the thumb of this hand across the crook of the ferret's elbow and apply gentle pressure.

   Rationale: This pressure will cause the cephalic vein to dilate and become more obvious.

4. **Action:** Gently rotate your thumb outwards.

   Rationale: This completes the dilation of the vein.

5. **Action:** The veterinary surgeon will clip a small area over the cephalic vein and prepare it aseptically.

Rationale: To prevent the introduction of infection into the vein.

6. **Action:** The veterinary surgeon will select a 23G needle and a small syringe filled with the drug to be administered and insert the needle through the skin and into the vein.

   Rationale: Use a small gauge needle as the vein has a narrow diameter.

7. **Action:** The veterinary surgeon will draw back on the syringe.

   Rationale: To check that the needle is in the lumen of the vein.

8. **Action:** If blood appears at the hub of the needle, inject the drug slowly into the vein.

   Rationale: Drugs given by the intravenous route are instantly absorbed.

9. **Action:** When the procedure is complete, you should apply gentle pressure over the injection site, while the veterinary surgeon slowly withdraws the needle.

   Rationale: This pressure prevents haemorrhage into the surrounding tissues.

10. **Action:** Dress the site appropriately.

    Rationale: To prevent infection and self-mutilation of the wound.

NB. The lateral saphenous vein running over the lateral aspect of the hock may also be used. If fluid therapy is to be given, place a catheter into the cephalic, saphenous or jugular vein. Blood samples can also be collected from these veins.

GENERAL ANAESTHESIA

Procedure: Induction of anaesthesia

1. **Action:** Starve the ferret for 6–12 hours before anaesthesia but allow free access to water.

   Rationale: Ferrets are able to vomit so it is important to ensure that the stomach is empty. Older ferrets should not be starved for longer than 4 hours, as there is a risk of an insulinoma precipitating a hypoglycaemic attack. Access to water should minimise dehydration.

2. **Action:** Weigh and examine the animal before giving the anaesthetic.

Rationale: This provides an accurate weight from which to calculate your dose and guarantees that there are no underlying problems that may affect the anaesthetic.

3. **Action:** Atropine given subcutaneously or intramuscularly can be used as a premedicant.

    Rationale: Atropine reduces salivation and gastrointestinal secretions and minimises cardiac arrhythmias.

4. **Action:** Induce anaesthesia by using an inhalation agent such as isoflurane given by mask or by placing the ferret in an induction chamber.

    Rationale: The response to inhalation anaesthesia is similar to that of the cat and the dog. Isoflurane provides rapid induction and recovery.

5. **Action:** Induction can also be achieved by using an appropriate injectable agent, e.g. ketamine, given by the correct route.

    Rationale: Do not use injectable agents in sick or debilitated patients.

6. **Action:** Once the ferret is anaesthetised, intubate with a 1.5–3.0 uncuffed endotracheal tube.

    Rationale: This is an easy procedure as the ferret is able to open its mouth wide for visualisation of the larynx. Ferrets do not seem to suffer from laryngospasm.

Procedure: Maintenance and monitoring of anaesthesia

1. **Action:** To maintain the anaesthetic use a non-rebreathing circuit delivering isoflurane.

    Rationale: The type of circuit must be appropriate to the size of the animal.

2. **Action:** During anaesthesia make sure that the ferret is kept warm by placing on a heat pad or wrapping in 'bubblewrap' or a 'space blanket'.

    Rationale: Hypothermia may be a problem as the ferret has a large surface area in relation to its bodyweight so it loses heat very rapidly.

3. **Action:** Monitor the hydration status of the patient.

Rationale: Give intravenous fluids to sick or debilitated animals during surgery.

4. **Action:** Monitor the depth of anaesthesia by assessing respiratory rate and depth, heart rate, jaw tone, withdrawal and palpebral reflexes.

    Rationale: Response to anaesthesia is similar to that of the cat.

5. **Action:** If the procedure is painful or likely to be painful, provide analgesia, e.g. buprenorphine or flunixin.

    Rationale: Pre-emptive analgesia is the most effective, i.e. that given before the onset of pain. The use of analgesics reduces the dose of anaesthetic required and increases the rate of recovery postoperatively.

Procedure: Postoperative care

1. **Action:** After the surgical procedure is complete, place the patient in a secure, warm cage in a quiet, warm and darkened room and cover with a towel, blanket, 'bubblewrap' or a 'space blanket' as appropriate.

    Rationale: Hypothermia during recovery can be fatal. Any noise or bright light will over-stimulate a recovering animal.

2. **Action:** Observe the patient quietly and unobtrusively.

    Rationale: Ferrets do not appreciate being touched or talked to. Look at the animal from a distance and only interfere if it is really necessary.

3. **Action:** Monitor the core temperature.

    Rationale: To be aware of hypothermia before it becomes critical.

4. **Action:** Monitor respiration.

    Rationale: Respiratory depression or arrest may also occur during the recovery period.

5. **Action:** If the patient shows signs of pain, e.g. vocalisation, aggression, hunched position, provide analgesia.

    Rationale: Any procedure that would cause pain in any other species should be considered to cause pain in the ferret and would warrant the use of analgesics. Correct use of analgesics, e.g. flunixin or buprenorphine, will do no harm.

6. **Action:** Continue to monitor the patient after it has regained consciousness.

    Rationale: Observe whether the animal is eating or drinking. Note the production of faeces and urine.

7. **Action:** Instruct the owner of the warning signs to watch out for when the patient is taken home.

    Rationale: The owner should monitor the patient for at least 24 hours after the surgical procedure.

CAGE AND AVIARY BIRDS

HANDLING AND RESTRAINT

Procedure: To capture and restrain a bird

1. **Action:** Make sure that all doors and windows are closed and that the extractor fans are turned off.

    Rationale: If the bird escapes from its cage, it will not be able to get out of the room or be injured in the extractor fan.

2. **Action:** Remove all movable objects from the cage, e.g. perches, feeding bowls, toys.

    Rationale: This makes capture quicker and easier and therefore less stressful for the bird.

3. **Action:** Turn the lights off or if possible dim them. Use a small hand torch covered in a red or blue filter for illumination.

    Rationale: Most common species of cage and aviary birds are active in daylight. A dim light will simulate night and induce quiet behaviour. Birds do not see well in red or blue light.

4. **Action:** Tip the cage on its side.

    Rationale: This enables you to approach the bird from the bottom of the cage and provides more room for manoeuvre.

5. **Action:** Approach the bird slowly.

    Rationale: This avoids causing air movement, which will startle the bird.

6. **Action:** Quickly grab the bird around its neck or close your hands around the wings and body (Fig. 12.13).

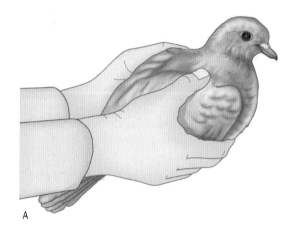

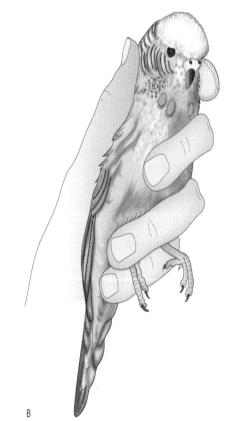

Figure 12.13 Handling small birds. A, A pigeon held in the hands. Note how the two hands encompass the wings and prevent the bird from flapping. B, A budgerigar in the hand. Note how the fingers form a 'net' around the bird: undue pressure must not be applied.

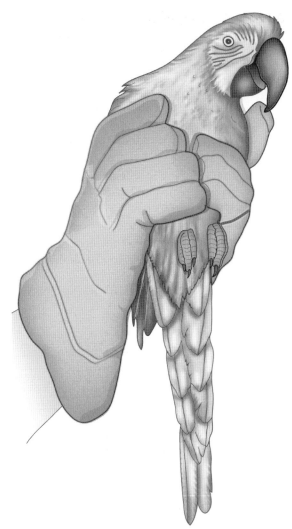

Figure 12.14   Handling large birds.

Rationale: These birds have vicious beaks. The use of gloves reduces your sense of touch when handling small birds.

Procedure: To capture a bird using the towel method

1. **Action:** Select a suitable towel.

    Rationale: A hand towel is about the right size.

2. **Action:** Drape the towel over one hand.

    Rationale: This disguises your hand.

3. **Action:** Advance your towelled hand towards the bird and trap it in a corner of the cage.

    Rationale: Trap the bird as quickly as possible. Making several attempts to catch the bird causes fear and distress and may damage the wings and plumage (Fig. 12.15).

4. **Action:** Catch hold of the bird by the neck.

    Rationale: The bird cannot bite you if the head and neck are controlled. There is very little chance of you strangling the bird because your hand is covered in the towel, which reduces the pressure you are able to apply.

5. **Action:** Taking your hand out of the towel, place your thumb and forefinger over the temporomandibular joint on either side of the head.

    Rationale: This prevents the bird from biting you.

    Rationale: It is important to catch the bird quickly, firmly and gently to avoid causing distress. Closing your hands around the body holds the wings closed and prevents them flapping and possibly breaking. This method can be used to catch small psittacine birds, e.g. budgerigars and lovebirds, and others such as canaries and finches.

7. **Action:** Wear clean, strong gloves if catching larger birds such as cockatoos and macaws (Fig. 12.14).

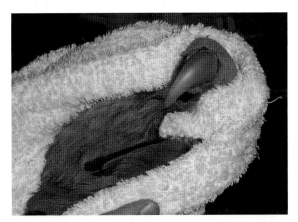

Figure 12.15   Restraining a bird in a towel.

6. **Action:** Take care with larger psittacines, e.g. macaws and cockatoos.

   Rationale: These species can deliver a nasty bite.

   NB. If you are bitten you can try:

- Blowing on the bird's face.
- Squeezing the top of the bird's head.
- As a last resort open the beak with whelping forceps – take care as you may damage the beak.

   Avoid pulling your finger out of the beak as this is curved and you may lose a chunk of flesh!

   It is often better if owners are not present during capture and treatment, as the more intelligent species will associate their experience with the owner.

Procedure: To clip the wings (Fig. 12.16)

This is performed in ducks, geese, chickens and guinea fowl to prevent them from escaping by flying over fences, but it may also be used in more exotic species such as large free-flying parrots.

1. **Action:** Ask an assistant to restrain the bird by placing the body under his or her arm and extending one of the wings.

   Rationale: Clipping is only done on one wing so that when the bird tries to fly it becomes aerodynamically unstable and is forced to land.

2. **Action:** Using sharp scissors, cut through the main part of the primary feathers (Fig. 12.16).

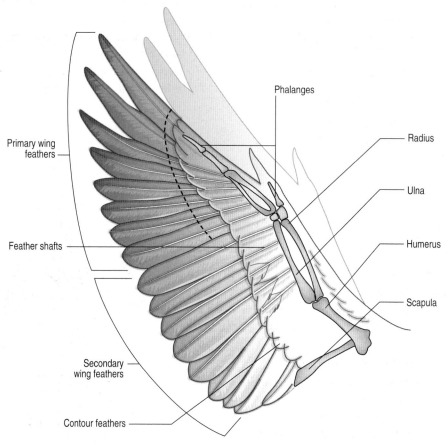

Figure 12.16 Where to clip the wings of a bird. Redrawn from Aspinall and O'Reilly (2004), Butterworth-Heinemann. Dotted line (---) indicates line of cutting.

Rationale: Cutting through the main part of the feathers does not cause any pain but do not cut into the shaft where it inserts into the skin as this will be painful and may cause bleeding. Wing clipping correctly done is no more painful than cutting hair.

Wing clipping must be repeated annually, usually after the late summer or autumn moult when the primary feathers will regrow. The procedure should not be confused with pinioning in which newly hatched birds have the bony tip of the wing removed. This is often done in captive bird collections and is not recommended unless it is really necessary as it causes permanent disfigurement.

ADMINISTRATION OF MEDICINES

Procedure: To administer fluid via a crop tube

1. **Action:** Select some form of metal catheter or crop tube and attach to the end of a syringe filled with warmed fluid.

    Rationale: Metal crop tubing catheters are available, but a Spreull needle can be used. Plastic and rubber tubing may be bitten through.

2. **Action:** Place the crop tube against the bird and mark the approximate area of the crop with a felt or ballpoint pen.

    Rationale: This measures the length of crop tube that must be inserted down the oesophagus to reach the crop. Ingesta travels from the mouth down the oesophagus into the crop, which is a diverticulum of the oesophagus, lying outside the body cavity in the ventral part of the neck (Fig. 12.17).

3. **Action:** Lubricate the crop tube.

    Rationale: To facilitate the passage of the crop tube down the oesophagus. KY jelly is a suitable lubricant.

4. **Action:** Restrain the bird by the neck.

    Rationale: You may need an assistant to hold the wings close to the body.

5. **Action:** Insert the crop tube on the left side at the junction of the upper and lower beak (Fig. 12.17). Extend the neck as you advance the tube.

Rationale: Extending the neck stretches the oesophagus, making placement easier.

6. **Action:** Direct the tube upwards towards the roof of the oropharynx and then down towards the oesophagus.

    Rationale: This ensures that the tube does not enter the glottis and trachea of the bird. Birds have a poor cough reflex and may asphyxiate or develop pneumonia if fluid enters the lungs or air sacs. Using a tube that is wider than the glottis may help to prevent incorrect positioning.

7. **Action:** Advance the crop tube down the right dorsal side of the oesophagus until it enters the crop.

    Rationale: The crop lies on the right side of the neck. The end of the tube can be palpated when it enters the crop. In fledglings, the tube can be seen passing down the oesophagus.

8. **Action:** Slowly administer an appropriate volume of fluid.

    Rationale: Slow infusion prevents the fluid refluxing up the oesophagus.

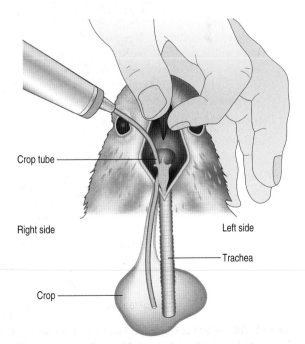

Figure 12.17   Crop tubing a parrot.

9. **Action:** Slowly withdraw the crop tube and observe the patient.

   Rationale: Slow withdrawal prevents damage to the tissues. It is important to observe the patient for adverse reactions.

Procedure: Intramuscular injection

1. **Action:** Restrain the bird so that it cannot struggle, holding its wings close to the body.

   Rationale: Small birds such as finches can be restrained and injected single-handedly, but be aware of the pressure that you are applying around the chest as this may restrict respiration. You may need an assistant to restrain larger species while you inject.

2. **Action:** Identify the pectoral muscles forming the breast of the bird. Select an area in the caudal part of the muscle group.

   Rationale: The pectoral muscles form the largest area of muscle in the bird.

3. **Action:** Using a sterile 21–23G needle and a syringe of an appropriate size, part the feathers and introduce the needle into the muscle.

   Rationale: Feathers should never be plucked unless it is essential. They will only grow back at the next moult and this may take months. Lack of feathers may affect insulation, flight and appearance depending on the site and the species.

4. **Action:** Draw back on the syringe.

   Rationale: To check that you have not penetrated a blood vessel.

5. **Action:** If no blood appears in the hub of the needle, inject the drug.

   Rationale: Drugs are rapidly absorbed from this site. Absorption from subcutaneous injections is slow so intramuscular injections are more commonly performed.

6. **Action:** Withdraw the needle and apply pressure over the site.

   Rationale: To prevent haemorrhage into the surrounding tissues. Birds bleed readily from injection sites.

Procedure: Intravenous injection

1. **Action:** Restrain the bird in the appropriate position to expose the vein. Ask an assistant to hold the head or hold the mask if the patient is anaesthetised.

   The following veins may be used for venepuncture:

   - Brachial (or basilic) vein – on the medial side of the elbow within the wing (Fig. 12.18).
   - Jugular vein – on either side of the neck. The right jugular vein is larger than the left (Fig. 12.19).
   - Medial metatarsal – on the caudal aspect of the leg. Easily visualised in larger species.

2. **Action:** Wet the feathers to enable the vein to be more easily visualised.

   Rationale: Avoid plucking the feathers to expose the vein. New feathers will not grow back until the next moult. Loss of feathers may affect the bird's ability to fly or to keep warm. In show birds it may affect their appearance.

3. **Action:** Prepare the site aseptically.

   Rationale: To prevent the introduction of infection.

4. **Action:** Raise the vein by applying pressure at the base of the right side of the neck (jugular), proximal to the injection site on the upper wing (brachial) or around the lower leg (median metatarsal).

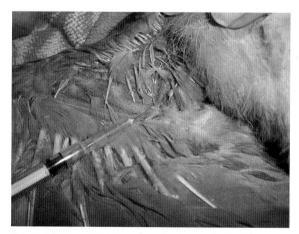

Figure 12.18 Method of using the brachial vein in the wing to give an intravenous injection.

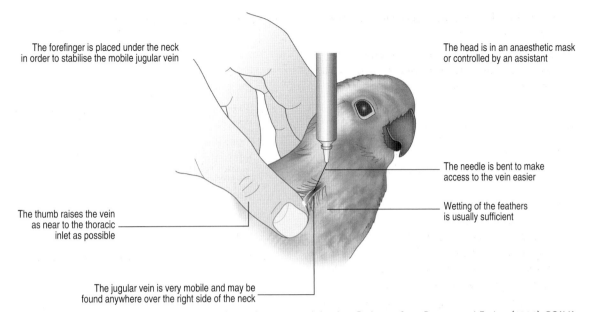

The forefinger is placed under the neck in order to stabilise the mobile jugular vein

The head is in an anaesthetic mask or controlled by an assistant

The needle is bent to make access to the vein easier

Wetting of the feathers is usually sufficient

The thumb raises the vein as near to the thoracic inlet as possible

The jugular vein is very mobile and may be found anywhere over the right side of the neck

Figure 12.19   Using the right jugular vein to give an intravenous injection. Redrawn from Beynon and Forbes (1996), BSAVA.

Rationale: Veins carry blood towards the heart. Pressure applied between the chosen site and the heart will prevent venous return and cause the vein to dilate or be 'raised'.

5. **Action:** Insert a small needle at an angle into the vein and draw back on the syringe. If using the jugular vein you may need to bend the needle (Fig. 12.19).

    Rationale: To check that the needle has penetrated the vein. Bending the needle facilitates access to the jugular vein.

6. **Action:** If blood appears in the hub of the needle, inject the drug slowly.

    Rationale: If the drug is injected too quickly, the pressure may cause it to spurt out of the hub of the needle.

7. **Action:** If the injection is to be repeated or if fluid is to be given intravenously, an indwelling 20G catheter can be inserted into the jugular vein.

    Rationale: This prevents damage to the vein by repeated injection.

8. **Action:** Suture or glue the catheter in place and cover with a light dressing.

Rationale: It is important that the catheter does not become dislodged by the bird's movement or by self-mutilation.

Procedure: Intraosseous injection

1. **Action:** Restrain the bird with a wing or leg extended.

    Rationale: The optimum site for an intraosseous injection is the distal radius or the proximal tibiotarsus. These bones have a medullary cavity from which fluid can be rapidly absorbed.

2. **Action:** Prepare the site aseptically.

    Rationale: To prevent the introduction of infection. Avoid plucking the feathers to expose the site. New feathers will not grow back until the next moult. Loss of feathers may affect the bird's ability to fly or to keep warm. In show birds it may affect their appearance.

3. **Action:** Select a 20–22G needle.

    Rationale: This size will be able to enter the medullary cavity.

4. **Action:** Introduce the needle into the bone and flush with heparinised saline.

Rationale: The saline will flush out any blood or bony tissue that accumulates as the needle is pushed through the cortex of the bone.

5. **Action:** Connect to a syringe or to a giving set and bag of fluid.

   Rationale: This procedure can be used to administer a bolus of fluid or for continuous infusion.

6. **Action:** Calculate the fluid requirement:

   Maintenance volume = 75 ml/kg bodyweight
   Fluid deficit of 4–10% = 40–100 ml/kg bodyweight replaced over 48 hours.

   Rationale: The majority of ill birds are dehydrated. Birds that are dehydrated and anorexic may suffer from a metabolic acidosis – correct this with lactated Ringer's (Hartmann's) solution.

7. **Action:** Set the fluid running at the required drip rate.

   Rationale: Volumes required are usually small.

8. **Action:** Cover the site with a bandage.

   Rationale: It is important that the needle or catheter is not dislodged by the bird's movement or by self-mutilation.

Procedure: To collect a blood sample

1. **Action:** Restrain the bird on its back on a soft surface with one wing extended – if you are right handed use the right wing.

   Rationale: The site for collecting a reasonable sample of blood is the brachial vein, which lies on the ventral aspect of the wing, distal to the elbow. A small sample can be collected by clipping a toenail. Small samples can be used for sexing the bird, but the cells are often distorted which may affect haematological studies.

2. **Action:** Wet the feathers over the site.

   Rationale: This enables you to see the vein more clearly. Avoid plucking the feathers to expose the vein. New feathers will not grow back until the next moult. Loss of feathers may affect the bird's ability to fly or to keep warm. In show birds it may affect their appearance.

3. **Action:** Prepare the site aseptically.

Rationale: To prevent the introduction of infection.

4. **Action:** Place the first and second finger of the left hand on the mid-distal humerus with the palm on the carpus of the wing.

   Rationale: This keeps the wing extended and restrained.

5. **Action:** Raise the vein with the thumb of your left hand.

   Rationale: Your right hand is free for sample collection.

6. **Action:** Select a 23–27G needle and a 1 ml syringe.

   Rationale: The needle must be able to enter the vein but must not be so small that it impedes the flow of blood and damages the red cells, leading to haemolysis of the sample.

7. **Action:** Flush the needle and syringe with dilute heparin (1:100) before use.

   Rationale: This prevents the blood from clotting if the sample collection is slow.

8. **Action:** Introduce the needle into the vein and draw back on the syringe.

   Rationale: If blood appears at the hub of the needle, the needle is correctly positioned in the vein.

9. **Action:** Collect the blood sample.

10. **Action:** Withdraw the needle applying gentle pressure over the site for 2–3 minutes as you do so.

    Rationale: This prevents haematoma formation.

NB. The jugular vein can also be used for blood sampling.

GENERAL ANAESTHESIA

Procedure: Induction of anaesthesia

1. **Action:** Do not starve birds that are less than 120 g in weight. Large psittacines may be starved for 1–2 hours. Fruit-eaters and waterfowl should be starved for 4–10 hours.

Rationale: Starvation in small birds may cause a fatal hypoglycaemia and increase the anaesthetic risk. Grain-eaters, e.g. psittacines, seldom regurgitate.

2. **Action:** Make sure that all equipment is ready before you start the procedure.

   Rationale: The procedure should run as smoothly and as quickly as possible to reduce stress to the patient and thus reduce anaesthetic risk.

3. **Action:** Handle the bird as little as possible.

   Rationale: To reduce stress.

4. **Action:** Induce anaesthesia by using a mask and an inhalation agent, e.g. isoflurane, or by using an injectable agent, e.g. ketamine.

   Rationale: For dose rates see Table 12.7.

5. **Action:** Intubate the bird. This should be done for all but very short procedures.

   Rationale: Use an uncuffed tube as birds have complete tracheal rings that may be ruptured by inflation of the cuff. Intubation protects the airway and allows intermittent positive pressure ventilation to be performed if necessary. Psittacines have large fleshy tongues that obscure the view of the glottis, making intubation difficult – use a tongue depressor.

6. **Action:** Attach to an appropriate type of anaesthetic circuit.

   Rationale: The circuit should provide low resistance, particularly for small birds.

Procedure: Maintenance and monitoring of anaesthesia

1. **Action:** Maintain anaesthesia using an inhalation agent, e.g. 2% isoflurane (Table 12.7).

   Rationale: If an injectable agent has been used, supplement with oxygen via a mask or endotracheal tube.

2. **Action:** Flow rate through the circuit should be three times the minute volume.

   Rationale: Flow rate is approximately 3 ml/g bodyweight and should not be less than 0.75 l/min. A high flow rate prevents hypercapnia.

3. **Action:** At all times ensure that the patient is warm. Use a heat pad or wrap in 'bubblewrap' or a 'space blanket'.

   Rationale: Birds have a high core temperature of 40–44 °C due to a high metabolic rate.

4. **Action:** Assess the need for fluid therapy. If necessary give intravenously or by intraosseous injection as previously described.

Table 12.7 Anaesthetic agents for use in birds

Anaesthetic agent	Dose rate (mg/kg)	Comments
Isoflurane	Induction 4%; maintenance 2%	Swift induction, rapid recovery
Halothane	Induction 1% increase to 3%, maintain at 1.5–3%	If induction is too rapid, cardiac failure may occur
Ketamine/diazepam or midazolam	Ketamine – 25; diazepam or midazolam – 2.5 IM	20–30 min of deep sedation
Ketamine/medetomidine	Raptors 3–5 ketamine/50–100 medetomidine IM Psittacines 3–7 ketamine/75–150 medetomidine IM	Reversed by atipamezole 250–380 µg/kg IM
Propofol	3–5 IV	Wears off very quickly. Care with transfer to gaseous anaesthetic

Source: Hotston-Moore (1999).

Rationale: Ill birds are often dehydrated and provision of fluid will increase the chances of recovery.

5. **Action:** Monitor the depth of anaesthesia using appropriate reflexes.

   Rationale: Toe, cere and wing reflexes are lost on a medium plane, palpebral reflex is lost on a deeper plane and the corneal reflex is lost when the bird is very deeply anaesthetised.

6. **Action:** Monitor respiration.

   Rationale: The rate and depth of respiration decrease as anaesthesia deepens. The rate should not fall below half the normal resting rate. The respiratory pattern should remain stable.

7. **Action:** Monitor the heart rate.

   Rationale: Use a cardiac monitor or an oesophageal stethoscope. Heart rate is a good indicator of pain – it increases when the bird feels pain.

8. **Action:** Place ECG leads over the distal tarsometatarsus and carpal joints of each wing.

   Rationale: To monitor the rate and pattern of the heart.

Procedure: Postoperative care

1. **Action:** After the surgical procedure is complete, remove the endotracheal tube and wrap the bird in a towel.

   Rationale: This keeps the bird warm and prevents the wings from flapping during recovery, causing possible damage. If isoflurane is used, the bird can be allowed to recover slowly in your hands before being placed in its cage.

2. **Action:** Place the bird into its own cage to recover in a warm, quiet, darkened room.

   Rationale: Remove all portable object such as toys, feeding bowls and perches to facilitate handling of the bird if necessary. If the bird is placed in a normal recovery cage, it will have to be caught to place it back into its own cage – this increases the stress to the bird.

3. **Action:** Keep the bird under discreet observation.

Rationale: Many problems can develop during the recovery period. Birds do not need to be talked to or touched.

4. **Action:** Continue to monitor the bird's progress for a few days after the operation.

   Rationale: It is important that the bird begins to eat and drink. Small birds cannot survive for long without a source of energy.

5. **Action:** If necessary feed the bird using a crop tube as previously described.

   Rationale: To prevent the onset of dehydration and hypoglycaemia.

REPTILES

Zoonoses   All species should be handled with care as many reptiles are known to carry zoonotic diseases. *Salmonella* is the most common disease. It is difficult to determine whether or not an individual is infected as the bacteria may be shed intermittently in the faeces and bacterial culture may not detect all species. *Salmonella* is spread by ingestion of the faeces, so although careful handling is not a risk, you must wash your hands after touching any reptile species.

As a general rule, the species of reptile most commonly kept as pets can be handled safely. However, precautions should be taken when handling venomous species. Large constrictors such as pythons should not be handled on your own, as you might need assistance if they wind themselves around your arm or your neck.

Snakes

Procedure: To restrain a snake

1. **Action:** Ask the owner if the snake is used to being handled.

   Rationale: This gives an indication of the response the snake may make to being handled and examined.

2. **Action:** A snake should be transported in a soft bag, which is closed securely by doubling over the top and then tying it.

Rationale: Bumping against the hard surfaces of a cage or box can easily damage a snake. Snakes are very good at pushing through loosely tied knots. A pillowcase makes a good snake bag.

3. **Action:** Avoid wearing gloves when handling snakes.

    Rationale: Wearing gloves makes it difficult to appreciate the pressure you are putting on the snake and may result in damage to the animal.

4. **Action:** Open the bag or vivarium and look inside.

    Rationale: This helps you to locate the position of the snake's head.

5. **Action:** If the snake is tame, pick it up gently around the body and lift it from the bag or the vivarium. Snakes over 2 metres in length must be lifted by two people.

    Rationale: Handle gently but positively. Snakes bruise easily but as they have a slow metabolism, the injury may not show for several weeks. A snake may die from severe bruising.

6. **Action:** Avoid making sudden movements or waving your hand in front of the snake.

    Rationale: This may cause the snake to strike.

7. **Action:** As soon as possible, support the body and allow the snake to move around.

    Rationale: Never suspend the body by the head – snakes have a single occipital condyle and the neck is easily broken. Use minimal restraint. Snakes do not like being held tightly or being stretched out.

8. **Action:** If further restraint is needed, place a finger and thumb on either side of the head and one finger on the top of the head (Fig. 12.20). Support the body with your other hand.

    Rationale: In this position the snake is prevented from biting.

9. **Action:** To handle more aggressive or vicious snakes use a towel. Move the towel towards the snake and catch the snake behind the head with your towel-covered hand.

    Rationale: If the snake strikes it will hit the towel. Snake hooks can be used.

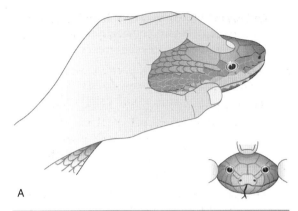

A

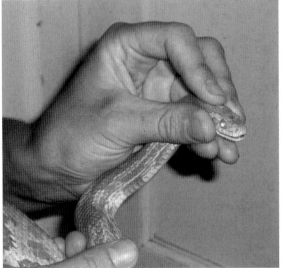

B

Figure 12.20   Restraining the head of a snake.

Procedure: To administer fluids or liquid medication

1. **Action:** Select and lubricate a 5–8F catheter.

    Rationale: The type used for dogs and cats is appropriate. Lubrication aids the introduction of the catheter.

2. **Action:** Lay the catheter along the outside of the snake. Mark the approximate position of the stomach on the catheter using a ballpoint pen.

    Rationale: The stomach lies approximately halfway down the length of the snake.

3. **Action:** Select an appropriate size of syringe and fill with fluid.

Rationale: It is good practice to have all equipment ready before you begin to handle the snake as this reduces the stress caused by the procedure.

4. **Action:** With the snake on a table restrain the head and open the mouth using a blunt metal spatula.

    Rationale: Snakes' teeth are very sharp and may point backwards in some species. They are also very dirty and any bite may become infected. Take steps to avoid being bitten.

5. **Action:** Use a mouth gag if necessary.

    Rationale: Most snakes will open their mouths quite easily when gentle pressure is applied. Make a gag by folding a small piece of radiographic film and cutting a hole in the centre. The catheter is passed through the hole.

6. **Action:** Support the weight of the body on the table or ask an assistant to help you.

    Rationale: Never suspend the body by the head – snakes have a single occipital condyle and the neck is easily broken.

7. **Action:** Slowly insert the catheter into the back of the mouth and down the oesophagus.

    Rationale: The glottis, leading to the trachea and lungs, sits forward in the oral cavity to avoid asphyxiation when the snake is swallowing prey. It is easy to see and there is little risk of the catheter entering it.

8. **Action:** Insert the catheter to the level of the stomach.

    Rationale: The ballpoint pen mark will lie at the level of the mouth.

9. **Action:** Introduce the fluid in the syringe slowly.

    Rationale: If you introduce the fluid too quickly the pressure applied may cause the fluid to spurt out of the junction with the syringe.

10. **Action:** Gently withdraw the catheter and observe the snake.

    Rationale: To check that there are no adverse effects.

Procedure: Intravenous injection or blood sampling

1. **Action:** Restrain the snake appropriately.

    Rationale: The site for intravenous injection is the ventral venous sinus in the midline of the ventral tail (Fig. 12.21). The jugular vein can be used but may require a surgical cut-down. The palatine veins can be seen when the mouth is open, but the snake must be anaesthetised or sedated if these are used.

2. **Action:** Prepare the site aseptically using povidone-iodine or 70% ethanol.

    Rationale: To prevent the introduction of infection.

3. **Action:** Select a small needle and syringe.

    Rationale: The needle must be small enough to enter the vein.

4. **Action:** Insert the needle between the paired caudal scales distal to the cloaca. Angle the needle at right angles to the tail. Draw back on the syringe.

    Rationale: In the male, care must be taken to avoid damaging the hemipenes, which lie here. If blood appears in the hub of the needle, the needle is correctly positioned in the vein.

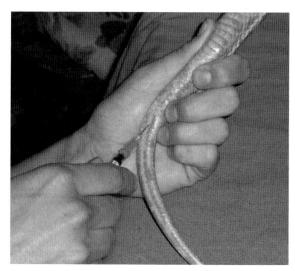

Figure 12.21 Method of using the ventral venous sinus in the tail to give an intravenous injection.

5. **Action:** Collect the sample into a lithium heparin tube.

    Rationale: EDTA lyses the cells.

6. **Action:** A drop of blood can be used to make a blood smear.

    Rationale: This is useful for haematology.

7. **Action:** If injecting intravenously, slowly give the drug into the vein.

8. **Action:** Withdraw the needle.

NB. The total volume of blood is approximately 5–8% of bodyweight. This is about 70 ml/kg and of this 10% can be collected in one withdrawal.

Sites for the administration of parenteral drugs:
- Subcutaneous – under the loose skin over the ribs.
- Intramuscular – into the intercostal muscles.

Injections may be given into the tail, but snakes have a renal portal venous system in which blood flows from the hind end of the body to the kidneys before returning to the heart. Any drug injected into the hind end may be eliminated by the kidneys without being absorbed. Nephrotoxic drugs must not be injected into the hind end.

Chelonians

These are the shelled reptiles, e.g. tortoises and terrapins.

Procedure: To restrain a tortoise or terrapin

1. **Action:** Consider the species you are to handle.

    Rationale: Most tortoises are non-aggressive and used to being handled. They may withdraw into their shells. Some species of terrapin, and particularly the snapping turtle, are aggressive and may bite rather than withdraw into their shells.

2. **Action:** Pick a tortoise up by placing both hands around the middle of the shell or carapace and support the whole body.

    Rationale: Some individuals can be heavy. Watch out for the hind legs, which may push against your hands and push the body out of your grip.

3. **Action:** If handling a terrapin, wear plastic gloves.

    Rationale: Terrapins are known to carry *Salmonella* and you should take precautions to protect yourself from this zoonosis. This is important if you have to remove the animal from water.

4. **Action:** Pick a terrapin up by placing your hands at the rear of the carapace just cranial to the hind legs. To achieve a better grip, place your fingers into the inguinal area.

    Rationale: This will prevent the terrapin from biting your fingers. If the terrapin has been in water it will be slippery. Some terrapins also have long claws, which can scratch.

5. **Action:** More aggressive individuals, e.g. snapping turtle, can be restrained in a towel while you move your hands towards the back of the carapace.

    Rationale: The towel will cover the head, preventing the animal from biting.

6. **Action:** Soft-shelled terrapins should be handled wearing leather gloves.

    Rationale: To prevent damage to the carapace and to prevent you being bitten.

7. **Action:** In any species of chelonian, extend the head by placing your finger and thumb behind the occipital condyle and pulling slowly against the action of the retractor muscles of the neck.

    Rationale: Gentle but firm and constant pressure must be applied. The muscles will become tired and relax. Holding a tortoise with its forelegs against the shell and its body downwards may induce the head to come out far enough for you to grasp it.

8. **Action:** Forcing the hind legs into the inguinal region may bring the head and forelegs out.

    Rationale: The use of padded forceps may help extraction of the head but be careful not to cause any damage.

Procedure: To administer fluids or liquid medication

1. **Action:** Select an appropriate type of stomach tube and lubricate it.

   Rationale: Tubes designed for use in chelonians can be obtained, but small dog catheters can be used.

2. **Action:** Calculate the required dose of fluid or medication and fill a syringe of an appropriate size.

   Rationale: It is good practice to have all equipment ready before you begin to handle the tortoise as this reduces the stress caused by the procedure.

3. **Action:** Holding the tortoise on its back for a short time, place the tube along the length of the plastron and mark the approximate position of the stomach on the tube using a ballpoint pen (Fig. 12.22).

   Rationale: The stomach lies under the abdominal scute of the plastron. Lay the tube from the gular notch to the caudal border of the abdominal scute (Fig.12.22).

4. **Action:** Restrain the tortoise so that it is resting on its caudal scutes and extend the head and neck.

   Rationale: If the patient withdraws into its shell you may need to ask for assistance.

5. **Action:** Pull the mandible down with one finger and insert your index finger into the commissure of the lips.

   Rationale: Your index finger acts as a gag. Tortoises have a beak but no teeth and placing your finger at the angle of the lips is unlikely to be painful.

6. **Action:** Slide the lubricated tube towards the back of the mouth, down the oesophagus and into the stomach (Fig. 12.23).

   Rationale: The glottis is easy to see and to avoid. You will feel the tube pass through the cardiac sphincter into the stomach. The ballpoint pen mark will lie at the mouth.

7. **Action:** Introduce the fluid in the syringe slowly.

   Rationale: If you introduce the fluid too quickly the pressure applied may cause the fluid to spurt out of the junction with the syringe.

8. **Action:** Gently withdraw the catheter and observe the patient.

   Rationale: To check that there are no adverse effects.

NB. This method is suitable for all types of chelonian.

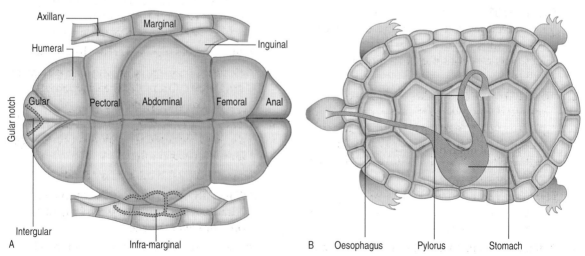

Figure 12.22 The position of the stomach in relation to the scutes of the plastron (A) and the carapace (B) of a tortoise.

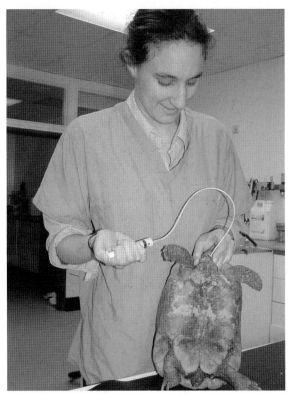

Figure 12.23 Administration of anthelmintics to a tortoise via a stomach tube.

Procedure: Intravenous injection or blood sampling

1. **Action:** Restrain the tortoise appropriately. You may need an assistant to hold the body.

   Rationale: The sites most commonly used in chelonians are the jugular and the dorsal venous sinus. If an assistant is not available, you can hold the shell between your knees.

2. **Action:** To use the jugular vein, extend the head and extend the neck fully by placing your finger and thumb behind the occipital condyle and pulling slowly against the action of the retractor muscles of the neck.

   Rationale: The jugular vein runs from the level of the eardrum to the base of the neck and may be visible (Fig. 12.24).

3. **Action:** Ask your assistant to raise the vein by applying pressure at the base of the neck.

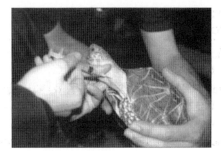

Figure 12.24 Intravenous injection in a tortoise using the jugular vein.

   Rationale: The jugular vein carries blood from the head and neck towards the heart.

4. **Action:** Insert a small needle parallel to the neck pointing towards the body (Fig. 12.24) and draw back on the syringe.

   Rationale: If blood appears in the hub of the needle, the needle is correctly placed.

5. **Action:** To use the dorsal venous sinus extend the tail fully.

   Rationale: The vein is located in the dorsal midline of the tail. This is the site of choice in the Mediterranean tortoise.

6. **Action:** Insert a small needle in the exact midline at an angle of 45° and advance the needle until it touches the bone. Aspirate the syringe and withdraw the needle slightly until blood appears in the hub of the needle.

   Rationale: At first the needle goes through the sinus but as you withdraw the needle, it re-enters the sinus and blood is aspirated.

7. **Action:** At both sites inject the drug slowly.

   Rationale: If you apply too much pressure, the drug may spurt out of the junction between the needle and syringe.

8. **Action:** If blood is to be collected, withdraw the required amount of blood and place in a lithium heparin tube.

   Rationale: EDTA lyses the blood cells.

9. **Action:** After the procedure is complete, withdraw the needle and apply gentle pressure over the site.

   Rationale: To prevent the formation of a haematoma.

NB. The total volume of blood is approx. 5–8% of bodyweight. This is about 70 ml/kg and of this 10% can be collected in one withdrawal.

Sites for the administration of parenteral drugs:
- Subcutaneous – use the loose skin around the neck.
- Intramuscular – triceps muscle in the forelimb; pectoral muscles at the angle of the forelimb and neck; muscles of the hindlimb.

Injections may be given into the hindlimb, but chelonians have a renal portal venous system in which blood flows from the hindlimbs to the kidneys before returning to the heart. Any drug injected into the hindlimbs and tail may be eliminated by the kidneys without being absorbed. Nephrotoxic drugs must not be injected into the hindlimb.

Lizards

Procedure: To restrain a lizard

1. **Action:** Identify the species of lizard and ask the owner whether it is used to being handled.

    Rationale: There are many species of lizard commonly kept as pets. They vary in size and in nature. Most are amenable to handling but some, notably the Tokay gecko, are aggressive. There are only two venomous lizards – *Heloderma suspectum* (the gila monster) and *Heloderma horridum* (the beaded lizard) – but neither is particularly aggressive.

2. **Action:** Place your hand around the shoulders and lift the animal clear of the cage.

    Rationale: Never lift a lizard by the tail. Many species are able to shed their tails as a means of defence – a process known as autotomy. The tail will regrow but it never looks the same again.

3. **Action:** Restrain the lizard by placing one hand around the pectoral girdle and the other around the pelvic girdle and hind legs. Hold the hind legs against the tail.

    Rationale: In this position the lizard is unable to struggle or to thrash its tail around.

4. **Action:** You may need to wear gloves when handling larger lizards.

    Rationale: Some species may bite or scratch, lash out with their tails or graze you with their scales.

5. **Action:** More aggressive specimens can be induced to lie still by placing a towel over the head.

    Rationale: If the head is in the dark, the lizard will remain motionless so that the body can be examined.

Procedure: To administer fluids or liquid medication

1. **Action:** Select a 5–8F catheter and lubricate it.

    Rationale: The type used for dogs and cats is appropriate. Lubrication aids the introduction of the catheter.

2. **Action:** Lay the catheter along the outside of the lizard. Mark the approximate position of the stomach on the catheter using a ballpoint pen.

    Rationale: The stomach lies at a point just caudal to the caudal border of the ribs.

3. **Action:** Select an appropriate size of syringe and fill with fluid.

    Rationale: It is good practice to have all equipment ready before you begin to handle the lizard as this reduces the stress caused by the procedure.

4. **Action:** With the lizard on a table restrain the body and open the mouth using a blunt metal spatula.

    Rationale: Take steps to avoid being bitten.

5. **Action:** Use a mouth gag if necessary.

    Rationale: Most lizards will open their mouths quite easily when gentle pressure is applied. Make a gag by folding a small piece of radiographic film and cutting a hole in the centre. The catheter is passed through the hole.

6. **Action:** Slowly insert the catheter into the back of the mouth and down the oesophagus.

    Rationale: The glottis, leading to the trachea and lungs, sits forward in the oral cavity.

It is easy to see and there is little risk of the catheter entering it.

7. **Action:** Insert the catheter to the level of the stomach.

    Rationale: The ballpoint pen mark will lie at the level of the mouth.

8. **Action:** Introduce the fluid in the syringe slowly.

    Rationale: If you introduce the fluid too quickly, the pressure applied may cause the fluid to spurt out of the junction with the syringe.

9. **Action:** Gently withdraw the catheter and observe the lizard.

    Rationale: To check that there are no adverse effects.

Procedure: Intravenous injection or blood sampling

1. **Action:** Restrain the lizard appropriately.

    Rationale: The site most commonly used in large lizards is the ventral venous sinus lying in the midline of the ventral surface of the tail. In smaller species a toe nail can be clipped to provide enough blood to fill a capillary tube.

2. **Action:** Prepare the site aseptically using povidone-iodine or 70% ethanol.

    Rationale: To prevent the introduction of infection.

3. **Action:** Select a small needle and syringe.

    Rationale: The needle must be small enough to enter the vein.

4. **Action:** Introduce the needle in the exact midline of the ventral surface of the tail distal to the vent, at an angle of 45°. Advance the needle until you touch bone.

    Rationale: The needle will go through the sinus and touch the underlying vertebra.

5. **Action:** Slowly withdraw the needle and aspirate the syringe at the same time until blood appears in the hub of the needle.

    Rationale: As you pull the needle back it will re-enter the sinus and blood will be aspirated into the syringe.

6. **Action:** Collect the sample into a lithium heparin tube.

    Rationale: EDTA lyses the cells.

7. **Action:** A drop of blood can be used to make a blood smear.

    Rationale: This is useful for haematology.

8. **Action:** If giving medication, slowly introduce the drug into the vein.

9. **Action:** Withdraw the needle.

NB. The total volume of blood is approx. 5–8% of bodyweight. This is about 70 ml/kg and of this 10% can be collected in one withdrawal.

Sites for the administration of parenteral drugs:
- Subcutaneous – under the loose skin of the ribs.
- Intramuscular – into the caudal muscles of the forelimb, the hindlimb (Fig. 12.25) or into the tail but care must be taken in those species that show autotomy as they may slough their tails.

Injections may be given into the hindlimb, but lizards have a renal portal venous system in which blood flows from the hindlimbs and tail to the kidneys before returning to the heart. Any drug injected into the hindlimbs may be eliminated by the kidneys without being absorbed. Nephrotoxic drugs must not be injected into the hindlimb.

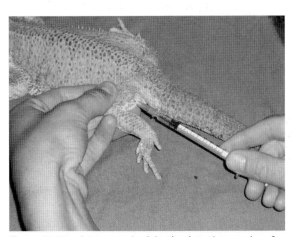

Figure 12.25   Intramuscular injection into the muscles of the hindlimb of a lizard.

GENERAL ANAESTHESIA

(General points to be considered for all species of reptile.)

Procedure: Induction of anaesthesia

1. **Action:** Have all anaesthetic equipment ready, organise assistance if required and be familiar with all the procedures involved before you get the patient from the cage.

   Rationale: This will minimise the stress caused to the patient. Reptiles are not as used to being handled as dogs and cats and this increase in stress will increase the risk of anaesthesia.

2. **Action:** Small species of reptile do not need to be starved before an anaesthetic. Starve larger lizards and chelonians for 18 hours and large snakes for 72–96 hours. Avoid feeding live insects just before an anaesthetic.

   Rationale: The presence of live insects in the stomach may cause a problem. Vomiting does not occur in reptiles.

3. **Action:** Weigh the animal accurately.

   Rationale: This enables you to calculate an accurate dose of anaesthetic and the replacement fluid requirement.

4. **Action:** Sedatives may be used as premedication, but the use of atropine to reduce the production of saliva is unnecessary.

   Rationale: The use of sedatives will facilitate handling and reduce the stress caused to the patient. Salivary secretions do not cause a problem in reptiles.

5. **Action:** Induce anaesthesia using injectable agents administered by the appropriate method.

   Rationale: For drugs and dose rates see Table 12.8.

6. **Action:** Induce anaesthesia by inhalational agents using a mask for large lizards and for snakes, but not for chelonians.

   Rationale: The use of a mask may be difficult in chelonians. For drugs and dose rates see Table 12.8.

7. **Action:** Induction chambers can be used to deliver inhalational agents for most reptiles except terrapins.

   Rationale: Terrapins are aquatic chelonians and are able to hold their breath and revert to anaerobic metabolism for up to 27 hours. This delays the uptake and activity of the anaesthetic agent.

8. **Action:** Reptiles can be intubated relatively easily using an uncuffed tube. The glottis is easily visualised in snakes but the large fleshy tongue of some lizards and chelonians may obscure the view.

   Rationale: Reptiles have complete tracheal rings, which may be ruptured by inflation of a cuff. Use a gag to keep the mouth open. Dog and cat intravenous catheters can be used to intubate small reptiles.

9. **Action:** Dehydration may increase the risks of anaesthesia.

   Rationale: Correct fluid imbalance before anaesthesia.

10. **Action:** Reptiles should be kept at their preferred body temperature throughout the anaesthetic and during the recovery period.

    Rationale: All reptiles have their own preferred body temperature (PBT) at which the metabolic rate is at its most efficient. If the PBT is too low the rate of recovery and healing will be reduced.

Procedure: Maintenance and monitoring of anaesthesia

1. **Action:** Closed anaesthetic circuits are commonly used in reptile anaesthesia.

   Rationale: The respiratory rate required to maintain an adequate level of anaesthesia is often greater than the rate shown by a conscious animal. A closed circuit will keep gas concentration higher than a semi-closed circuit.

2. **Action:** Intermittent positive pressure ventilation (IPPV) may be used as a continuous means of ventilation during the anaesthetic.

Table 12.8   Anaesthetic agents for use in reptiles

Anaesthetic agent	Dose rate (mg/kg)	Site
Alfaxalone/alfadolone (Saffan)	6–9 9–15	IV IM
Ketamine	20–100 (larger dose to smaller animals)	SC, IM, IP
Propofol	Tortoises 14 Lizards 10 Snakes 10	IV (agent of choice for induction)
Halothane	1–4%	Inhalation
Isoflurane	1–6%	Inhalation (agent of choice for maintenance)

Source: Hotston-Moore (1999).

Rationale: Reptiles have a low respiratory rate and apnoea is common. Administer at the rate of 2 breaths/min.

3. **Action:** Monitor the respiratory rate by observation.

    Rationale: Observation of the respiratory rate may be difficult as the rate is often slow.

4. **Action:** The corneal and palpebral reflexes may be used to monitor the depth of anaesthesia except in the snake.

    Rationale: Snakes have no eyelids and the cornea is covered in a transparent skin scale known as a spectacle. The palpebral reflex is lost when the surgical plane of anaesthesia is reached.

5. **Action:** The tongue withdrawal reflex is a useful means of monitoring the depth of anaesthesia in snakes and in some lizards.

    Rationale: Pull out the tongue gently and note whether it flicks or is withdrawn. This is lost when the surgical plane of anaesthesia is reached.

6. **Action:** Monitor jaw tone, pedal and tail reflexes.

    Rationale: The pedal and tail reflexes are lost when the surgical plane of anaesthesia is reached.

7. **Action:** Monitor the heart rate by oesophageal stethoscope, Doppler ultrasound or electrocardiography.

Rationale: During deep anaesthesia the heart rate slows and the pupils become fixed and dilated.

Procedure: Postoperative care

1. **Action:** If a reptile has been induced with an injectable anaesthetic agent it may take hours to regain complete consciousness.

    Rationale: Reptiles have a slow metabolic rate so anaesthetic drugs are broken down slowly and recovery will be slow.

2. **Action:** Continue to give oxygen by IPPV until the reptile has begun to breathe spontaneously.

    Rationale: To maintain adequate levels of oxygen to the tissues.

3. **Action:** Keep the patient warm at all times. Once the surgical procedure is complete, transfer it to its vivarium maintained at its preferred body temperature (PBT). Monitor the environmental temperature to avoid overheating.

    Rationale: Reptiles are cold-blooded and the environmental temperature influences their metabolic rate. If the reptile is kept at its PBT, the recovery will occur more quickly than if the reptile is cold.

4. **Action:** Monitor the respiratory rate until the patient is fully conscious and moving around.

    Rationale: Respiratory stimulants, e.g. doxapram, can be used.

5. **Action:** Give replacement fluid therapy orally, intravenously or intraperitoneally – up to 4% of bodyweight.

   Rationale: Dehydration can lead to visceral gout – the build-up of urates in the visceral organs.

6. **Action:** Monitor the patient until it is fully conscious.

   Rationale: Problems may occur during the postoperative period. Appetite is often difficult to measure as many reptiles eat infrequently.

REFERENCES AND FURTHER READING

Anderson R S, Edney A T B (eds) 1991 Practical Animal Handling. Pergamon, Oxford

Aspinall V 2006 The Complete Textbook of Veterinary Nursing. Elsevier, Oxford

Aspinall V, O'Reilly M 2004 Introduction to Veterinary Anatomy and Physiology. Butterworth-Heinemann, Oxford

Beynon P H (ed) 1991 Manual of Exotic Pets. BSAVA, Gloucester

Beynon P H (ed) 1994 Manual of Reptiles. BSAVA, Gloucester

Beynon P H (ed) 1996 Manual of Psittacine Birds. BSAVA, Gloucester

Debmark Rabbit Education Resource. Online. Available: http://www.debmark.com/rabbits/sexing.htm 13 May 2006

Hillyer E V, Quesenberry K E 1997 Ferrets, Rabbits and Rodents, Clinical Medicine and Surgery. WB Saunders, Philadelphia

Hotston-Moore A (ed) 1999 Manual of Advanced Veterinary Nursing. BSAVA, Gloucester

Laber-Laird K, Swindle M, Flecknell P 1991 Handbook of Rodent and Rabbit Medicine. Pergamon, Oxford

O'Malley B 2005 Clinical Anatomy and Physiology of Exotic Species. Elsevier Saunders, Oxford

Chapter 13

Preparing for the veterinary nursing exams

Justine Dunstone and Sarah Cottingham

CHAPTER CONTENTS

Advanced preparation for the practical
   tasks 323
Why your portfolio is relevant to the practical
   exams 324

Learning and memory 324
Short- and long-term memory 324
How to remember information 325
Why do I need to revise? 325
How do you learn? 325
Hemispheres of the brain and learning 326
Putting learning styles to practical use 326
Methods of revising 327

Revision 330
The study environment 330
Time management 330
Practising tasks 330
Revision schedules 331

Final practical exam 331
General practical exam techniques 331
Advanced preparation checklist for the
   exam 332
Final preparation for the practical tasks – one
   week before the practical exams 333
Planning your journey to the practical
   exams 333
The night before the practical exam 333
The day of the practical exam 334

The exam process – what to expect 334
After the exam 335

Although not the primary aim of this book, the first edition has been widely used by student nurses to prepare for their exams, so, to help, this chapter has been added to the new edition.

The professional exams for veterinary nurses (VN) are awarded by the Royal College of Veterinary Surgeons (RCVS) and consist of the NVQ level 2 theory papers and the NVQ level 3 theory papers and practical exams.

Advanced preparation for the practical tasks

Be prepared – this is the most important factor if you want to pass.

1. **Action:** Ensure that you have printed off all the tasks that are available on the RCVS website (www.rcvs.org.uk) well in advance.

    Rationale: We would advise that you have this available right at the start of your level 3 programme. This will mean that you can refer to them throughout the year, practising them when you complete relevant case studies and when you cover the areas at college. This will mean that by your final

term at college you will be extremely familiar with the tasks and can then dedicate
additional time to practising them.

2. **Action:** Tasks should be practised so that you
feel you can do them in your sleep.

   Rationale: It is no good doing something once
   or twice and then expecting to complete it
   perfectly under very nerve-racking conditions. During this final term, use your time
   at college, work and home to repeat tasks
   that you find more difficult or challenging.
   So if that means conducting each radiography position as if you were under exam
   conditions or gloving up while watching
   television, then do so. Repetition is the best
   way to ensure competence.

3. **Action:** Get as many people involved with
your practical revision as you can.

   Rationale: Get people observing you, testing
   you and even grading you. You should also
   test or grade other level 3 trainees; this is
   a great way to learn. It is no good feeling
   nervous about being watched or graded,
   you have to get used to this and the more
   you do it the less of an issue it will be on
   the day.

4. **Action:** Receive any feedback constructively
and use the variety of books and DVDs
available to you for your revision.

   Rationale: Feedback is designed to help you
   improve your practical skills.

If you feel that you will never get the hang of
certain tasks, just think of something that you
never thought you would be able to master but
now do as if it were second nature. It is human
nature to avoid doing something that we do not
particularly enjoy or that we find difficult; however, this is all the more reason to spend extra time
going over these areas. See it as a challenge to master these tasks and not to be beaten!

Why your portfolio is relevant to the practical exams

If you have completed all of your level 3 portfolio, prior to the exams, then you should be able
to demonstrate extensive practical competence.

Completion of the portfolio is there to ensure
that throughout the year you are practising all of
the practical areas involved with the award. The
assessments that you undertake are to ensure
that you are able to complete these practical areas
to the level of the VN occupational standards.
Therefore do not look upon the portfolio as something tedious and time-consuming, that you just
want to get completed as soon as possible. It is a
crucial part of your practical training and assessment. Try to enjoy the learning that it involves and
remember that completion of it will mean that by
the time your practical exams arrive you will have
the competence needed to pass.

LEARNING AND MEMORY

As a level 3 student veterinary nurse you must
prepare for both a written multiple choice exam
and a practical exam in order to qualify. Both types
of exams can be approached in a similar way and
tailored to fit the particular task. To begin with
it is important to understand how you learn in
order to understand how you as an individual can
best revise. Once you have identified these areas,
you can then move on to different revision and
practical techniques to ensure you are successful
in your exams.

Short- and long-term memory

Memory is an interesting phenomenon – you will
forget 80% of what you have learnt unless you
reread the information within 24 hours and then
at regular intervals after that period. We must
therefore ensure that we are able to store the information. Research has shown that it is essential to
understand the information completely as this
allows your brain to remember the information
better, and then recall it when you need to apply
it. Memory works on two main levels – short-term
and long-term.

Short-term memory is for very recent information. The brain is only able to hold approximately
seven items in short-term storage. After this
point, the brain needs to transfer this information somewhere else in order to make sure that
there is room for the next input of information.

To be able to learn and recall information, the brain needs to move it into long-term memory. Once the information is stored in your long-term memory, you are able to recall it easily. However, we need to get it there in the first place. The main two methods of storing information in long-term memory are:

- rote learning, i.e. learning through repetition
- understanding the information.

By reviewing information continually, you are able to strengthen the neurological pathway in your brain, and your memory of the information will be much better. The less you review the information, the more the neural pathway becomes weakened, to the point where you forget the information.

Some scary facts A study of memory recall showed that information fades unless it is reviewed:

- After 1 day, 54% was remembered.
- After 63 days, 17% was remembered.

It is important therefore to review information within the first 24 hours, otherwise you may lose it. This means that effective revision should actually start after your very first lesson!

How to remember information

It is important to find a method that best allows you to file information into your long-term memory. There are different ways that you can do this:

- Be interested in the subject; it is much more effective if you are actually interested in the subject and engage in what you are studying.
- Make sure you have decided what you want to gain; having a goal will make learning and revising so much easier and once you care about the outcome, you are so much more likely to succeed.
- Visualise the information. Some people are able to create a picture in their mind as to what the information looks like written down, or what a practical task should look like during and at its completion.
- Try to link or group information into compartments – file information into related areas that follow on from each other or relate easily.

- Repeat information in order to store it in your long-term memory. This can involve saying information aloud, writing it in your own words, or performing the task repetitively.

Why do I need to revise?

- The reason is probably clear by now! Revision is important to ensure that during an exam you are able to recall the information and either answer a question or perform a task in the correct sequence of events and with confidence.
- It also increases your memory and deepens the level of learning and understanding that you already have of the task.
- Revision is also immensely important in increasing self-confidence and self-belief that you will succeed. Entering an exam knowing that you are prepared is half the battle.

How do you learn?

In order to make sure you learn effectively and how best you should revise, you need to understand how your brain works. There are many factors involved with learning and you may be able to identify yourself in more than one. Once you have decided which one(s) you are most like, you can then start to use the strategies that will work best for you.

For example:

- Are you organised and systematic in your approach to work and enjoy routine?
- Do you study when you feel like it, if you have time, and what you want to research at that moment in time?
- Do you enjoy working on your own?
- Do you enjoy working with others?
- Do you find it easy/preferable to work with lots going on around you?
- Do you find it preferable to work in a quiet environment?
- Do you prefer to hear information being given (able to recall information in the form of speech)?
- Do you prefer to visualise information (see information as a picture in your mind)?
- Do you prefer to recall information in the way that it feels, moves or by touch?

Hemispheres of the brain and learning

The way in which your brain works also has a bearing on how you learn. The brain is divided into two main hemispheres, the left and the right (Fig. 13.1). The two sides handle information quite differently even though they are not discrete and are linked by many, many millions of nerve fibres. Each hemisphere controls the opposite side of the body, so the left hemisphere controls the right side of the body and vice versa. There are some activities that involve using both sides of the brain together.

Depending on the hemisphere of the brain that you predominantly use, certain learning styles will be more appropriate. From the information below, see if you show a preference for one hemisphere more than another. If you do, try employing the learning methods below to see if they improve your retention of knowledge.

Right hand preference – try these methods

- Diagrams, pictures – such as mind maps.
- Personalise information – own notes using phrases.
- Add colour to your work, decorate and personalise.
- Highlight work and topics.
- Try to sing your notes and information.
- Be active when learning – move around the room and do something when trying to recall what you have recently learnt.

Left hand preference– try these methods

- Rewrite your own notes by hand.
- List and bullet point information and facts.
- Write information into a sequence, e.g. from 1 to 10.
- Use headings and subheadings to split and highlight information and locate it easily.
- Use flow diagrams to visualise progression and logical sequences.

In addition to these methods of learning, Honey and Mumford (1992) developed a questionnaire that categorised learners into four classes. These are:

- *Activist* – enjoys new experiences, generating ideas and trying things out, group discussions, active 'doing' tasks rather than passive activities.
- *Reflector* – enjoys having time and space to consider facts, listen, observe and spend time making a decision.
- *Theorist* – enjoys facts and performing tasks logically. Theorists also enjoy assimilating new information into a model format. They prefer facts to opinions or creative ideas.
- *Pragmatist* – these learners enjoy activities that are practical and like to test out theories in a practical manner rather than through discussion.

Putting learning styles to practical use

Once you have identified your learning strategy, consider the following methods to help you revise and become an effective learner:

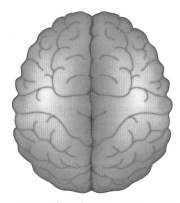

Preference to use left side of brain	Preference to use right side of brain
• Logical thinking style	• Seeing the whole
• Sequence	• Imagination
• Logic	• Pattern recognition
• Analysis	• Emotion
• Numbers	• Faces
• Language	• Intuition
• Names	• Image
• Sense of time	• Colour

Figure 13.1 The human brain. Redrawn from Cottrell (2003), Palgrave Macmillan.

- *Visual learners* – mapping, drawings, colour-coded notes, and note-taking strategies that include visual designs.
- *Auditory learners* – tape the information and play it back in the car or at home. Also tape lectures at the time of delivery.
- *Step-by-step learners* – use an outline format for recording information that will help put information into a linear format.

Methods of revising

These methods of revision can be used for both theory and practical tasks.

1. Flash cards/revision cards

Use index cards with key words, phrases or points written down on them (Fig. 13.2). These are small enough to be carried around and pulled out for revision of practical tasks when you get stuck on a point. They are particularly useful for practical exam tasks that you may be practising on a daily basis (rather than having to get your textbooks or task sheets out).

2. Post it notes and sticky paper

These are particularly good for reinforcing small chunks of information that you have problems remembering. The key points, phrases or sections of tasks can be written down on colourful paper and stuck anywhere around your house or areas of the practice that are out of bounds to clients!

3. Writing your notes

Rewrite your notes before you start revision. In this way they will be in your own language, a format that you understand, a layout that you can read and absorb facts from to gain the best amount of information. This should be done at the end of each lecture so you avoid having a whole year's notes to rewrite and condense. Imagine how good it will feel to get to the revision stages and have a full set of revision notes ready for you.

4. Mind maps

Mind maps are very useful for remembering practical tasks as each section can be added to the next to build up a picture. A mind map starts with a central point from which sub-topics or related words branch out to create a tree-like diagram. Key areas to remember are:

- start in the centre of the page with the main concept (Fig. 13.3)
- use key words rather than sentences
- be colourful
- use your own words that you can remember (tailor your learning)
- create links where necessary
- use a picture or diagram where necessary (Fig. 13.4).

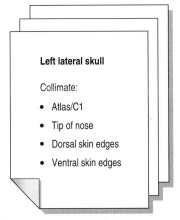

Left lateral skull

Collimate:

- Atlas/C1
- Tip of nose
- Dorsal skin edges
- Ventral skin edges

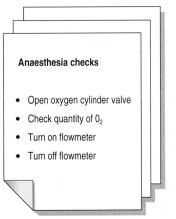

Anaesthesia checks

- Open oxygen cylinder valve
- Check quantity of O_2
- Turn on flowmeter
- Turn off flowmeter

Figure 13.2   Examples of short notes or flash cards used to revise information that you are not able to recall easily.

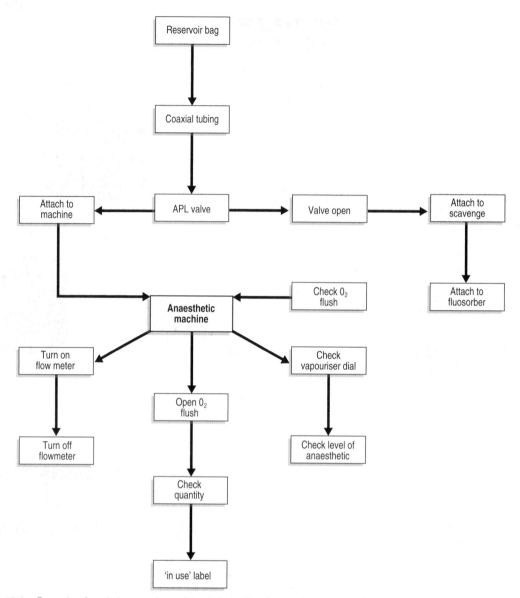

Figure 13.3 Example of a mind map using written information for an anaesthetic task.

5. Mnemonics and acronyms

These work for some people and not for others. A mnemonic is a device to help the memory and may take the form of patterns of words or phrases written in a sentence or rhyme that helps the recall of information. It may also be an acronym, which is a word formed from the first letters of a useful phrase. For example, an acronym used in first aid is:

- **A CRASH PLAN** = Airway Cardiovascular Respiration Abdomen Spine Head Pelvis Limbs Arteries Nerves

When creating mnemonics or acronyms, the ones that are most easily remembered are the simple, funny (or rude!) ones, and ones with symbols, pictures and diagrams.

6. Discuss the topics with friends

Talking to friends and other nurses is an invaluable aid to revision. Ask questions; request that people ask you questions; discuss information that you have read; summarise the information and discuss your findings. All discussions, questions and

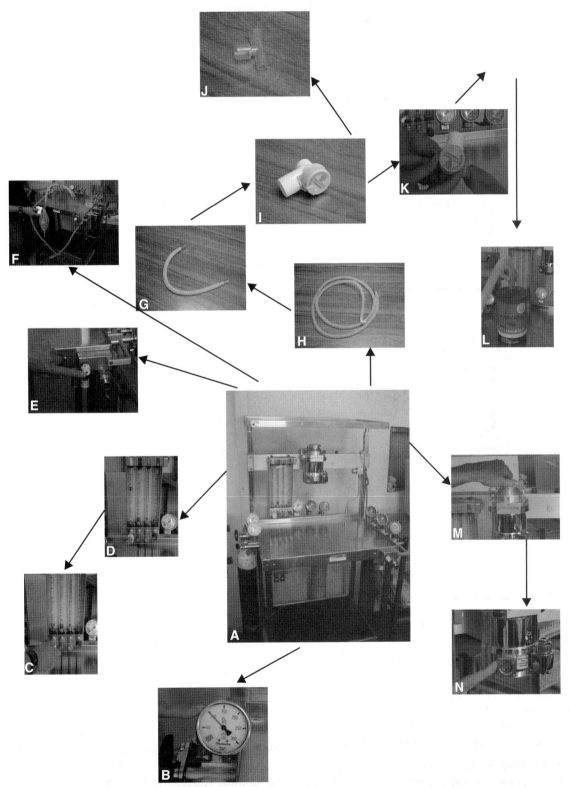

Figure 13.4 Example of a mind map using pictures to illustrate an anaesthetic task.

answers will directly increase your understanding and deepen the level of learning.

REVISION

The study environment

The study environment must be suitable for learning. Think about these factors and what would work best for you:

- Create a relaxed environment.
- Make sure you are feeling positive at the time of studying.
- Listen to music played on string instruments with a bass rhythm of 60 beats/min as this stimulates learning areas of the brain, e.g. Baroque classical music, New Age or Indian music.
- Revise when you are most alert – not when you are tired.
- Study in pairs, groups or on your own – choose your preference.
- Choose a position that is most comfortable for you – walking around, lying on the sofa, sitting on a chair at a table.
- Ensure that lighting is adequate and comfortable for your eyes.
- Ensure that you are at a comfortable body temperature.

Time management

Time management is important in any course and particularly during revision. You need to be clear as to what you want from the course and set yourself realistic goals. Give yourself rewards when you achieve them.

Consider your time management in the 8 weeks prior to the examinations. Be prepared to give up on a social life for this period! You must organise your life to allow enough time for both theory and practical revision. It is not enough to cram all of your practical revision into a week before the written and practical exams – this is not enough time to ensure competence on the day.

The following points may help you to manage your time effectively:

- Identify your work schedule and commitments over the three months leading up to the exams.

- Work out how many hours you can put aside each week for your revision schedule.
- Motivate yourself by visualising the end goal – being qualified!
- Prioritise what needs to be done and when it needs to be done.
- Strike a balance between theoretical revision and practical revision.
- Devise a schedule with work colleagues that will allow all practical tasks to be performed, repeated and practised as many times as possible before the exams.
- Make sure that you understand fully all the tasks that you will be required to perform.
- Break down the tasks into related chunks. This will make learning easier as some tasks have generic areas.
- Do not expect to be able to cram revision for practicals in the last week – they need to be thoroughly learnt if you are to perform them and feel confident.
- The practical task does not have to be perfect – remember you only have to pass 50% of the criteria (including the essential elements) in order to pass the task. Have realistic expectations but do not be lazy.

Practising tasks

It is important to practise the actual tasks as these are what you will be required to perform in the exam. They can be downloaded from the RCVS website (rcvs.org.uk). The tasks should be practised in front of an 'examiner' and completed within 6 minutes but the final 2 minutes may be for questions or related calculations.

1. **Action:** You should practise completing the tasks under conditions that resemble the actual practical exam as closely as possible.

   Rationale: In this way, you will be able to perform the tasks in a logical pattern that is already familiar to you.

2. **Action:** Describe why and what you are doing during the procedure.

   Rationale: This will consolidate your understanding.

3. **Action:** Ensure you are timing yourself.

Rationale: This will enable you to get used to the 6 minute period that is allocated for each task.

4. **Action:** Repeat a part if you miss it out or perform it incorrectly.

   Rationale: This will ensure that you learn to do all parts equally correctly.

5. **Action:** Ask the 'examiner' to be critical of your performance and give you constructive feedback.

   Rationale: This will teach you what you have done wrong and provide guidance as to how you can improve.

6. **Action:** Practise at work as much as possible.

   Rationale: This ensures that you have all the equipment required for the task and that you have another nurse present to give you the feeling of being watched.

7. **Action:** Practise at home.

   Rationale: Take equipment home if you have permission. Practise during every spare moment.

8. **Action:** Teach someone else how to perform the task.

   Rationale: This is a very good way of consolidating your own knowledge. By teaching them you have to think through the task in a logical manner and you also need to know what you are talking about. An ideal person to teach is a level 2 student as they will already have a basic idea and understanding of what you require them to do.

9. **Action:** Practice 'examining' and marking someone else's performance.

   Rationale: This will help as you are able to observe both good techniques and any mistakes so that you are less likely to make them yourself. The person being 'examined' will benefit from your feedback and constructive criticism.

10. **Action:** Ask your head nurse if she/he will set up a mock practical.

    Rationale: This can be carried out after work in your own time if necessary – remember, it is for your benefit! The more times you practise tasks under exam conditions the

more confident and comfortable you will be in the actual exam. Ask the 'examiner' to complete a mark sheet for each task while you are performing it. This adds authenticity to the mock exam and later will allow a thorough debriefing of the performance.

Continually practising under exam conditions will ensure that your memory recall will be effective as the surroundings in which you are performing will be familiar and non-threatening.

Revision schedules

Devise a revision schedule that will work for you. It is important to build a schedule that can be tailored to your day and includes revision that can be carried out at work within your normal duties. Try to fit appropriate tasks into your daily schedule when the opportunity arises. As most training practices have a varied workload that includes radiography, laboratory, anaesthesia and fluid therapy on a daily basis, there are always important tasks to try and cover during working hours. The schedule in Table 13.1 provides you with an idea as to how you can arrange each week of your revision to suit the practice case load. The radiography and laboratory tasks can be repositioned depending on the type of cases in on that day. The contingency periods are needed if for any reason you were unable to perform a scheduled task the previous day.

In addition to a schedule, it is a good idea to have some form of checklist that can be designed to work in conjunction with your revision scheme. In this way you can ensure that all tasks are covered at least once during the week while you are at work. As it is impossible to predict the cases that will be coming into the practice, you should be flexible; ticking off the tasks when they are completed will ensure all tasks are practised. The checklist will also give you a visual overview of the areas that you have covered and the areas that need extra time and attention.

FINAL PRACTICAL EXAM

General practical exam techniques

Expect to feel nervous on the day. Everyone experiences nervousness when put into that sort of

Table 13.1   An example of a practical task revision schedule identifying the numbers of the relevant RCVS practical tasks

	Monday	Tuesday	Wednesday	Thursday	Friday	Saturday	Sunday
7 am	Read through tasks for the day	Read through tasks for the day	Read through tasks for the day	Read through tasks for the day	Read through tasks for the day		
During work hours	Administration of fluids SF01 Laboratory tests SL01; SL02 Radiographic positioning SR01; SR02 Use of anaesthetic equipment SA01	Administration of medicines SP01 Laboratory tests SL03; SL04 Radiographic positioning SR03; SR04 Use of anaesthetic equipment SA02	Administration of fluids SF01 Laboratory tests SL05; SL06 Radiographic positioning SR05; SR06 Use of anaesthetic equipment SA03	Administration of medicines SP02 Laboratory tests SL07 Radiographic positioning SR07; SR08; SR09 Use of anaesthetic equipment; SA04	Administration of fluids SF02 Laboratory test (contingency time) Radiographic positioning SR09 Use of anaesthetic equipment (contingency time)	Cover tasks that have been omitted during the week	Cover tasks that have been omitted during the week
Evening	Dressing, bandaging and splinting SB01; SB02	Dressing, bandaging and splinting SB04; SB05	Dressing, bandaging and splinting, SB06; SB07	Dressing, bandaging and splinting (contingency time)	Dressing, bandaging and splinting (contingency time)		
Evening	Aseptic technique and theatre practice ST01	Aseptic technique and theatre practice ST02	Aseptic technique and theatre practice ST03	Aseptic technique and theatre practice ST04	Aseptic technique and theatre practice ST05		

situation. However, going into your exams well prepared will mean that you feel less nervous and far more confident. With luck this should mean that you make fewer mistakes.

When you enter the exam room there are a few simple steps that you can take to ensure that you perform to the best of your ability and that you recall the information easily and quickly. These include:

- Smile at the examiner – this will put you at ease.
- Breathe evenly – do not hold your breath as this will cause you to panic.
- Listen to the instructions being read to you.
- Read the instructions on the task sheet if you find this easier.

- Put the task sheet in front of you so you can refer back to it.
- Visualise the details required by the task.
- Visualise performing the task.
- Speak as you perform the task; this will reinforce and help you to recall the information.
- If there is a calculation, ensure that it is laid out so that the examiner can clearly understand the steps that you have taken.

Advanced preparation checklist for the exam

- Obtain a copy of the practical exam tasks at the start of your level 3 course (available on RCVS website www.rcvs.org.uk).

- Refer to the tasks throughout the year.
- Try to complete your level 3 portfolio prior to the exams and use it in conjunction with the practical tasks.
- Eight weeks prior to your exam, make a revision plan.
- Concentrate more on the areas you find difficult.
- Stick to your revision plan.
- Practise, practise, practise.

Final preparation for the practical tasks – one week before the practical exams

Once your theory examinations are over, forget about them and focus solely on your practicals. If you felt you did not do well in your theory exams, this is all the more reason to put them out of your mind and anyway no one knows definitely how they did until they receive the results. Negative thoughts surrounding your written papers will only interfere with the concentration and confidence needed for your practical exams.

You may not have sufficient time left to repeat further practice of all the tasks, but you will know the ones that you are completely confident about and the ones that would benefit from further practice. Focus on these and ensure you do them under exam conditions including being timed. You must ensure that you can perform them well and that you can perform them in the 6 minutes allowed.

Again our best advice is practise, practise, and practise!

Planning your journey to the practical exams

1. **Action:** Consider how to get to the exam in good time with the minimum amount of stress.

   Rationale: The RCVS will let you know well in advance which centre you have been allocated for your exam and at what time.

2. **Action:** The exams are carried out in groups of four students so you may be able to travel with some of your work colleagues or college friends.

   Rationale: This is a big advantage, so having someone to chat to on the journey will calm your nerves.

3. **Action:** Decide whether it is best to travel by train or car.

   Rationale: Depending on the location of the exam centre it may be easier and more restful to travel by train. Travelling by car may be more flexible but allow time to park when you get there.

4. **Action:** If your exam is very early you may have to travel the day before and stay overnight.

   Rationale: Ensure that you plan this well in advance as accommodation at the exam centre may be limited.

5. **Action:** Ensure that if you travel by car that you have studied the route well and have estimated accurately how long the journey will take.

   Rationale: Remember to allow for traffic jams! Always add an hour to your estimated travel time. It is much better to arrive early and to wait around for a while than to arrive late or with only minutes to spare, which will result in you feeling stressed.

6. **Action:** If you arrive a little early, take this time to try and relax yourself, take a little stroll, get yourself a drink and the all important one, spend a penny!

   Rationale: All these activities will calm your nerves and give you time to get used to the surroundings.

The night before the practical exam

The last thing that you want to feel on the morning of your exam is tired, so try to relax the night before and do not cram in any last minute revision. What you do not know by then you are unlikely to take in and you will only frighten yourself.

Take some time to ensure that you have everything prepared for the morning; for example:

- your uniform
- your exam entry card and identification
- any food or drink you wish to take with you
- your mobile phone and the exam centre's telephone number, just in case you encounter a problem while getting there

- if going by car, ensure the car is filled with fuel and that you have the directions and map
- if going by train make sure that you have double checked the train times and ensured that arrangements are in place to get you to and from the station.

When all of this is in place and your alarm clock is set, try to get to sleep early, so that you will feel alert the following day.

The day of the practical exam

1. What to wear

- Ensure you are wearing an appropriate uniform, not a qualified VN's uniform.
- Ensure long hair is tied back and do not wear excessive jewellery or long, painted fingernails.
  You will not get marked down for your dress, but you are expected to dress appropriately for the tasks that you may be asked to perform.

2. What to take with you

Make sure that you have with you:

- your exam entry card
- your identification.
  You may want to take a packed lunch as food is not always available at the exam centre.

The exam process – what to expect

1. Dispelling the myth

Whatever horror stories you may have heard from other VNs, remember the examiners are not there to try and catch you out. They are human beings and not ogres and although they expect you to perform to a standard they are fair and friendly and will do their best to put you at ease. There are no trick questions and everyone is marked to the same grading criteria for each individual task. A second examiner is present in order to ensure that you are treated fairly and equally. External verification to ensure consistency is also undertaken at each exam centre by an RCVS external verifier. The examiner is there to assess safe, effective nursing practice and really does want you to pass.

2. On arrival

Make your way to the reception area and you will be given directions or escorted to the examination area. Once your group of four is assembled you will be given a briefing by the head examiner. Stay focused and listen carefully, remaining as calm and relaxed as possible. Do not be afraid to ask any questions if you are not clear about any area covered.

3. On entry into the exam room

There will be eight practical tasks. When you approach the first task, the examiner will give you a brief introduction; a second examiner will also be present. Do not let it unnerve you if the examiner appears a little brusque; remember they have to maintain a degree of detachment. This is not a reflection on you, everyone will be treated the same. The examiner will read the task out for you. The task will remain there for you to refer to during your 6 minutes. Refer back to it as many times as you need to, so that you can check any details as you go along. Silly mistakes can be made by carelessly reading the task, e.g. bandaging the wrong limb!

4. The equipment provided

Have a good look at what equipment is available and think carefully and logically about what you will need. Prepare it prior to starting the task if appropriate. All of the equipment you need will be provided but if you think you need something else that you are unable to see, ask the examiner.

5. Talk and do

You will not gain any marks for explaining what you are doing, only for actually doing it. Remember it is a practical exam. The oral part comes with the questions you will be asked at the end of the task. However, if talking through what you are doing will help you to think logically and methodically, then talk. It may also make you appear more knowledgeable and confident as well as creating a less nervous atmosphere. Stone cold silence will not help your nerves!

6. The speed of the task

Remember you only have 6 minutes to complete each task and answer questions related to that area. There is no time for uncertainty; you need to start straight away and proceed at an industrial speed. However, there is a thin line between that and rushing it, which may cause you to make silly mistakes or overlook something important. You will be told when you have 2 minutes remaining and you may ask how you are doing for time at any other point.

7. What if I make a mistake?

If you realise you have done something incorrectly or have forgotten to do something, you must assess if you have enough time to change it. Check what time you have left, with the examiner. If you feel you have enough time, then tell them your mistake and rectify it; if you do not have enough time, then you can still explain your mistake. It may cause you to lose more marks if you go back and try to rectify it and run out of time. Remember you may also have some questions to answer.

8. On completion of the task

Ensure you have completed everything you need to and are happy with how you have done it before confirming to the examiner that you have finished. Just check the task sheet once more. Once you have been asked the oral questions, even if you have time spare you will not be permitted to go back to the task.

9. The oral questions

You will probably have limited time to answer these. If you do not know the answer immediately, give yourself a few seconds to think about it. If the answer still does not come to mind then move on to the next question if there is one. If you have time remaining you will be permitted to go back to any questions you have passed on. If your time is running out and you are stuck on a question, then it is worth giving it a guess. Do not worry that it may be a silly or a wrong answer, it may be correct. You would not leave a question unanswered on your written exam paper.

10. Focus on the next task

Once you have come away from one practical task, forget about it. Do not ponder on how you did. You must focus straight away on the next one. If you feel upset or frustrated by your previous performance, this will only put you in a bad state of mind for the next one. Remember you only have to achieve 50% on each task to pass it and you must pass five out of eight tasks to pass the whole exam. It is better to have failed one task than the whole lot because you got yourself into a state. Just take a deep breath and remain calm, positive and focused.

11. How to conduct yourself in the exam

Your attitude: When entering the room and performing the tasks try to appear positive and confident and smile; it will make you feel much better. If you have prepared well there is no reason why you should not be able to perform competently any of the tasks asked. So go in there with a positive attitude; negativity will show in your performance.

A methodical approach: If you have practised the tasks as advised, you will have devised a methodical approach to performing them. Remember this and follow it on the day. Do not let the fact that you are in a different environment with slightly different equipment put you off. Perform the task as you would if your assessor were watching you because if you deviate from the routine you are used to this may confuse you or put you off.

After the exam

Once you have completed your exams, however you felt you performed, you will not be able to change it, so it is pointless to be upset about your performance or to keep going over it. You have about a 4-week wait until the results are out, so try not to spend this time in despair or depression. Remember you do not have to achieve 100% to pass. You have worked extremely hard to gain your qualification and you should be proud of yourself whatever the outcome. Now is the time to give yourself some rest from revision and exams and have some time off. This is the perfect time to book your summer holiday.

If you are unfortunate enough to have failed the practical exams, do not see this as a complete failure. Take notice of the feedback provided and the areas you did not pass and use that to make you more determined to practice even more before the resits.

Take the advice given in this chapter and always keep a positive attitude and of course practise, practise, practise!

REFERENCES

Cottrell S 2003 The Study Skills Handbook, 2nd edn. Palgrave Macmillan, Basingstoke

Honey P, Mumford A 1992 The Manual of Learning Styles. Peter Honey Publications, Maidenhead

Index

Note: Page number in *italics* refer to figures and page numbers in **bold** refer to tables.

A

Abdomen radiography, 218–19, *219*
Abrasions, **165**
Abscess, **165**
Absorbable sutures, **182**
Acepromazine (ACP)
  general description, **113**
  misuse, **197**
Acronyms, 328
Activated charcoal, **197**, **202**
Active scavenging, 133
Activists, 326
Adrenaline, **129**
Agar plates, 268, *268*
Aggressive cats, 15, *15*
Airway obstruction, **130**
Alcohol poisoning, **200**
Alfadolone, **115**, **321**
Alfaxalone, **115**, **321**
Alginates, **167**
Allergic-type response
  to medication, **197**
Allis tissue forceps, 232
Alphachloralose poisoning, **200**
Amino acids, 98, 102
Ammonium urate, *275*
Anaesthesia, 105–33
  admitting the patient, 109–10, **110**
  anaesthetic machines, 106–7, *107*, **108**
  birds, 310–12, **311**
  circuits, 120–3, **124**

consent form, *111*
control of pollution, 132–3
drugs for, blood pressure and, 36
emergencies, 128–30, **129**, **130**
ferrets, 302–4
gas flow rate calculation, 123–7
heart rate changes, **126**
induction agents, **115**, **287**, **311**, **321**
induction methods, **116**
  birds, 310–11
  ferrets, 302–3
  rabbits, 285–7
  reptiles, 320
  small rodents, 297
inhalation agents, **117**
masks, 119–20
monitoring, 125, **125–6**
birds, 311–12
  ferrets, 303
  rabbits, 287
  reptiles, 320–1
  small rodents, 298
patient preparation, 107–12
pre-anaesthetic
  check, 110–12
  instructions, 107–9
premedicant drugs, **113**
rabbits, 285–8, **286**
recovery, 127–8
reptiles, 320–2
respiratory pattern changes, **126**
small rodents, 297–8
specialised techniques, 130–2
stages of, 112–19, **114**
Anaesthetics circuits, 120–3
Anaphylactic reaction, **197**
Anaphylactic shock, **204**

Anions, 68
Anticoagulants poisoning, **200**
Anticonvulsants, 58
Antidiuretic hormone (ADH), 64
Antifreeze poisoning, **201**
Anus injuries, **207**
Apex beat palpation, **125**
Apnoea, **125**, **126**, **130**
Apomorphine, **201**
Arrhythmias, 32
Arterial blood pressure *See* Blood
  pressure
Arterial haemorrhage, **190**
Artificial respiration
  intubated patient, 194, *194*
  no endotracheal tube, 194
Ascites, 61
Asepsis, 139–40, **140**
Asphyxia, **189**, *192*, 192–3
Aspirin poisoning, **197**
Atipamezole, **129**, **287**
Atracurium, **132**
Atropine, **113**, **129**
Atropine sulphate, **199**
Attire, theatre, **143**, 143–8, *144–7*, *149–51*
Autoclaves, 136, **137**
  care and use of, 245
Automatic pipettes, 250–1
Automatic processing of radiographs,
  237–9
Avulsion, **165**

B

Bacterial culture, 267–8, *268*
Bacterial smears, 266

Bain circuit, modified, 121, *122,* **124**
Balances, care and use of, 245–6
Band neutrophils, **258**
Bandaging techniques, 167–76, **169,** *170–1, 173–5*
Barbiturate, **199, 200**
Barium sulphate, 227–30
    enema, *229,* 229–30
    meal/follow through, 228–9
    swallow, 228
Barrier nursing, 42–3
Basophils, normal ranges for dogs and cats, **258**
Battlement technique of counting cells, 261, 264, *265*
BCK granules, **202**
Bee sting, **203**
Behaviour, natural
    rabbits, **279**
    small rodents, **279**
Beta-blockers, **198**
Biological data
    ferrets, **299**
    rabbits, **379**
    small rodents, **379**
Biopsy techniques, 181–3, **182**
Bipolar diathermy, 159
Birds, 304–12
    anaesthesia, 310–12
    capture and restraint, *304,* 304–6, *305*
    drug administration, *307,* 307–10, *308, 309*
Birth, difficult, 205–10, **210**
Bitches, catheterisation, 45–6
Bites to patients, 202, **203**
Bladder manual expression, *48,* 48–9
Blood
    loss in anaesthesia monitoring, **126**
    parasites, 262–3
    products, 69
    smear preparation, 261, *261*
    transfusion, 83–5, *84*
        reactions, 85 *See also* Whole blood
Blood pressure
    anaesthesia monitoring, **125**
    measuring, *35,* 35–6, *36*
        cuff positioning sites, 36, *36*
    normal in cats and dogs, **26**
Blood sample collection
    birds, 310
    chelonians, 317–18
    lizards, 319
    small rodents, **296,** 296–7
    snakes, 314–15
    for transfusion, 80–3
Body temperature *See* Temperature, body

Bodyweight
    enteral feeding, 98
    ferrets, **299**
    fluid therapy monitoring, 80
    parenteral feeding, 102
    rabbits, **279**
    small rodents, **279**
Bone plates and screws, **179**
Borax poisoning, **199**
Boric acid, 273
Bowie-Dick indicator tape, **138**
Boyle's bottle vaporiser, **108,** *109*
Brachial vein injection, *308,* 308–9
Brachycephalic dogs, tape muzzles, 2–3
Bradycardia, **126, 130**
Bradypnoea, **126**
Braided nylon, **182**
Braided silk, **182**
Brain hemispheres, 326
Browne's tubes, **138**
Buprenorphine, **113**
Burns, 191
Butorphanol, **113**

C

Cage rest, fracture fixation, **179**
Calciferol poisoning, **200**
Calcipotriol poisoning, **198**
Calcium carbonate, *275*
Calcium oxalate, *275*
Calculus, tooth, **185**
Capillary haemorrhage, **190**
Capillary refill time (CRT)
    anaesthesia monitoring, **125**
    assessing, 30
    fluid therapy monitoring, 80
    normal in cats and dogs, **26**
Capnographs
    mainstream, 36–7
    sidestream, 37, *38*
Carapace, 316, *316*
Carbamate poisoning, **199**
Carbon dioxide concentration
    measuring using a mainstream capnograph, 36–7
    measuring using a sidestream capnograph, 37, *38*
    normal in cats and dogs, **26**
Cardboard cartons, sterilisation packing, **139**
Cardiac arrest, **130**
Cardiac failure, 59
Cardiac massage, 195–6
Cardiac monitor, anaesthesia monitoring, **125**
Cardiogenic shock, **204**

Caries, **185**
Carprofen, **113**
Carrying
    cats, 15–16, *16*
    rabbits, 278–81, *280*
Cassettes, radiography
    light leakage, 239–40
    poor film/screen contact, 240–1
Cast, **169,** 176, **179**
Catgut, chromic, **182**
Catheters
    cats
        equipment, *44*
        queen, 47–8
        tom, 46–7, *47*
    dogs, 43–6
        bitches, 45–6
        equipment, *44*
        male, 43–5
    equipment, *44, 71*
    rabbits, 285
    urinary, 38, **177**
Cations, 68
Cats
    carrying, 15–16, *16*
    catheterisation, *44,* 46–8, *47*
    endotracheal intubation, 117, *118*
    general examination of, 16–17, 42
    handling and restraint, 14–24
        for drug administration, *17,* 17–24, *18, 20, 21, 23*
        for general examination, 16–17
    hypertension in, 36
    lifting
        aggressive/frightened, 15, *15*
        friendly, 14–15
    normal clinical parameters, **26**
    normal haematology ranges, **258**
Caudal end of body restraint, 6
Central venous pressure (CVP)
    measuring, 32–5, *34*
    normal in cats and dogs, **26**
Centrifuges, 252
    care and use of, 246–7
Cephalic vein
    intravenous fluid therapy, 74–5
    intravenous injection
        cats, *21,* 21–2
        dogs, *11,* 11–12
Cerclage wire, **179**
Cerebrospinal fluid (CSF) collection, 233–5
Chamber induction, **116**
Charcoal, **197, 202**
Cheatle forceps, 155
Chelonians, 315–18

Chemical indicator strips, **138**
Chest
    auscultation
        anaesthesia monitoring, **125**
        fluid therapy monitoring, 80
    bandaging, **169**, 172–3, *173*
    injuries, **205–6**
    palpation to measure
        pulse rate, 28
Cheyletiella spp., *271*
Chinchillas
    biological data, **279**
    blood sampling, **296**
    drug administration, **295**
    restraint, 288–9
    sexing, 289
Chlorate poisoning, **198**
Chocolate poisoning, **200**
Chromic catgut, **182**
Cimetidine, **197**
Circle anaesthetic breathing system,
    122, *122*, 124, **124**
Circuit factor, 124
Circulating nurse, 156
Circulation assessment, 30
Cisternal puncture, 233–5, *235*
Cleaning
    automatic processors, 238–9
    instruments, 156–7
    regime, theatre, 139–40, **140**
Clinical parameters
    enteral feeding, 98
    fluid therapy, 80
    measuring, 25–40
    normal, **26**
    parenteral feeding, 102–3
Clipping hair, 150–1
Closed drains, **177**
Closed gloving, 148, *149*
Closed wounds, **166**
Coat
    clipping, 150–1
    examination of brushings, 270
Collapse, **189**
Colloids, 69
Coma, **189**
Congestive heart failure, 59
Contrast media, 227–35, *229*
Contusions, **166**
Convulsions, 58–9
Coplin jar, 263
Corneal reflex
    anaesthesia monitoring, **126**
    rabbits, 287
    reptiles, 321
Counting chambers, 259, *259*, 260
Coupage, 51
Cranial end of body restraint, 6

Craniocaudal radiography views
    limbs, 223–4, *224*
    shoulder, 225–6, *226*
Crop tubing, *307*, 307–8
Cross-infection avoidance, 42–3
Crown (tooth), fractured, **185**
Cryosurgery, 159–60
Crystalloids, 69
Cultures
    bacterial, 267–8, *268*
    ringworm fungus, 269–70
Curette, **185**
Cystocentesis, 49–50
Cystography, 233
Cytology, *252*, 252–3

D

Death, **189**
Deciduous teeth, retained, **185**
Decubitus ulcers, 58
Degloving wound, **165**
Dehydration, 54, 56
    assessing level of, 69
Demodex spp., *271*
Demulcent agents, **202**
Dental mirror, **185**
Dental probe, **185**
Dentistry, 183–6, *184*, **185**, *186*
Depolarising muscle relaxants, **132**
Dermanyssus gallinae, *271*
Dexamethasone, **129**
Dexon, **182**
Dextrose, 69
Diabetes insipidus, 64
Diabetes mellitus, 62–4
Diagnostic imaging, 213–42
Diagnostic laboratory techniques, 243–75
Diagnostic ultrasound, 241–2
Dialysis, peritoneal, 50–1
Diaphragm injuries, **206**
Diarrhoea, 53–6
Diathermy, 159
Diazepam, **113**, **287**, **311**
Diet
    ferrets, **299**
    rabbits, **279**
    small rodents, 279
Diff-quik stain, 264
Digestive system injuries, **206–7**
Digital pressure, direct, **190**
Dinitro compounds poisoning, **198**
Dipstick testing urine, 274–5
Direct digital pressure, **190**
Disinfectants
    poisoning, **200–1**
    using, 251

Dobutamine, **129**
Dogs
    catheterisation, 43–6, *44*
    enema, 43
    general examination of, 6–7, *7*, 42
    handling and restraint, 2–14, *3*
        for drug administration,
            8, 8–14, *11*, *12*, *14*
        for general examination,
            6–7, *7*
    hydrotherapy, 52–3
    lifting, *4*
        large, with spinal damage,
            5–6, *6*
        over 20 kg, 4
        small, with spinal damage,
            4–5, *5*
        up to 15 kg, 3–4
    normal clinical parameters, **26**
    normal haematology ranges, **258**
    supported exercise, 51–2, *52*
Dorsopalmar/dorsoplantar radiogra-
    phy views, limbs, 223–4, *224*
Dorsoventral radiography views
    intraoral view of nasal chambers,
        222, *222*
    thorax, 217–18, *218*
Double contrast cystogram, 233
Doxapram, **129**
Drainage systems, **177**, 177–8
Drapes
    draping a trolley, 155
    draping the patient, 152–4, *153*
    fenestrated, 154
    folding, *153*
    limb draping, 154, *154*
    packing for sterilisation, 152
    types of, **152**
Dressings, **167** *See also* Bandaging
Drip rate calculation, 77–8
Drug administration
    birds, *307*, 307–10, *308*, *309*
    cats, *17*, 17–24, *18*, *20*, *21*, *23*
    dogs, *8*, 8–14, *11*, *12*, *14*
    ferrets, 300–2
    rabbits, 281–5, *284*
    small rodents, 294–7
Drug poisoning, **197–8**
Dry eye, 39
Drying hands, 142–3, *143*
Dynamic compression
    bone plate, **179**
Dyspnoea, **126**
Dystocia, 209–11
    fetal, **210**
    maternal, **210**
    parturition stages, **209**
    types of, **210**

E

Ear(s)
bandaging, **169**, 172, *173*
injuries, **207**
medication administration for
cats, *18*, 18–19
dogs, 9
mites, 272
Ectoparasites
burrowing, 270–2
common, *271*
surface-living, 270
EDTA (sodium ethylene diamine
tetraacetic acid), 256
Ehmer sling, **169**, 169–72, *171*
Electrocardiography (ECG), 30–2, *31*
anaesthesia monitoring, **125**
Electrocautery, 159
Electrocution, 203
Electrolytes, 54, 68, 101
parenteral feeding, 102–3
Electronic impedance technology, 244
Elevator, **185**
Embolism, 34
Emergency patient evaluation, 187–8
Emetic agents, **201**
Endoscopy, 159–60
Endotoxic shock, **204**
Endotracheal intubation, 112–19,
118, 119
care of tubes, 119
removal of, 119
Enema
barium, *229*, 229–30
dogs, 43
Energy requirement, 87, 88, 98
See also Resting energy
requirement (RER)
Enflurane, **117**
Enteral nutrition, 87–8, 88–98
calculation of energy needs, 88
calculation of food quantities, 88–9
forced feeding, *89*, 89–90
gastrostomy tube placement and
feeding, 94–7, *95, 96*
maintenance of feeding tubes, 97
monitoring, 97–8, *99–100*
naso-oesophageal tube placement
and feeding, 90–2, *91, 92*
nasogastric tube placement and
feeding, 90–2
pharyngostomy tube placement
and feeding, 92–4, *93, 94*
selection of food, 89
Enzyme-linked immunosorbent assay
(ELISA), 244
Eosinophils, normal ranges, **258**

Epidural anaesthesia, **131**
Epilepsy, 58–9
emergency first aid, **189**
Erythrocytes *See* Red blood cells
Ethanol, **201**
Ethilon, **182**
Ethylene glycol poisoning, **201**
Ethylene oxide, 137, **138**
Exam (nursing) preparation, 323–36
Examination
cats, 16–17, 42
dogs, 6–7, *7*, 42
Excisional biopsy, **182**
Exercise, supported (dogs), 51–2, *52*
Exocrine pancreatic insufficiency
(EPI), 62
trypsin digest test, 255
Exotic species, 277–322
See also specific species
External fixators, **179**
External haemorrhage, **190**
Extracellular fluid (ECF), 68
Extraction forceps, **185**
Extubation, 119
Eye(s)
general surgical kit, 158
injuries, **207**
medication administration for
cats, 19
dogs, 9–10

F

Face masks, **143**
Faecal examination, 253–6, *254*
Fat in faeces, 255–6
Felicola subrostratus, *271*
Femoral artery, pulse rate
measurement, 27, 27–8
Fenestrated drapes, 154
Fentanyl, **287**
Ferrets, 299–304
biological data, **299**
drug administration, 300–2
handling and restraint, *299*,
299–300
sexing, 300, *300*
Fetal dystocia, **210**
Fine needle aspiration (FNA), 181–3,
182, 252–3
First aid, 187–210, **189**
suspected fracture, 178–80
Fistula, **166**
Fits, 58–9
Fleas, 270, *271*
Flexible endoscopes, 159–60
Fluanisone, **287**

Fluid therapy, 67–85
calculation of fluid deficit and
maintenance requirements, 77
drip rate calculation, 77–8
equipment, *71*
intraperitoneal, 72
intravenous *See* Intravenous fluid
therapy
monitoring
chart, *81, 82*
essential parameters, 80
general guidelines, 80
oral, 70
subcutaneous, 70–2
Flunixin, **113**
Flurbiprofen poisoning, **197**
Foam dressing, **167**
Foam wedges, radiography
positioning, **216**
Foley catheter, *44*, 45
Food
placing in mouth, *89*, 89–90
quantity calculation, 88–9
selection for enteral feeding, 89
types, 87
Footwear, **143**
Forced feeding, *89*, 89–90
Formol saline, 265
Fracture management, 178–80, **179**
crowns (dental), **185**
Free skin graft, **166**
Frostbite, 191–2
Furosemide, **198**

G

Gamgee, **167**
Gastrointestinal tract barium studies,
227–30, *229*
Gastrostomy tube placement and
feeding, 94–7, *95, 96*
Gauze, **167**
Gelofusine, 70
General anaesthesia *See* Anaesthesia
General surgical kit, 158
Gerbils
biological data, **279**
blood sampling, **296**
drug administration, **295**
restraint, 289
sexing, 290
Gestation period
ferrets, **299**
rabbits, **279**
small rodents, **279**
Giemsa stain, 262–3
Gingivitis, **185**

Glassware, care and cleaning of, 246, 250
Glaucoma, 40
Gloves, surgical, **143**, 148, *149, 150, 151*
Glucose, 62, 63
 enteral feeding, 98
 parenteral feeding, 98, 102, 103
Glycogen, 62
Gower's solution, **259**, 260
Gowns, surgical, **143**, 144–7, *144–7*
Gram's stain
 cytology, 253
 microbiology, 266–7
Guinea pigs
 biological data, **279**
 blood sampling, **296**
 drug administration, **295**
 restraint, 290, *290*
 sexing, 291

H

Haemaccel, 70
Haematology, 256–65
 analysers, 244
 normal ranges for dogs and cats, **258**
Haematoma, **166**
Haemocytometer, 258–60, *260*
Haemorrhage, **130**, 188–91
 first aid treatment of, **190**
 types of, **190**
Hair/coat
 brushings examination, 270
 clipping, 150–1
Halothane, **117**, **311**, **321**
Hamsters
 biological data, **279**
 blood sampling, **296**
 drug administration, **295**
 restraint, 291, *291*
 sexing, *289*, 291–2
Handling
 birds, *304, 305*
 dogs, 2–14, *3*
 ferrets, *299*, 299–300
 lizards, 318
 rabbits, 277–81, *280*
 small rodents, 288–94
 snakes, 312–13, *313*
Handwashing routine, 141, *142, 143*
Hartmann's solution, 54, 69, *71*, **198**
Headwear, **143**
Health and safety, laboratory, 244–5
Heart
 blocks, 32
 chamber size irregularities, 32

failure, 59
 measuring electrical activity of, 30–2, *31*
 rate changes during anaesthesia, **126**
Heimlich manoeuvre, 192, *192*
Heimlich valve, **177**
Hemispheres, brain, 326
Hepatic disease, 60–1
Herbicide poisoning, **198–9**
Hernia, **166**
Hippuric acid, *275*
Histopathology, 265–6
Hospitalisation kennel chart, 55
Hot-air oven, 136, **136**
Household chemicals poisoning, **200–1**
Humphrey ADE system, 122–3, *123*
Hydrocolloids, **167**
Hydrogels, **167**
Hydrotherapy (dogs), 52–3
Hypercapnia, 37
Hyperglycaemia, 62
Hypertension in cats, 36
Hyperthermia, **208**
Hypertonic fluid, 69
Hypocalcaemia, **208**
Hypocapnia, 37
Hypochlorite disinfectants, 251
Hypoglycaemia, 63, **208**
Hypostatic pneumonia, 58
Hypotension, **130**
 anaesthetic drugs, 36
Hypothermia, **130**, **208**
Hypotonic fluid, 69
Hypovolaemic shock, **204**

I

Ibuprofen poisoning, **197**
Ictal phase, epilepsy, **189**
Idiopathic epilepsy, 59
Illness energy requirement (IER), 88
 See also Resting energy requirement (RER)
Incised wounds, **165**
Incisional biopsy, **182**
Incubators, care and cleaning of, 246–7
Induction agents, **115**, **321**
 birds, **311**
 rabbits and small rodents, **287**
Induction of anaesthesia, 112, **116**
 birds, 310–11
 ferrets, 302–3
 gas flow rates, 124–5
 rabbits, 285–7
 reptiles, 320
 small rodents, 297

Infection
 barrier nursing, 42–3
 care of patients with, 41
Infiltration anaesthesia, **131**
Infusion set, *71*
Inhalation agents, **117**
Injections *See specific route; specific species*
Injuries to the body systems, **205–8**
Insecticide poisoning, **199**
Insensible water loss, 68
Instrumentation, surgical, 155–61
 assisting during surgery, 155–6
 care and maintenance of, 156–7
 care of specialist equipment, 159–61
 surgical kits, 157–9, *158*
 trolley preparation, 155
Insulin, 62, 63
Intensifying screens, 239
Intermittent positive pressure ventilation (IPPV), 129–30
Internal fixators, **179**
Internal haemorrhage, **190**
Intestines, injuries, **206**
Intracellular fluid (ICF), 68
Intramedullary pins, **179**
Intramuscular induction, **116**
Intramuscular injection
 birds, 308
 cats, *20*, 20–1
 chelonians, 318
 dogs, 10–11
 ferrets, 301
 lizards, 319, *319*
 rabbits, 283
 small rodents, **295**
 snakes, 315
Intraocular pressure (IOP)
 measuring, *39*, 39–40
 normal in cats and dogs, **26**
Intraosseous catheters, rabbits, 285
Intraosseous injection, birds, 309–10
Intraperitoneal injection
 ferrets, 301–2
 fluid therapy, 72
 rabbits, *284*, 284–5
 small rodents, **295**
Intravenous anaesthesia, **131**
Intravenous fluid therapy, 71, 72–4, *73*
 cephalic vein access, 74–5
 general maintenance, 78
 jugular vein access, 76–7
 removal of equipment, 79
 replacement/changing of bags, 78–9
 saphenous vein access, 75–6
 types of catheter, 74

Intravenous induction, **116**
Intravenous injection, *308*, 308–9
  cats
    cephalic vein, *21*, 21–2
    jugular vein, 22–4, *23*
    lateral saphenous vein, 22
  chelonians, *317*, 317–18
  dogs
    cephalic vein, *11*, 11–12
    jugular vein, 13–14, *14*
    lateral saphenous vein, *12*, 12–13
  ferrets, 302
  lizards, 319
  rabbits, 283–4
  small rodents, **295**
  snakes, *314*, 314–15
Intravenous urography, *230*, 230–1
Iodine, 234
  stain, 255
Ions, 68
Isoflurane, **117**, **311**, **321**
Isospora spp, *254*
Isotonic fluid, 69

J

Jackson Rees modified T-piece circuit, 120, *120*, **124**
Jackson's cat catheter, *44*, 46, 47, *71*
Jaundice, 61
Joint movement, passive, 53
Jugular vein injection
  birds, 308–9, *309*
  cats, 22–4, *23*
  chelonians, 317, *317*,
  dogs, 13–14, *14*
  intravenous fluid therapy, 76–7
  parenteral feeding, 101–2

K

Kaolin, **202**
Keratoconjunctivitis sicca (KCS), 39
Ketamine, **115**, **287**, **311**, **321**
Ketoacidosis, 62
Ketones, 62, 63
Ketoprofen, **113**
Kirschner wire/nail, **179**

L

Laboratory
  care of equipment, 245–52
  health and safety in the, 244–5

Laboratory techniques *See* Diagnostic laboratory techniques
Lacerations, **165**
Lack circuit, 120–1, *121*, **124**
Lag screws, **179**
Laryngeal injuries, **205**
Laser flow technology, 244
Lateral radiography views
  abdomen, 218, *218*
  pelvis, 219, *220*
  shoulder, 224–5, *225*
  spine, 226, *226*, *227*
  thorax, 215–16, *217*
Lateral saphenous vein injection
  cats, 22
  dogs, *12*, 12–13
  fluid therapy, 75–6
Learning, 324–30
Left hand brain preference, 326
Left-sided heart failure, 59
Leishman's stain, 263–4, *265*
  cytology, 253
Leptospirosis, 60
Leucocytes *See* White blood cells
Lice, 270
Lidocaine, **129**, 131
Lifespan
  ferrets, **299**
  rabbits, **279**
  small rodents, 279
Lifting
  cats
    aggressive/frightened, 15, *15*
    friendly, 14–15
  dogs, *4*
    large, with spinal damage, 5–6, *6*
    over 20 kg, 4
    small, with spinal damage, 4–5, *5*
    up to 15 kg, 3–4
Light beam diaphragm, 240
Limbs
  bandaging, **169**, 173–4, *174*
  draping, 154, *154*
  radiography, 223–6, *223*, *224*
  splinting, **169**, 176
Linen drapes, sterilisation packing, **139**
Linognathus setosus, *271*
Lint, **167**
Liquid feed/medication administration
  cats, 18, *18*
  chelonians, 316, *316*, *317*
  dogs, 8–9
  ferrets, 300–1
  lizards, 318–19
  rabbits, 281–2
  small rodents, 294
  snakes, 313–14

Litter size of ferrets, **299**
Lizards, 318–19, *319*
Local anaesthesia, 106, 130–1, **131**
Long-term memory, 324–5
Lumbar puncture, 233–5
Lung injuries, **205–6**
Luxator, **185**
Lymphocytes, **258**

M

Magill circuit, 120, *121*, **124**
Maintaining instruments, 156–7
Manual expression of the bladder, *48*, 48–9
Manual processing of radiographs, 235–7, *235*
Marginal ear vein, 283–4
Mask induction, **116**
Masks, anaesthetic, 119–20
Massage, 51
Maternal dystocia, **210**
Medetomidine, **113**, **287**, **311**
Medicine administration. *See* Drug administration
Medicines poisoning, **197–8**
Mediolateral radiography views, limbs, 223, *223*
Meloxicam, **113**
Memory, 324–30
Mersilk, **182**
Metabolic acidosis, 54, 69
Metabolic alkalosis, 69
Metabolic disorders, 54, 69, **208**
Metal tins, sterilisation packing, **139**
Metaldehyde poisoning, **199–200**
Methanol, 261
Methionine, **198**
Methohexital, **115**
Methoxyflurane, **117**
Methylene blue
  injection for poisoning, **198**
  stain, 262, 267
Mice
  biological data, **279**
  blood sampling, **296**
  drug administration, **295**
  restraint, *292*, 292–3
  sexing, *289*, 293
Microbiology, 266–8
Microscopes, care and use of, 247–9, *248*
Microsporum spp., 269–70, *270*
Midazolam, **287**, **311**
Mind maps, 327, *328*, *329*
Minute volume, 123–4

Mites, 272
Mixed haemorrhage, **190**
Mnemonics, 328
Molluscicide poisoning, **199–200**
Monitoring, anaesthesia,
    125, **125–6**
  birds, 311–12
  ferrets, 303
  rabbits, 287
  reptiles, 320–1
  small rodents, 298
Monocytes, normal ranges, **258**
Monofilament nylon, **182**
Monopolar diathermy, 159
Mouth injuries, **206**
Mouth to nose resuscitation,
    194–5, *195*
Mucous membranes
  anaesthesia monitoring, **125**
  changes during anaesthesia, **127**
  fluid therapy monitoring, 80
Muscle fibres in faeces, 255
Muscle relaxation, 131–2, 132
Mustard, 201
Muzzles, tying tape, 2–3, *3*
Myelography, 233–5, *234*

N

N-acetyl cysteine, **197–8**
Naloxone, **129**
Naproxen poisoning, **197**
Nasal chambers, radiography,
    222, *222*
Naso-oesophageal tube placement
    and feeding, 90–2, *91*, *92*
  rabbits, 282
Nasogastric tube placement and
    feeding, 90–2
Nasopharynx, radiography,
    222–3, *222*
Needle core biopsy, **182**
Neurogenic shock, **204**
Neuromuscular blocking agents,
    131–2
Neutrophils, normal ranges, **258**
Newton's rings, 259, 260
Nitrous oxide, 124
Non-absorbable sutures, **182**
Non-depolarising muscle relaxants,
    132
Non-steroidal anti-inflammatory
    drugs (NSAIDs) poisoning, **197**
Nose injuries, **205**
Nurolon, **182**
Nursing exam preparation, 323–36
Nutrition support, 87–103

Nylon
  braided, **182**
  film, sterilisation packing, **139**
  monofilament, **182**

O

Oedema, peripheral, 80
Oesophageal injuries, **205**
Oesophageal stethoscope
  measuring pulse rate
    using an, 28–9
  measuring respiratory rate
    using, 29–30
Oestrus cycle
  ferrets, **299**
  rabbits, **279**
  small rodents, **279**
Oocysts, 254, *254*
Open drains, **177**
Open gloving, 148, *150*
Open wounds, **165**
Oral fluid therapy, 70
Organochlorine poisoning, **199**
Organophosphate poisoning, **199**
Orthopaedic pinning kit, 158–9
Oryctolagus cuniculus See Rabbits
Osmosis, 68
Osmotic pressure, 68
Otodectes spp., *271*, 272
Oxygen during anaesthesia, 124
Oxygen saturation
  measuring, 32, *33*
  normal in cats and dogs, **26**

P

Packed cell volume (PCV)
  hydration status, 54, 57
  normal ranges for dogs
    and cats, **258**
  procedure for, 256–8, *257*
Packing materials for sterilisation,
    138–9, **139**
Palatine veins, 314
Palpebral reflex
  anaesthesia monitoring, **125**
  rabbits, 287
  reptiles, 321
Pancreatic disease, 61–2
Paper drapes, sterilisation
    packing, **139**
Paracetamol poisoning, **197–8**
Parallel Lack circuit, 120–1, *121*
Paraphimosis, **207**
Paraplegic patient, 57–8

Paraquat poisoning, **199**
Parasites, 268–72
  blood, 262–3
  surface-living *See* Ectoparasites
Parenteral feeding, 87–8,
    98–103
  calculation of nutrition
    requirements, 98–101
  jugular vein access, 101–2
  monitoring, 102–3
Parturition stages, **209**
Passive joint movement, 53
Passive physiotherapy, 51–3
Passive scavenging, 133
Patient evaluation, emergency,
    187–8
Pedal reflex
  anaesthesia monitoring, **125**
  rabbits, 287
  reptiles, 321
Pedicle skin graft, **166**
Pelvis radiography, 219–21, *220*
Penis injuries, **207**
Penrose drain, **177**, *177–8*, *178*
Pentobarbital, **115**
Perforated film dressing, **167**
Perineum injuries, **207**
Perineural anaesthesia, **131**
Periodontal disease, **185**
Periodontal probe, **185**
Periodontitis, **185**
Periosteal elevator, **185**
Peripheral oedema, 80
Peritoneal dialysis, 50–1
Pethidine, **113**
Petroleum gauze, **167**
Petroleum products poisoning, **201**
Pharyngostomy tube placement
    and feeding, 92–4, *93*, *94*
Pharynx
  anatomy of, *118*
  injuries, **205**
Phenylbutazone, **113**, **197**
Phosphorus, 60
Physiotherapy, passive, 51–3
Pipettes
  automatic, 250–1
  glass, 250
  volumetric, 250–1
Plaque, tooth, **185**
Plasma, 69, 70
Plaster of Paris, **169**, 176
Plastron, 316, *316*
Platelets, normal ranges, **258**
Platinum loop, 266
Plunge method of gloving,
    148, *151*
Pneumocystogram, 233

Pneumonia, hypostatic, 58
Poisoning, **196**, 196–202, **197–202**
Polishing the teeth, 183–6, *184*
Pollution control, anaesthesia, 132–3
Polydioxanone, **182**
Polyglactin, 910, **182**
Polyglycolic acid, **182**
Polyps, uterine, **207**
Polythene bags, sterilisation packing, **139**
Positive contrast cystogram, 233
Post-ictal phase, epilepsy, **189**
Postoperative care
  birds, 312
  ferrets, 303–4
  rabbits, 287–8
  reptiles, 321–2
  small rodents, 298
Poultice, **167**
Pragmatists, 326
Pre-ictal phase, epilepsy, **189**
Pressure bandage, **190**
Pressure points, **190**
Prolapsed uterus, **207**
Propofol
  birds, **311**
  general description, **115**
  rabbits, **287**
  reptiles, **321**
  small rodents, **287**
Protein, 60
  parenteral feeding, 98
Puberty, age at
  ferrets, **299**
  rabbits, **279**
  small rodents, **279**
Pulse oximetry, 32, *33, 38*
  anaesthesia monitoring, **125**
Pulse rate
  changes during anaesthesia, **127**
  enteral feeding, 98
  ferrets, **299**
  fluid therapy monitoring, 80
  general examination, 42
  measuring
    by chest palpation, 28
    by femoral artery palpation, *27*, 27–8
    using a stethoscope, 28
    using an oesophageal stethoscope, 28–9
  normal in cats and dogs, **26**
  parenteral feeding, 102
  rabbits, **279**
  small rodents, **279**

Punch biopsy, **182,** 183
Puncture wounds, **165**

Q

QBC Autoread (IDEXX), 244
Queens, catheterisation, 47–8

R

Rabbits, 277–88
  biological data, **379**
  blood sampling, **296**
  drug administration, 281–5, *284*
  general anaesthesia, 285–8, **286, 287**
  handling and restraint, 277–81, *280*
  sexing, 281, *281*
Radiation sterilisation, 137
Radiography, 214–42
  maintenance of equipment, 239–41
  patient positioning, 215–27, **216**
  patient preparation, 215
  processing, 235–9, *236*
  room preparation, 214–15
  use of contrast media, 227–35, *229*
Raising the vein, 13, 22, 33
Rats
  biological data, **279**
  blood sampling, **296**
  drug administration, **295**
  restraint, *293*, 293–4
  sexing, 294
Recovery, 127–8
  gas flow rates, 125
  position, 194, *194*
Rectum
  injuries, **206**
  taking the temperature in dogs, 6
Recumbent patient, 57–8
Red blood cells
  count, 260–1
  counting fluid, **259,** 260
  normal, **258**
Reflectors, 326
Reflexes *See specific reflex*
Refractometer, *273*, 273–4
Regional anaesthesia, **131**
Renal disease, 60
Reptiles, 312–22
Respiratory failure, **189**
Respiratory rate
  anaesthesia, 123
    changes during, **126**
    monitoring, **125**
  enteral feeding, 98
  ferrets, **299**

fluid therapy monitoring, 80
general examination, 42
measuring
  by direct observation, 29
  using a stethoscope, 29
  using an oesophageal stethoscope, 29–30
normal in cats and dogs, **26**
rabbits, **279**
small rodents, **279**
Respiratory system injuries, **205–6**
Resting energy requirement (RER), 88
Restraint
  birds, *304, 305*
  cats, 14–24
  chelonians, 315
  dogs, 2–14
  ferrets, 299–300, *300*
  lizards, 318
  rabbits, 277–81, *280*
  small rodents, 288–94
  snakes, 312–13, *313*
Resuscitation, mouth to nose, 194–5, *195*
Reticulocyte count, 262, *262*
Retrograde urethrography, 231–2
Retrograde vaginourethrography, 232–3
Revision, 327–31, **332**
Right atrium, pressure of blood entering *See* Central venous pressure (CVP)
Right hand brain preference, 326
Right-sided heart failure, 59
Rigid endoscopes, 159–60
Ring bandage, **169,** *175*
Ringer's solution, 69–70
Ringworm fungus, *270*
  culture for, 268–9
  Wood's lamp detection, 269–70
Robert Jones bandage, 168, **169,** *170,* **179**
Rodenticide poisoning, **200**
Rodents, small *See* Small rodents
Romanowsky stain, 264
Rostrocaudal radiography views, tympanic bullae, *221,* 221–2
Rupture, **166**
Rush pin, **179**

S

Safelight function, 239
Salbutamol poisoning, **198**
Saline solution, 69, *71*
Saliva, anaesthesia monitoring, **126**
Salmonella, 312, 315

Salt, dietary, 59
Sandbags, radiography positioning, **216**
Sarcoptes spp., *271*
Scalds, 191
Scaler, **185**
Scaling the teeth, 183–6, *184*, **185**
Scavenging, 132–3
Schiotz tonometer, 39–40
Schirmer tear measurement strips, 38–9, *39*
Scrub nurse, 156
Scrub suits, **143**
Scutes, 316, *316*
Sedistain, 275
Self-seal pouches, sterilisation packing, **139**
Semi-permeable film dressing, **167**
Sensible water loss, 68
Seton drain, **177**
Sexing
    chinchillas, 289
    ferrets, 300, *300*
    gerbils, 290
    guinea pigs, 291
    hamsters, *289*, 291–2
    mice, *289*, 293
    rabbits, 281, *281*
    rats, 294
Shearing wound, **165**
Sherman plate, **179**
Shock, 203–5
    clinical signs of, **204**
    types of, **204**
Short-term memory, 324–5
Shoulder radiography, 224–5, *225*, *226*
Silk, braided, **182**
Sinus, **166**
Site preparation, surgical, 148–52
Skin
    fluid therapy monitoring, 80
    grafts, **166**
    preparation for surgery, 151–2
    scrapings, 270–2
Skull radiography, *221*, 221–3, *222*
Small rodents, 288–398
    biological data, **379**
    blood sampling, **296**, 296–7
    drug administration, 294–7
    general anaesthesia, **287** *See also specific type*
Smears
    bacterial, 266
    blood, 261, *261*
    cytology, *252*, 252–3
    mites, 272
Snake bite, **203**
Snakes, 312–15
Soda lime, 123

Sodium bicarbonate, 54, **129**
Sodium chloride (NaCl), 68, 69
Sodium ethylene diamine tetraacetic acid (EDTA), 256
Spinal anaesthesia, **131**
Spine
    damage, lifting dogs with, 4–6, *5*, *6*
    radiography, 226–7, *226*, *227*
Splint, **169**, 176, **179**
Spore strips, **138**
Squash prep, 252, *252*
Starch in faeces, 255
Status epilepticus, 58
Steinmann pin, **179**
Sterilisation, 136–9
    autoclaves, 136, **137**
    ethylene oxide, 137
    hot-air oven, 136, **136**
    monitoring the efficacy of, 137, **138**
    packing materials for, 138–9, **139**
    radiation, 137
Stethoscopes
    measuring pulse rate using, 28
    measuring pulse rate using an oesophageal, 28–9
    measuring respiratory rate using, 29
    measuring respiratory rate using and oesophageal, 29–30
Stings, 202, **203**
Stomach injuries, **206**
Struvite, *275*
Stupor, **189**
Subcutaneous fluid therapy, 70–2
Subcutaneous injection
    cats, 19–20, *20*
    chelonians, 318
    dogs, 10
    ferrets, 301
    lizards, 319
    rabbits, 282–3
    small rodents, **295**
    snakes, 315
Sudan 3 stain
    cytology, 253
    fat in faeces, 255–6
Sump drain, **177**
Superficial artery palpation, **125**
Supported exercise (dogs), 51–2, *52*
Surface anaesthesia, **131**
Surgery, assisting during, 155–6
Surgical gloves, **143**, 148, *149*, *150*, *151*
Surgical gowns, **143**, *144*, 144–7, *145*, *146*, *147*
Surgical kits, 157–9, *158*
Surgical scrub, 141–3, *142*, *143*
Surgical site preparation, 148–52

Suturing
    materials, **182**
    techniques, *180*, 180–1
Swabbing, 156
Syringe forced feeding, 90

T

Tablet administration
    cats, *17*, 17–18
    dogs, 8, *8*
Tachycardia, **126**
Tachypnoea, **126**
Taenia spp., *254*
Tail
    bandaging, **169**, *174*, 174–6
    reflex, 321
Tape muzzles, tying, 2–3, *3*
Tapes, radiography positioning, **216**
Tears
    anaesthesia monitoring, **126**
    volume produced
        measuring, 38–9, *39*
        normal in cats and dogs, **26**
Tec and Penlon type vaporisers, **108**, *109*
Teeth
    retained deciduous, **185**
    scaling and polishing, 183–6, *184*
Temperature, body
    anaesthesia monitoring, **125**
    enteral feeding, 98
    ferrets, **299**
    fluid therapy monitoring, 80
    general examination, 42
    measuring, 26–7
    normal in cats and dogs, **26**
    parenteral feeding, 102
    rabbits, **279**
    small rodents, **279**
    taking from the rectum in dogs, 6
Terrapins, 315–18
Theatre attire, **143**, 143–8, *144–7*, *149–51*
Theatre practice, 135–61
Theorists, 326
Thermocouples, **138**
Thermometers, 26–7
Thiopental, **115**
Thorax
    drain, **177**
    radiography, 215–18, *217*. *See also* Chest
Tidal volume, 123
Tieman's catheter, *44*, 45
Ties, radiography positioning, **216**
Time management, 330

To and fro circuit, 121–2, *122*, 124, **124**
Toad skin venom, **203**
Tomcats, catheterisation, 46–7, *47*
Tongue withdrawal reflex, 321
Tono-Pen, *39*, 40
Tonometers, *39*, 39–40
Tortoises, 315–18
Touch prep, 252
Tourniquet, **190**
Towel walking, 51–2, *52*
Toxascaris spp., *254*
Toxic agents, **197–201**
Toxocara spp., *254*
Trachea
    injuries, **205**
    placement of endotracheal tube,
        119
Tracheotomy, 193, **193**
Transfusion, 83–5, *84*
    reactions, 85
Trauma, **205–8**
Trephine biopsy, **182**
Trichodectes canis, *271*
Trichophyton spp., *270*
Trichuris spp., *254*
Trochar, 50
Trombicula autumnali, *271*
Troughs, radiography positioning,
    216
True-cut biopsy, **182**
Trypsin digest test, 254–5
Tumour, **166**
Tympanic bullae radiography,
    221, 221–2

U

Ulcers, **166**
    decubitus, 58
Ultrasonic scaler, 184, *186*
Ultrasonography, 214
Ultrasound, 241–2
Uncinaria spp., *254*
Unconsciousness, **189**
Uraemia, **208**
Urates, *275*
Urea, parenteral feeding
    monitoring, 103

Urethrogram
    female, 232–3
    male, 231–2
Urine
    dipstick testing, 274–5
    examination, 272–5
    gross examination, 273
    output
        enteral feeding monitoring, 98
        fluid therapy monitoring, 80
        parenteral feeding
            monitoring, 103
    preservation, 272–3
    sedimentation examination,
        275, *275*
    specific gravity, *273*, 273–4
    volume produced
        measuring, 38
        normal in cats and dogs,
            26, 38
Urogenital system injuries, **207**
Urography, intravenous, *230*,
    230–1
Uterus
    polyps, **207**
    prolapsed, **207**

V

Vaginourethrography, retrograde,
    232–3
Vaporisers, **108**, *109*
Vasculogenic shock, **204**
Vecuronium, **132**
Velpeau sling, 168, **169**, *171*
Venables plate, **179**
Venous haemorrhage, **190**
Ventral venous sinus, 314
Ventrodorsal radiography views
    abdomen, 218–19, *219*
    pelvis, 219–21, *220*
    skull, 221, *221*
    spine, 226–7, *227*
Vernier scale, *249*, 249–50
Veterinary nursing exam preparation,
    323–36
Vicryl, **182**
Vitamin B complex, 101

Volumetric pipettes, 250–1
Vomiting, 56–7

W

Washing soda crystals, **201**
Wasp sting, **203**
Waste disposal and decontamination, 251
Water, body, *68*
    balance, 68–9
    content, 67, 68
Water bath care, 251–2
Water trap, **177**
Weaning age
    ferrets, **299**
    rabbits, **279**
    small rodents, **279**
Wedge biopsy, **182**
Weight *See* Bodyweight
White blood cells, **259**
    count, 258–60, **259**, *259*
        differential, 264–5
        parenteral feeding, 102
    normal ranges for dogs and cats, **258**
Whole blood, 69, 70
Wing clipping, *306*, 306–7
Wooden blocks, radiography
    positioning, **216**
Wood's lamp, 269–70
Worm egg count, 253–4, *254*
Wound(s)
    classification, **165–6**
    dressings, **167**
    management, 164–7.
        See also Bandaging

X

X-ray machine set up, 214
X-ray tube leakage, 240
Xylazine, **113**, **201**

Z

Zoonotic diseases, 42
    reptiles, 312

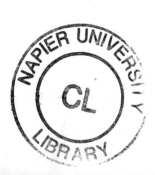